T0314063

Microsurgery

Microsurgery

Applied to Neurosurgery

By

M. G. Yaşargil

Foreword by H. A. Krayenbühl

With Contributions by
R. M. P. Donaghy, U. P. Fisch, J. Hardy,
L. I. Malis, S. J. Peerless and M. Zingg
and Engineers
W. J. Borer, H. Littmann and H. R. Voellmy

316 Illustrations

1969

Georg Thieme Verlag · Stuttgart

Academic Press · New York and London

Library of Congress Cataloging-in-Publication Data is available from the publisher.

This volume is a reprint of the classic 1969 edition of
Microsurgery—Applied to Neurosurgery.

© 2007 Georg Thieme Verlag,
Rüdigerstrasse 14, 70469 Stuttgart, Germany
http://www.thieme.de
Thieme New York, 333 Seventh Avenue,
New York, NY 10001, USA
http://www.thieme.com

Typesetting and printing in Germany by primustype hurler GmbH, Notzingen

ISBN-10: 3-13-453502-5 (GTV)
ISBN-13: 978-3-13-453502-0 (GTV)
ISBN-10: 1-58890-575-6 (TNY)
ISBN-13: 978-1-58890-575-8 (TNY)

1 2 3 4 5 6

Acknowledgements

During the past two years, the interest and enthusiasm of surgeons from all over the world for microsurgical techniques applied to neurosurgery has resulted in many surgeons visiting our clinic. This monograph represents an attempt to compile the experience, techniques, suggestions and unresolved problems of all the surgeons of our acquaintance who are involved in the development of the exciting field of microsurgery.

I am greatly indebted to Prof. R. M. P. Donaghy for introducing me to the techniques of microvascular surgery of peripheral arteries and to Prof. H. A. Krayenbühl my chief and teacher for 17 years, for his support of the development of clinical microsurgery. I am grateful to the Hartford Foundation, the Sandoz Co., and the Swiss National Funds for their generous financial support.

It is a pleasure to acknowledge the great help of Dr. V. Elsasser (Director of the Kantonsspital Zürich), Mr. F. Höchli (Chief Foreman of the Kantonsspital Zürich), and Mr. W. Vetterli (Superintendent of Experimental Animals).

The German text was translated by Dr. H. H. Burrows and Dr. P. Levin, Dr. S. J. Peerless and Dr. P. Lipron assisted in the organization of the English version.

Prof. K. C. Bradley, Dr. R. Crowell, Prof. T. Dinning, Dr. A. N. Guthkelch, Dr. J. Keith and Dr. G. S. Merry have been very kind to read and correct the galley proofs.

Mr. H. P. Weber is credited with the art work and Mr. A. Würth for the photographic reproduction. Miss M. Traber typed the manuscript and checked the bibliography.

I am gratefull to Dr. R. Stursberg, Mr. H. G. Hildebrand, Mr. F. Hilzinger (Aesculap), Mr. R. Berger and Mr. H. Sutter (Fischer), Mr. M. C. Hollander (Holco) for their great help to develop microsurgical instruments.

The interest and cooperation of Thieme Publisher and especially Dr. G. Hauff is greatly appreciated.

Finally, this monograph is dedicated to Miss Esther Roberts, Senior Theatre Sister of Prof. R. M. P. Donaghy, and to the nurses of the Neurosurgical Department Kantonsspital Zürich, whose interest, assistance and enthusiasm encouraged my intention to microsurgery.

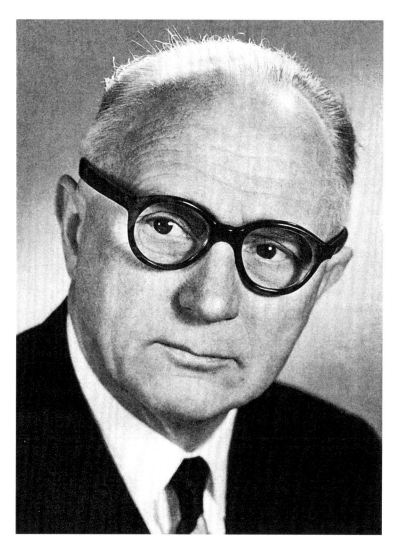

Prof. H. A. KRAYENBÜHL, my esteemed chief and teacher whose forethought and encouragement made possible the application of the microtechnique in its broadest sense to clinical neurosurgery.

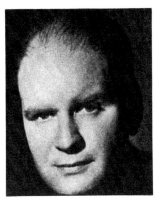

Julius H. Jacobson, II, M. D.
Prof. of Vascular Surgery
Mount Sinai Hospital, New York, N. Y.

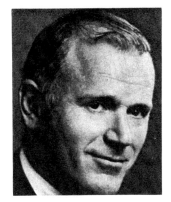

Harry J. Buncke, Jr. M. D.
Prof. of Plastic and Recontructive Surgery
Univ. of Stanford, Palo Alto, California

Pioneers
of Microsurgery

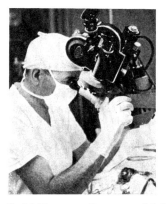

R. M. Peardon Donaghy, M. D.
Prof. of Neurosurgery
Univ. of Vermont, Burlington

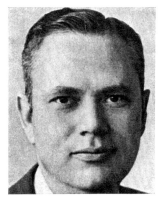

William F. House
Prof. of Otolaryngology
Univ. of Southern California, Los Angeles

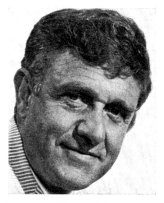

Theodor Kurze, M. D.
Prof. of Neurosurgery
Univ. of Southern, California, Los Angeles

Contributing Authors

BORER, W. J., Ingenieur, Autophon, Zürcherstraße 137, CH-8952 Schlieren, Zürich, Schweiz.

DONAGHY, R. M. P., M. D., Professor of Neurological Surgery, University of Vermont, College of Medicine, Mary Fletcher Hospital, Burlington, Vermont, USA.

FISCH, U., Priv.-Doz. Dr. med., Oberarzt, Otolaryngologische Universitätsklinik, Kantonsspital Zürich, Rämistraße 100, CH-8006 Zürich, Schweiz.

HARDY, J., M. D., F. R. C. S. (C) F. A. C. S., Neurochirurgien de l'Hôpital Notre Dame, Professeur Agrégé à l'Université de Montréal, 1386 Est, Rue Sherbrooke, Montréal 24, P. Q., Canada.

KRAYENBÜHL, H. A., Prof. Dr. med., Direktor der Neurochirurgischen Universitätsklinik, Kantonsspital Zürich, Rämistraße 100, CH-8006 Zürich, Schweiz.

LITTMANN, H., Dr. sc. nat., Carl Zeiss, D-7082 Oberkochen, Württ., Deutschland.

MALIS, L. I., M. D., Professor of Neurological Surgery, Neurosurgical Service, The Mount Sinai Hospital. 1176 Fifth Avenue, New York City, N. Y., USA.

PEERLESS, M. D., F. R. C. S. (C), Assistant Professor of Surgery (Neurological Surgery), Faculty of Medicine, University of British Columbia, Vancouver, Canada.

VOELLMY, H. R., Dr. Ing., Contraves A.-G., Schaffhauserstraße 580, CH-8052 Zürich, Schweiz.

YAŞARGIL, M. G., Prof. Dr. med., Neurochirurgische Universitätsklinik, Kantonsspital Zürich, Rämistraße 100, CH-8006 Zürich, Schweiz.

ZINGG, M., Frau Dr. med., Oberärztin, Institut für Anästhesiologie der Universität Zürich, Kantonsspital Zürich, Rämistraße 100, CH-8006 Zürich, Schweiz.

Table of Contents

CHAPTER 4

Reconstructive and Constructive Surgery of the Cerebral Arteries in Man   82

A. The Cerebral Vasculature (S. J. Peerless)   82

B. Diagnosis and Indications for Operations in Cerebrovascular Occlusive Disease (M. G. Yaşargil)   95

C. Aneurysms, Arteriovenous Malformations and Fistulae (M. G. Yaşargil) . 119

CHAPTER 5

A. Intracranial Tumors (M. G. Yaşargil) 150

B. Cranial Nerve Lesions (M. G. Yaşargil) 164

CHAPTER 6

A. Vertebral Column and Spinal Cord Lesions (M. G. Yaşargil) 167

B. Peripheral Nerve Lesions (M. G. Yaşargil) 179

CHAPTER 7

Transnasal-transsphenoidal Approach to the Pituitary Gland (J. Hardy) 180

CHAPTER 8

Oto-neurosurgical Operations: Transtemporal Extralabyrinthine Operations on the Internal Auditory Canal, the Eighth and the Seventh Cranial Nerves (U. P. Fisch) 195

CHAPTER 9

Anesthesia in Microsurgical Operations on the Central Nervous System (M. Zingg) 211

Appendix (M. G. Yaşargil) 217

Foreword

This work is concerned with the micro-surgical approach to cerebrospinal lesions and its authors are men whose previous publications in recent years have been directed to the improvement of surgical technique. I am greatly pleased to be able to write a few words of introduction for this work which will stimulate the younger generation of Neurosurgeons.

The principles of Neurological Surgery were laid down by Harvey Cushing in an address on "The Special Field of Neurological Surgery" published as early as March 1905, in which he said: "It seems clear that in order to advance surgical measures, specialization or, better, concentration of thoughts and energics along given lines, is necessary." From these premises there has developed over the last fifty years the special field of neurosurgery and, surprisingly, the tools for the operative skills have remained practically unchanged for many decades. Dr. Cushing's guiding principle was avoidance of injury to the brain by the introduction of manipulations whose gentleness would, in general surgery, be regarded as excessive. Every device has been employed to protect the brain during its retraction. Besides this, painstaking hemostasis was achieved by application of cotton-wool pledgets or fragments of muscle to the bleeding area, by the introduction of the silver clip in 1911 and of coagulation of vessels by means of high-frequency electric current in 1927. And, finally, special equipment for irrigation and suction was developed to keep the operative field clear and clean, which is just as necessary when working on the surface or in superficial parts of the brain as it is when working at deeper levels.

Gentleness in manipulation, elaborate hemostasis and an accurate closure of the wound were therefore recognized as the basic principles in neurological surgery. In spite of this knowledge, no attempt has been made to improve this careful and meticulous operative technique down to nearly the pre-sent time. It is astonishing that the operating microscope came to be employed so late in the field of neurosurgery, since it has been an indispensable tool in routine otologic surgery for four decades. The development of the binocular surgical microscope with stereoscopic vision, the objective magnifications from six to forty times and great illuminating power made this instrument an extremely useful adjunct to surgery. The instrument is also equipped with photo, motion picture and television cameras; the assistants are able to follow in detail all the operative manipulations of the surgeon.

In the field of otology since 1961 House and his associates have developed the surgical approaches to acoustic tumors, and Kurze discussed for the first time in 1963 the micro-techniques in neurological surgery. Pool and Colton (1965) were the first to use the microscope for intracranial aneurysmal surgery. Knowing of this new development, I decided to have my associate Yaşargil trained by Dr. Peardon Donaghy in Burlington, Vermont, who was already a pioneer in reconstructive vascular surgery, which was initiated at his clinic by J. H. Jacobson in 1960.

For success in microsurgery, however, micro-instruments and micro-suture material still had to be developed, and these were demonstrated by Yaşargil during a course in microsurgery which was held at my clinic from November 14 to 20, 1968. The particular anatomical and physiological features of the central nervous system call not only for specially designed surgical microscopes but also for new surgical techniques, and at present microsurgery is still in the developmental phase.

Furthermore, the construction of the bipolar coagulator by Malis is a milestone in operative neurosurgery. As early as 1940, Greenwood introduced the two-point coagulation as a new principle and instrument for applying coagulation current in neurosurgery. With the use of fine forceps, extremely small structures may be grasped, isolated, and coagulated. There is negligible heat damage to surrounding structures as the high-frequency current passes only from one forceps tip to the other. Such coagulation can be carried out with the use of the dissecting microscope directly on important structures without damaging them.

The microtechnique therefore combines the use of the binocular microscope, micro-instruments, microsutures, microdrill, bipolar microcoagulation of Malis and the meticulous preparation of tissues. It is not the microscope alone but the combination of these elements that constitutes the great improvement in the classical neurosurgical techniques.

Finally, I wish to emphasize that the surgical microscope also has educative potentialities. As it can be coupled with television cameras, the surgical procedure can be followed not only by the assistant watching through the observer's eye-piece, but also by a large group of students and doctors viewing the screen. In this way, training in the art of surgery is promoted, and it should be possible by educative measures and incentives to encourage young surgeons to carry out original work.

In reviewing the history of neurosurgery, I admit that a number of different forms of treatment have been advocated and that each method has had its advocates at different times and in different places. Nevertheless, I believe in the necessity of this new technical approach for relief of certain cerebrospinal disorders. An authoritative work like this on the methods of applying it is invaluable. In conclusion I wish to emphasize, with Hugh Cairns, "that surgery is and must be always an art, but its progress and thus its vitality depend on the maximum application to it of the methods and discoveries of science."

HUGO KRAYENBÜHL

Zürich, Switzerland, Summer 1969

Introduction

Good illumination, unobstructed vision and a view of the whole operative field are of essential value to the surgeon. The better these conditions are, the greater the precision with which he can identify the structures of pathophysiological significance. Various types of magnifying spectacles introduced by ophthalmologists (von Zehender 1887, von Rohr and Stock 1913) and otologists (Lempert and Storz) have been employed in neurosurgery for the past 40 years (Riechert 1948). While all these spectacles permit free movement of the head they are uncomfortable by virtue of the unstable field. Furthermore the problem of adequate illumination in the depths of a neurosurgical wound remains unresolved. Modern technology has furnished the surgeon with an extremly valuable tool in the form of the binocular surgical microscope with stereoscopic vision, 6- to 40-fold magnification and intense illumination. To be precise, however, it is not a true microscope in that it simply provides magnification, with optimal illumination, of macroscopic structures. It is, therefore a sophisticated form of magnifying loupe and the instrument was designed primarily as a colposcope by Hinselmann in 1925.

The binocular operating microscope has been used for 46 years in otology. Holmgren (1923) replaced the monocular microscope of Nylén used in 1921/1922 by the binocular operating microscope for operations on the labyrinth in otosclerosis. Shambaugh, Simpson-Hall applied the operating microscope in 1940 to the one-stage fenestration operation. Cawthorne (Shambaugh 1967) had already used the microscope for operations on the facial nerve. The advantages of 6-to 25-fold magnification have caused otologic surgeons to adopt the operating microscope for fenestration, stapes operations, tympanoplasties and myringoplasties facial nerve surgery, labyrinth and endolymphatic sac operations and translabyrinthine removal of acoustic neurinomas. The operating micro-scope has only recently been introduced to ophthalmology (Perritt 1950, Barraquer 1956, Troutman 1964, De Voe 1964, Harms, Mackensen 1966).

It was not until the pioneer work of House (1961) in the exploration of the internal auditory canal and removal of acoustic neurinomas that most neurosurgeons became sufficiently stimulated and challenged to recognize the value of the microscope and microtechniques. Jacobson, Donaghy 1962, Kurze, Doyle 1962, Kurze 1964, Rand, Kurze 1965, Lougheed et al. 1965, Pool 1965, Pool, Colton 1966, Rand, Jannetta 1967, have reported on the use of the microscope in neurosurgery.

However, it should never be forgotten that there is much more to microtechnique in neurosurgery than the possession of a highly perfected optical instrument. This alone is of little value without special methods of bipolar coagulation, carefully adapted instruments, and, above all, atraumatic operation techniques.

The operating microscope has proven particularly useful in bloodless fields, in operations on avascular or poorly vascularized organs such as the middle ear, and on the cornea and the lens of the eye. However, before its use could be extended to fields rich in blood vessels or highly vascular organs it was necessary first to develop practical techniques of *microvascular* surgery. The pioneering work was done by Jacobson and Suarez (1960). They operated succesfully on blood vessels with a diameter less than 3 mm. using a binocular microscope, and they designed microinstruments and microsuture material for this purpose. The microsurgical technique has been of particular interest to vascular and plastic surgeons. The laboratory work concentrated on solving the technical problems associated with anastomosing vessels in the range 1 mm. in diameter (Buncke, Schulz 1965, Krizek et al. 1965, Fisher, Lee 1965). Buncke refined the suture technique and showed that the survival of tissues transplanted in this fashion is directly proportional to the mechanical efficiency of the anastomosis. Smith (1966) emphasized the significance of the vasa vasorum. This work had its clinical application in the use of the operating microscope for vascular surgery in the upper and lower limbs (Cobbett 1965, Jenning and Addison 1966, Goldwyn 1966, Buncke et al. 1967).

These new operative techniques and micro-instruments required modification for operations in the central nervous system. The approaches to the blood vessels at the skull base are funnel-shaped, narrow and deep; the close proximity of the cerebral vessels to the brain substance — which is easily damaged — called for additional techniques and instruments for dissection, isolation and mobilization of these vessels. The extreme sensitivity of the brain to hypoxia made it necessary to develop bypass techniques during temporary occlusion of the cerebral vessels. Donaghy (1967) redesigned De Bakey's large-caliber plastic T-tube for carotid surgery into a smaller tube with an outer diameter of only 1 mm. He used this tube for operations on smaller peripheral arteries in rabbits and dogs. Recognition of the particular value of the bipolar coagulation apparatus developed by Malis (1967) permitted the application of these techniques to the cerebral vasculature.

The special problems of cerebrovascular surgery were studied and systematized and a technique for the surgery of the brain arteries was developed by the author in the Research Laboratories of the Department of Neurosurgery, University of Vermont (1965/66). Since January 1967 these techniques have been applied to patients in the Department of Neurosurgery, University of Zürich. As a result of this experience, the microtechnique has been shown to be of value in the following fields of neurosurgery: Firstly for the improvement of operative techniques of known efficacy on large lesions. Such as the excision of cerebral and spinal tumors and angiomas, resection of sacculated aneurysms, sectioning of cranial and spinal nerves (trigeminal neuralgia, spasmodic torticollis,

Menière's disease). Cordotomy can be carried out with enhanced precision if a surgical microscope is used. Magnification and excellent lighting permit closer observation, clearer differentiation and gentler exposure of pathological tissues, and the normal structures in the vicinity can be spared injury. Moreover, the use of the microscope has opened up new possibilities by making some pathological conditions at the base of the brain and skull, which had previously been regarded as inoperable, accessible to the surgeon (e.g. transsphenoidal, transpetrosal, transmastoidal, translabyrinthine and trans-clival craniotomy).

Furthermore, the micro-technique has brought the surgery of the smaller cerebral structures within the realms of possibility. For instance, embolectomy and thrombectomy of cerebral vessels, the creation of collateral channels to improve the cerebral circulation. For the anastomosis of cranial and peripheral nerves and the plastic repair of the basal dura the use of the microtechnique will soon be regarded as essential.

The use of the surgical microscope in operations on animals allows the surgeon to acquire experience and practice in microtechniques, and to perform surgical experiments with a view to improving standard operative methods.

As the surgical microscope can be coupled with still, cine and television cameras it is also of value in teaching. The surgical procedures can be followed not only by the assistant through the observer's eyepiece, but also by large groups during the operation or at some later time. Moreover these methods of recording operative details afford the surgeon an opportunity to review and modify his technique.

This volume was compiled on the basis of a firm belief in the future of microtechniques in neurosurgery. This work is not presented as the final word on a subject as rapidly developing and untried as microsurgery. Rather it is intended to be an introduction and a stimulus to a new and rapidly developing field in surgery.

References

Barraquer, J. I.: The microscope in ocular surgery. Amer. J. Ophthal. 42 (1956) 6

Barraquer, J. I., J. Barraquer, H. Littmann: Nuevo microscopio para cirugia ocular. Arch. Soc. oftal. hisp.-amer. 5 (1966) 271

Buncke, Jr., H. J., W. P. Schulz: Experimental digital amputation. Plast. reconstr. Surg. 36 (1965) 62

Buncke, H. J., A. I. Daniller, W. P. Schulz, R. A. Chase: The fate of autogenous whole joints transplanted by microvascular anastomoses. Plast. reconstr. Surg. 39 (1967) 333

Cawthorne: Quoted by Shambaugh (1967)

Cobbett, J.: Microsurgery. Paper presented to the British Association of Plastic Surgeons, Dec. 2, 1965, London

Dekking, H. M.: Use of the binocular microscope in eye operations. Arch. Ophthal. (Chicago) 55 (1956) 114

Donaghy, R. M. P.: Patch and bypass in microangeional surgery. In: Micro-Vascular Surgery, Ed. by R. M. P. Donaghy, M. G. Yaşargil. Thieme, Stuttgart 1967, pp. 75-86

Fisher, B., S. Lee: Microvascular surgical techniques in research, with special reference to renal transplantation in the rat. Surgery 58 (1956) 904

Goldwyn: Quoted by Smith (1966)

Grünberger, V., R. Ulm: Diagnostische Methode in Geburtshilfe, Gynäkologie. Thieme, Stuttgart 1968

Harms, H., G. Mackensen: Augenoperationen unter dem Mikroskop. Thieme, Stuttgart 1966

Hinselmann: Quoted by Grünberger und Ulm (1968)

Holmgren, G.: Some experiences in surgery of otosclerosis. Acta oto-laryng. (Stockh.) 5 (1923) 460

House, W. F.: Surgical exposure of the internal auditory canal and its contents through the middle cranial fossa. Laryngoscope 71 (1961) 1363

Jacobson, J. H., R. M. P. Donaghy: Microsurgery as an aid to middle cerebral artery endarterectomy. J. Neurosurg. 19 (1962) 108

Jacobson, J. H., E. L. Suarez: Microsurgery in anastomosis of schmall vessels. Surg. Forum 11 (1960) 243

Jenning and Addison: Quoted by Smith (1966)

Krizek, T. J., T. Tani, J. D. Desprez, C. L. Kiehn: Experimental transplantation of composite grafts by microsurgical vascular anastomosis. Plast. reconstr. Surg. 36 (1965) 538

Kurze, T., J. B. Doyle Jr.: Extradural intracranial (middle fossa) approach to the internal auditory canal. J. Neurosurg. 19 (1962) 1033

Kurze, T.: Microtechniques in neurological surgery. In: Clinical Neurosurgery, Vol II. Williams & Wislkins, Baltimore 1964, pp. 129-137

Lempert and Storz: Quoted by Shambaugh (1967)

Lougheed, W. M., R. W. Gunton, H. J. Barnett: Embolectomy of internal carotid, middle and anterior cerebral arteries. J. Neurosurg. 22 (1965) 607

Malis, L. I.: Bipolar coagulation in microsurgery. In: Micro-Vascular Surgery. Ed. by R. M. P. Donaghy, M. G. Yaşargil. Thieme, Stuttgart 1967, pp. 126-130

Nylén, C. D.: The microscope in aural surgery, its first use and later development. Acta oto-laryng. (Stockh.) Suppl. 116 (1954) 226

Perritt, R. A.: Recent advantages in corneal surgery. Amer. Acad. ophthal. oto-laryng. Course Nr. 288, 1950

Pool, J. L.: New dimension in aneurysm surgery. P. S. Quart. (Columbia) 18-20 Sept. 1965

Pool, J. L., R. P. Colton: The dissecting microscope for intracranial vascular surgery. J. Neurosurg. 25 (1966) 315

Rand, R. W., P. J. Jannetta: Microneurosurgery for aneurysms. J. Neurosurg. 27 (1967) 330

Rand, R. W., T. Kurze: Microneurosurgical resection of acoustic tumors by a transmeatal posterior fossa approach. Bull. Los Angeles Neurol. Soc. 30 (1965) 17

Riechert, T.: Die Operationen an der WS und am Rückenmark. In: Chirurgische Operationslehre. Hrsg. Bier, Braun und Kümmel, Vol. 2, 7. Aufl., Barth, Leipzig 1948, p. 753

Rohr, M. von, W. Stock: Über eine achromatische Brillenlupe schwacher Vergrößerung. Klin. Mbl. Augenheilk. 51 (1913) 206

Shambaugh, Jr., G. E.: Modified fenestration technic. Arch. Otolaryng. 36 (1942) 23

Shambaugh, Jr., G. E.: Surgery of the Ear. 2nd. Ed. Saunders, Philadelphia. 1967 p. 179

Shillito, Jr., J.: Indications for surgery in cerebrovascular accidents. Postgrad. Med. 30 (1961) 537

Simpson-Hall: Quoted by Shambaugh (1967)

Smith, J. W.: Microsurgery: review of the literature and discussion of microtechniques. Plast. reconstr. Surg. 37 (1966) 227

Troutman, R. C.: Microsurgery. Highlights Ophthal. 7 (1964) 162

Troutman, R. C., J. Barraquer and J. Rutllan: Surgery of the Anterior Segment of the Eye, Vol. 1. McGraw-Hill, New York 1964

Voe, A. G. De: Microsurgery. Highlights Ophthal. 7 (1964) 212

Zehender, W. von: Beschreibung der binocularen Cornea-Lupe. Klin. Mbl. Augenheilk. 25 (1887) 496

CHAPTER 1

A History of Microsurgery

"If I have contributed the meanest foundations whereon others may raise nobler superstructures, I am abundantly satisfied, and all my ambition is, that I may serve to the great philosophers of this age, as the makers and the grinders of my glasses did to me; that I may prepare and furnish them with some materials, which they may afterwards order and manage with better skill and to far greater advantage."

Robert Hooke 1665

Any historian discovers that history has no beginning nor an end. No matter how diligent the search, sooner or later evidence is always discovered of a development anteceding what had been considered the earliest beginnings. Likewise between the writing and the publication or between the preparation and the telling a succession of days enters history during which advances are invariably made which make the latest presentation or publication a little out of date. Cognizant of this and aware of the fact that in microsurgery we are dealing with a discipline so new that most of the developers are still living, we realize that we lack the clarification that comes from distant appraisal. Yet an historical sketch has been deemed advisable because microsurgery has become a discipline of importance and a discipline of importance deserves to have its history known.

The term "microsurgery" has come to mean surgery performed upon small structures usually with the help of some form of magnification, in particular the dissecting microscope.

The term „Microscope" is derived from the Greek:

μιχρο (small)
σχοπέυω (I view)

The origin of this term is attributed by Quekett to Demisianus. Skinner attributes the term to Johannes Faber (1574—1629) of Bamberg. If Quekett is correct it is a little difficult to consider when microsurgery under magnification began, because the word "microscope" was coined before the compound microscope was invented. In its beginning the term probably meant only magnification.

Sir John Layard found what appeared to be a simple magnifying lens in the excavations at Nineveh believed to date from 700 B. C. Aristophanes, 500 years B. C. wrote of small globules of glass which were filled with water and used as burning spheres. It seems unlikely they were not likewise used for magnification.

Pliny, who died in 79 A. D., mentions "burning spheres" and Ptolemy of Alexandria also of the first century, uses the word refraction as related to optics.

Roger Bacon (1214—1294) is believed to have invented the telescope. It would seem incredible that he did not peer at small objects through the instrument with a variety of lenses, but no record is available of his having done so.

Nicolas Copernicus of Poland, in 1542 observed the sky and planets through an instrument with more than one lens. He thus discovered that the sun was the center of our Universe but that we were only one of many Universes.

Credit for the first use of the principle of compound lenses for viewing small objects is given by various authors to different individuals. Borelli states that Zacharias Janssen of Holland first invented and used the compound microscope in 1590. Galileo is said by Viviani to have invented a compound microscope in 1610, while Fontana of Naples claimed a similar discovery himself in 1618.

Huyghens gives credit for disvovery to a Dutchman, Drebbel, in 1621. At any rate, by the mid-seventeenth century much microscopic investigation was being carried out.

In 1665 Robert Hooke of England published his "Micrographia" "on some physiological descriptions of minute bodies made by magnifying glasses." This was an early and major work having to do with accurate scientific observations through the microscope.

Jan Swammerdam (1637–1680) of Amsterdam wrote "Book of Nature" considered by some to be the greatest compilation of data ever made through a microscope and recorded by one man.

Sir Isaac Newton in 1672 invented a compound reflecting microscope and in 1673 Anthony van Leuwenhoeck published "Philosophical Transactions," a major scientific treatise on observations through a microscope.

Malpighi, about this time, wrote of observations under magnification and in 1661 observed capillary circulation. In 1682 Mehemia Gren (1641–1712) of London wrote "The Anatomy of Plants." He noted that plants were sexual and traced the vascular patterns of plants under magnification.

Jean Zahn of Nuremberg in 1702 published the description of several compound microscopes, including two which were binocular, in a work entitled "Occulus Artificialis Teledoptricus."

The muscular coat of arteries and various portions of the brain as seen under the microscope were described in "Handbook of Systematic Anatomy," by Jacob Henle (1809 to 1885).

In 1886 F. E. Schulze, a zoologist in Berlin, used the device put together by Westien of Rostock to prepare zoological specimens more accurately. This consisted of binocular magnifying glasses. Zehender adapted this to ophthalmic surgery in what was known as "Zehender-Westiensches Doppelskop".

In 1899 Axenfeld reported an instrument with a headband giving 5–6-fold magnification but which had a prohibitive weight. The wide use of magnification in surgery, however, did not occur for some years yet.

The otorhinolaryngologists seem to have been about the first to realize the limitation

placed upon the human hand by the human eye.

Nylén in 1924 reported an apparatus which allowed for a microscope tube through which he could visualize a portion of his field. He obtained in his monoscope a magnification from 18–235 but complained of poor lighting at higher magnifications, a complaint not uncommon in microsurgical operating rooms 45 years later.

Cawthorne in "A Review of Surgery of Otosclerosis" written in 1946 says, "Holmgren soon abandoned the superior canal and turned his attention back to the lateral canal and even to the promontory, and in 1921 he was trephining the promontory, fashioning the mucoperiosteal flap, using magnifying spectacles and a binocular microscope. Holmgren was the first to advocate the use of a binocular dissecting microscope using 10 diopters of magnification."

In 1941 Cawthorne spoke of his own work with a Leitz dissecting microscope and gave credit to Professor Dohlman at Lund and Mr. C. H. Hallpike for having suggested its use to him.

Joseph A. Sullivan in 1952 stated "I particularly stress the importance of magnification in any procedure on the facial nerve. I have been using it now for years."

House and House in 1964 wrote "One of the pioneers of otologic surgery was George Shambaugh Jr. While Gunnar Holmgren had used a binocular dissecting microscope for his early operations for otosclerosis, Shambaugh was the first to use it consistently and routinely for the one stage Lempert fenestration operation, beginning as early as 1939."

Next the ophthalmologists evinced interest. Perritt of Chicago used the dissecting microscope for operating on the eye in 1946. Barraquer in 1956, Becker in 1956, Dekking and Troutman followed.

Beyond the field of otolaryngology and ophthalmology the first publication came from vascular surgeons Jacobson and Suarez of the University of Vermont, who in 1960 wrote an article in Surgical Forums entitled "Microsurgery in Anastomosis of Small Vessels." The time was ripe and a succession of articles from many disciplines in numerous centers and from all corners of the world have followed since that time.

There may have been earlier application, at least in the field of the nervous system, but they have not been published and so all agree that Jacobson and Suarez must be given the credit for directing the attention of so many to this intriguing technique.

It is interesting to note that although Jacobson has written much on microsurgery that he felt it important to advance first along vascular channels and that workers in most other disciplines since, that is in neurosurgery plastic surgery and cardiology, have followed this pattern.

Perhaps before embarking upon a summary of the history of surgery in such small vessels one should first recall a short history of vascular surgery in general because here, except for the size of the vessels involved, the pattern of advance has been very much the same and even the failures and frustrations have been very similar.

Apparently Lambert in England must have expressed the opinion that one might suture the wound in an artery sometime before 1759, because on June 15, 1759 Hallowell in England attempted to do this very thing, and this case was later discussed by Jassinowsky, at which time he stated that Hallowell had used the method of Lambert. Jassinowsky had this to say about the case "Der Puls war in dem verletzt gewesenen Arme um ein geringes schwächer als im gesunden, aber doch so stark, daß man an einer freien Zirkulation des Blutes in der genähten Arterie nicht zweifeln konnte".

This case was probably not succesful since in 1762 Lambert wrote "Upon the whole I was in hopes that suture of the wound of the artery might be successful and if so it would certainly be preferable to tying up the trunk of the vessel." Then he goes on prophetically to state, "If it should be found by experience that a larger artery when wounded may be healed up by this kind of suture, without becoming impervious, it would be an important discovery in surgery, it would make the operation for the aneurysm still more successful in the arm when the main trunk is wounded, and by this method, we might be able to cure the wounds of some arteries that would otherwise require amputation or be altogether incurable."

In 1773 Conradus Asman tried to perform such suturing on the femoral vessels of four dogs, apparently without success. "His factis ne gutta quidem sanguinis per arteriae vulnus effluebat." "Systole et diastole etiam infra arteriae vulnus admodum erant conspicuae." Asman contended with many hardships including lack of anesthesia, "vulnus vero propter motum canis non in loco arteriae, per quem acicula erat demissa, sed infra illum fuit inflictum, ita ut canis brevi ex hemorrhagia mortua fuisset."

Surgeons have always worried about beginning a new procedure because in their thinking brain they have known what they sought to develop but their doing brain had not reached the point of perfection to allow for success, and so they were likely to give the procedure a bad reputation before it had been established. This was true with appendectomy where, for some years, all patients with abdominal pain were observed. If they improved they were discharged. If they worsened, i. e. ruptured, they were given to the surgeon. Statistics definitely demonstrated a much lower mortality in those conservatively managed.

Likewise the vascular situation was misinterpreted by Broca in 1856 in his monograph on Aneurysm. "L'idée de Lambert ne prit cependant pas place dans la pratique; mais elle eut un grand succés dans les livres, jusqu'a ce qu'enfin Asman eût demonstré, par des experiences faites sur des animaux, que la suture oblitérait infailliblement les artères."

The first venous surgery of which we have record was suturing of a partially severed femoral vein by Travers in 1816.

In 1881 Czerny sutured a jugular vein which had bled in a suppurating wound. Schede in 1882, while operating upon an inguinal carcinoma, injured a femoral vein and repaired it. Also in 1882 Gluck experimentally sutured the common iliac artery and the aorta in the dog.

It was in 1889 that Alexander Jassinowsky wrote his remarkable treatise on Arterial Suturing in which he discussed comparisons of suture materials and size, needle size and shape, padding, patches, instruments etc.

His conclusions were:

1. Arterial sutures are safe for vessel wounds.

2. There is little bleeding after operation.

3. Even after time neither bleeding nor thrombosis nor aneurysm formation need be feared.

4. The arterial suture may be longitudinal, diagonal, or overlapping, and closure is indicated for transverse wounds of half the circumference.

5. Strict asepsis is a sine qua non of arterial suturing.

6. Arterial suturing is easily feasible.

The use of various prostheses either to replace the vessel wall or as a frame over which to suture, is likewise of long standing.

Robert Abbe used glass tubing in performing end to end anastomosis of femoral arteries in the dog in 1894.

An ivory prosthesis for help in intima-to-intima anastomosis of a divided vessel was used by Nitze in 1897. Likewise, in 1897 the first end-to-end anastomosis in man was performed by Murphy. In 1900 Payr used absorbable magnesium prostheses and in 1903 Jensen used bone as a prosthetic device. Carrel and Guthrie gave tremendous impetus to vascular surgery by their extensive work and publications dating from 1906 on, during which time not only did they experiment to find the most favorable methods of suturing both arteries and veins, but also experimented with suture types and tissue transplantation.

Matas pioneered in vascular surgery in the days before World War II, and with World War II new interest was kindled. Many names now famous began to enter the literature, Elkins, De Bakey, De Takats, Harken, Bailey, etc. Once large vessel techniques were reasonably well worked out improvement in small vessel techniques were naturally sought.

Microangeional or Microvascular Surgery

Although microsurgery is tremendously facilitated by the use of the surgical dissecting microscope and many of the advances in surgery of small structures have been dependent upon it, it would not be proper to exclude from the category, surgery upon small structures where magnification is not employed. In the field of blood vessels the term "microsurgery" has been limited to vessels under 4 mm. in outside diameter and in particular those with an outside diameter of 2 mm. or less.

The terms microangeional or microvascular are synonymous and are both included in this heading to point out the fact, so that future confusion may be avoided, since both terms are to be found in the literature. The term used is not important, and minor controversies are boring, but do deserve an explanation. In this case traditionalists such as Jacobson and Cobbett have felt that "microvascular" has been a widely used and well known term, that it is understood and deserves to be retained on the basis of precedent. It has to be pointed out that the origin of both parts of the word "microscope" are derived from the Greek, that this is likewise true of the word "microsurgery", but that the term "microvascular" is half Greek and half Latin in derivation, and that the term "microangeional", therefore, more nearly conforms to customary practice.

Schumacker and Lowenberg in 1948 conducted a study on various suture techniques on small vessels. A better understanding of flow patterns came from the beautiful work on microsurgery by Sven Bellman in 1953.

Crawford, Beall, Ellis and De Bakey, in 1960, presented experimental data to demonstrate the advisability of patching small vessels to prevent narrowing at the point of suture. Urschel and Roth attained a patency of 73 per cent in the ulnar arteries of dogs measuring 1.5 to 2 mm. in outside diameter, in 1960 even without the microscope.

Many techniques hitherto unknown were being added to the armamentarium to help insure an increased patency rate. Hedberg in 1961 forced dilatation of small vessels prior to suture in order to overcome spasm and noted a patency rate approaching 100 per cent in canine femoral arteries.

Casten, Sadler and Forman in 1962 reported a beneficial effect on patency rate of end-to-end anastomoses in small arteries if sympathectomy were performed prior to surgery.

Seidenberg, Hurwitt and Carton in 1958 described their meticulous technique for small vessel suture and advised "a flange method" of small arterial anastomosis of real value when vessels can be joined at points of branching. They also recorded experience with three successful human cases:

1. A spleno-renal arterial anastomosis.

2. The anastomosis of visceral arteries to an aortic homograph.

3. An end-to-end anastomosis between the radial branch of the superior mesenteric artery and the inferior thyroid artery in a case where jejunum was used to form a cervical esophagus.

Other contributions to methods of suturing have come from De Leon, Crane and Spencer in 1961; Man and Kohn of Haifa, Israel, in 1962; Stahl and Katsumura of Burlington in 1964; Khodadad and Lougheed of Toronto in 1966; Donaghy in 1966; and in veins, Carter in 1962, and Collins and Douglass in 1964.

Most, but not all, of the advances made in suturing after 1960 were made by use of the dissecting microscope. The history of the expanding use of the surgical microscope is worth reviewing. As previously mentioned,

Jacobson and Suarez deserve the credit for bringing to the attention of surgeons in general the possibilities of this instrument. Several other early workers with the microscope deserve mention.

Neurosurgery

In so far as the nervous system is concerned the first record of the use of the scope was that by Lougheed and Tom of Toronto. In 1961 they published a paper "A Method of Introducing Blood into the Subarachnoid Space in the Region of the Circle of Willis in Dogs." The work reported had been begun in the middle of 1950 and in the experiment the Zeiss dissecting microscope had been used.

The first clinical application to the nervous system was by Theodore Kurze of Los Angeles, as Rand states, "I know that Dr. Ted Kurze began to use the surgical microscope in August 1957 and thought of the idea of the subtemporal transmeatal approach to the internal auditory canal". Ernest Sachs in 1965 wrote, "Theodore Kurze of The University of Southern California, who started the microsurgical approach to the petrous bone in the middle fossa with Dr. House, showed a movie, with Robert Rand, of the suboccipital total removal of an acoustic neurinoma."

On August 4, 1960 Jacobson and Donaghy in Burlington performed an endarterectomy on the middle cerebral artery of a patient of Dr. George Schumacher, the craniotomy and vessel exposure having been done under the microscope by the latter surgeon, and the actual endarterectomy by the former. This case was reported by them in 1961. The procedure, of course, was not original, the first such procedure having been done by Keasley Welch in 1955 and by Scheibert in 1959, but without the aid of the microscope. Neither Welch's case nor that of Donaghy and Jacobson maintained patency, as noted on subsequent angiography. The case of

Dr. Scheibert remained open until he died of coronary thrombosis nine months later. The first totally successful case was reported by Shelley Chou in 1963. The first publication on the use of the microscope in intracranial aneurysm surgery was by Pool and Colton in 1966, although Adams and Witt had given a paper on this subject in 1964. Rand published his case in 1967 of the first cerebral aneurysm done under the operating microscope in 1964, Jannetta was the first to use the transtentorial approach in the exposure of the trigeminal nerve under the microscope (1966).

The outstanding contributions to surgery of blood vessels of all sizes in the nervous system by Krayenbühl and Yaşargil in Zürich have been well known for many years. Yaşargil had been somewhat concerned when dealing with smaller vessels because of the poor visibility, and had come to the United States to do experimental work in the micro-angeional laboratory of Burlington.

One point was still of concern. This was the control of bleeding of small vessels on the cord surface without damage to contiguous tissue. At this very time Leonard Malis of Mount Sinai Hospital in New York brought forth his bipolar coagulator.

Bipolar Electric Coagulation

Leonard Malis of New York in 1956 working in the animal laboratory found he could not successfully elevate the dura from an area previously operated and irradiated except under the dissecting microscope, and that even then bleeding could not be easily controlled without undue tissue damage, and so he developed a bipolar coagulator capable of coagulating fine vessels without damage to surrounding tissue, and this instrument has become widely used in working with vessels in an area surrounded by important tissues.

Microinstruments

Jacobson early on pointed out the necessity for special instruments with small tips for work under the microscope. His first instruments were borrowed from ophthalmologists, otorhinolaryngologists and from jewellers.

Scarcely an operator since has not devised some instrument of his own. Of special importance are such instruments as the pneumatic needle holder of Salmon and Assimacopoulos.

A further refinement has been the double hydraulic needle holder of Buncke and Schulz. The latest instruments to be designed in this line are the battery of very beautiful instruments recently designed by Yaşargil and the instruments designed by Hardy for transsphenoid hypophysectomy.

Peripheral nerves

The surgical microscope has proven to be a great advantage in the alignment and suture of nerves. Perhaps the outstanding clinical experience with the technique belongs to James W. Smith of New York. He has made a particularly complete and important study of the vascular supply of nerves as seen under the microscope and of the vaso vasorum.

Chaffee and Numoto in 1964 demonstrated a more complete return of motor units as demonstrated by EMG and muscles innervated by the sciatic nerves of rats when the nerves were sutured under the microscope than when they were sutured under normal vision.

Plastic Surgery

Almost all investigators in any field will state the development of their final concepts and techniques were gradual and began only as a faint idea which invariably came from stimulus or other.

In the field of plastic surgery the man who more than any other has been responsible for the development of micro methods is Harry

J. Buncke of San Mateo, California. He gives credit to Mr. Thomas Gibson of Glasgow for the idea that in transplanting, a temporary vascular hookup might be made to survive until a more permanent system had developed. This was in 1957, and in 1958 Dr. Buncke set out to do just this with the rabbit's ear. At once he learned he must deal with vessels with external limits of 0.8 to 1.2 mm. He gives credit to Jacobson for directing him to the dissecting microscope which he began using in 1962. His first published work in which he had used the microscope was in 1963. By 1964 he had transplanted a thumb and index finger in a monkey.

John R. Cobbett of London who saw the work of Buncke in California while a Moynihan Fellow in 1965 has used the technique to successfully transplant a great toe for use as a thumb in a human. He has added to the technique one of his own features for vascular surgery which he terms "eccentric biangulation".

In 1965 Krisek, Tani, Desprez, and Kiehn wrote a stimulating article on a transplantation of composite grafts by utilizing microsurgical anastomoses.

Clinical Application

There have been many clinical applications of the dissecting microscope in the human and this, after all, is the measure of the method.

These include approaches to problems concerning the ossicles of the ear, the facial nerve in its canal and the fenestration by the otorhinolaryngologists.

It has contributed to most of the procedures done upon the eye.

The approach to the acoustic neurinoma *via* the external auditory canal has been based on the use of the dissecting microscope. Other tumors of the nervous system, particularly in the posterior fossa and spinal canal have likewise been resected under such magnification.

Intracranial aneurysms can be more accurately ligated; if torn, the opening can be more accurately closed by this technique.

Operations for trigeminal neuralgia are commonly done with the microscope to guide the hand and there is evidence that by this method some function may be spared while relief is obtained.

Thrombectomies and embolectomies of intracranial vessels have been performed, extra-intracranial blood flow diversions have been made, communications between intracranial vessels have been created to provide circulation to a distal part where a proximal ligation has been necessary.

Digits have been replaced when amputated and a great toe has even been substituted for a thumb when the latter was lost.

The pituitary gland has been removed under the microscope and under the microscope it has been possible to selectively remove that part of the gland desired while leaving the remainder intact.

Peripheral nerves, the ureter and the coronary artery have all felt the benefit of more accurate surgery under magnification.

The road so far travelled has been short but broad and no man sees its end.

References

Allen, R. M.: The Microscope. Van Nostrand, New York 1940

Bellman, S.: Microangiography. Acta radiol. Suppl. 102 (1953)

Buncke, Jr. H. J., W. P. Schulz: Experimental digital amputation and reimplantation. Plast. reconstr. Surg. 36 (1965) 62

Buncke, Jr. H. J., A. I. Daniller, W. P. Schulz, R. A. Chase: The fate of autogenous whole joints transplanted by microvascular anastomoses. Plast. reconstr. Surg. 39 (1967) 333

Byron, F. X., J. Fields, R. Hood, A. Foster: The use of rigid prosthesis in vascular surgery. J. thorac. Surg. 34 (1957) 423

Carrel, A., C. C. Guthrie: Uniterminal and biterminal venous transplantations. Surg. Gynec. Obstet 2 (1906) 266

Carter, E., E. J. Roth: Direct nonsuture coronary artery anastomosis in the dog. Ann. Surg. 148 (1958) 212

Carter, P. D.: Suture and nonsuture methods of small vein anastomoses. Arch. Surg. (Chic.) 84 (1962) 350

Casten, D. F., A. H. Sadler, D. Forman: An experimental study of the effect of sympathectomy on patency of small blood vessels anastomoses. Surg. Gynec. Obstet. 115 (1962) 462

Chaffee, B.: Personal communication, 1965.

Clendenning, L.: Source Book of Medical History. Dover, New York 1942

Cobbett, J. R.: Microvascular surgery. Surg. Clin. N. Amer. 47 (1967) 521

Collins, R. E., F. M. Douglass: Small vein anastomosis with and without operative microscope. A comparative study Arch. Surg. Chicago 88 (1964) 740

Crawford, E. S., A. C. Beall, P. R. Ellis Jr., M. E. DeBakey: A technic permitting operation upon small arteries. Surg. Forum 10 (1960) 671

Donaghy, R. M. P.: Patch and by-pass in microangeional surgery. In: Micro-Vascular Surgery. Ed. by R. M. P. Donaghy, M. G. Yaşargil. Mosby, St. Louis, Thieme, Stuttgart 1967, pp. 75-86

Donaghy, R. M. P., J. H. Jacobson, III, L. J. Wallman, M. E. Flanagan, A. G. Mackay: Microsurgery: A neurological aid. Second Int. Congress of Neurological Surgeons (Washington, D.C.). No. 36, Excerpta Medica International Congress Series, 1961, E-175-176

Donaghy, R. M. P., M. G. Yaşargil: Extra-intracranial blood flow diversion. Presented to American Association of Neurological Surgeons, Chicago, Ill. 11 April, 1968

Guthrie, C. C.: Some physiological aspects of blood vessel surgery. J. amer. med. Ass. 51 (1908) 1658

Guthrie, D.: A History of Medicine. Lippincott, Philadelphia 1946

Harms, H., G. Mackensen: Augenoperationen unter dem Mikroskop. Thieme, Stuttgart 1966

Hedberg, St. E.: Suture anastomosis of small vessels following relief of spasm by hydrostatic pressure dilatation. Ann. Surg. 155 (1962) 51

House, H., W. House: Historical review and problem of acoustic neuroma. Arch. Otolaryng. 80 (1964) 601

Jacobson, J. H., II, D. B. Miller, E. Suarez: Microvascular surgery: a new horizon in coronary artery surgery. Abstr. Circulation 22 (1960) 767

Jannetta, P. J.: Transtentorial retrogasserian rhizotomy in trigeminal neuralgia by microneurosurgical technique. Bull. Los Angeles Neurol. Soc. 31 (1966) 93

Jannetta, P. J.: Gross (mesoscopic) description of the human trigeminal nerve and ganglion. J. Neurosurg. 26 (1967) 109

Jannetta, P. J. Arterial compression af the trigeminal nerve at the pons in patients with trigeminal neuralgia. J. Neurosurg. 26 (1967) 159

Jannetta, P. J.: The surgical binocular microscope in neurological surgery. Amer. Surg. 34 (1968) 31

Jannetta, P. J., R. W. Rand: Vascular compression of the trigeminal nerve at the pons in patients with trigeminal neuralgia. In Micro-Vascular Surgery. Ed. by R. M. P. Donaghy, and M. G. Yaşargil, Mosby, St. Louis, Thieme, Stuttgart 1967, p. 150

Jassinowsky, A.: Die Arteriennaht. Med. Diss. Mattiesen, Dorpat 1889

Khodadad, G., W. M. Lougheed: Stapling technique in segmental vein autografts and end-to-end anastomosis of small vessels in dogs. Utilization of the operating microscope. J. Neurosurg. 24 (1966) 855

Khodadad, G., W. M. Lougheed: Repair and replacement of small arteries, microsuture technique. J. Neurosurg. 24 (1966) 61

Kosse, K. H., E. L. Suarez, W. T. Fagan, P. R. Powell, J. H. Jacobson II.: Microsurgery in ureteral reconstruction. J. Urol. 87 (1962) 48

Krizek, T. J., T. Tani, J. D. Desprez, C. L. Kiehn: Experimental transplantation of composite grafts by microsurgical vascular anastomoses. Plast. reconstr. Surg. 36 (1965) 538

Leon, A. R. De, P. S. Crane, F. C. Spencer: Use of an autogenous vein patch in the performance of end-to-end anastomoses in small arteries. Surg. Forum 12 (1961) 258

Lougheed, W. M.: Surgery of intracranial vascular occlusion. In: Micro-Vascular Surgery. Ed. R. M. P. Donaghy, M. G. Yaşargil. Mosby, St. Louis, Thieme, Stuttgart 1967, pp. 142—147

Lougheed, W. M., R. W. Gunton, H. J. M. Barnett: Embolectomy of internal carotid, middle and anterior cerebral arteries. J. Neurosurg. 22 (1965) 607

Lougheed, W. M., M. Tom: A method of introducing blood into the subarachnoid space in the region of the Circle of Willis in dogs. Can. J. Surg. 4 (1961) 329

Malis, L. I.: Bipolar coagulation in microsurgery. In: Micro-Vascular Surgery. Ed. by R. M. P. Donaghy, M. G. Yaşargil. Mosby, St. Louis, Thieme, Stuttgart 1967, pp. 126—130

Man, B., Z. Kohn: Experiments on the anastomosis of small vessels. J. cardiovasc. Surg. 3 (1962) 195

Moody, R. A.: Some observations on the development of the new microangeional service. In: Micro-Vascular Surgery. Ed. by R. M. Donaghy, M. G. Yaşargil. Mosby. St. Louis, Thieme, Stuttgart 1967, pp. 19—24

Mozes, M., B. Man, M. Agmon, R. Adar: Small vessel anastomoses. Surg. 54 (1963) 609

Muñoz, F. J., H. A. Charipper: The Microscope and its use. Chemical Publishing, Brocklyn, 1943

Nylén, C. O.: An oto-microscope. Acta otolaryng. (Stockholm) 5 (1924) 414

Quekett, J.: A practical Treatise on the Use of the Microscope. Bailliere London 1955

Rand, R. W., P. J. Jannetta: Micro-neurosurgery for aneurysms of the vertebral-basilar artery system. J. Neurosurg. 27 (1967) 330

Schumacker, Jr., H. B., R. I. Lowenberg: Experimental studies in vascular repair. Surg. 24 (1948) 79

Scobie, D. H., T. K. Scobie, I. J. Vogelfanger: Venous autografts. Canad. J. Surg. 5 (1962) 471

Seidenberg, B., E. S. Hurwitt, C. A. Carton: The technique of anastomosing small arteries. Surg. Gynec. Obstet. 106 (1958) 743

Shillito, J.: Intracranial arteriotomy in three children and three adults. In: Micro-Vascular Surgery. Ed. by R. M. P. Donaghy, M. G. Yaşargil. Mosby, St. Louis, Thieme, Stuttgart 1967, pp. 138—142

Skinner, H. A.: The Origin of Medical Terms 2nd. Ed. Williams & Wilkins, Baltimore 1961 (Microscope p. 276 and surgeon p. 372)

Smith, J. W.: Microsurgery: Review of the literature and discussion of microtechniques. Plast. reconstr. Surg. 37 (1966) 227

Stahl, W. M., T. Katsumura: Reconstruction of small arteries. A study of methods. Arch. Surg. 88 (1964) 384

Stevenson, G. C.: Trans-clival exposure of the basilar artery: A case presentation of basilar artery embolectomy in man. In: Micro-Vascular Surgery. Ed. by. R. M. P. Donaghy, M. G. Yaşargil. Mosby, St. Louis, Thieme, Stuttgart 1967, pp. 148—149

Stevenson, G. C., R. J. Stoney, R. K. Perkins, J. A. Adams: A transcervical transclival approach to the ventral surface of the brain stem for removal of a clivus chordoma. J. Neurosurg. 24 (1966) 544

Tiscornia, O. M., J. H. Jacobson II, D. A. Dreiling: Microsurgery of the canine pancreatic duct: experimental study and review of previous approaches to the management of pancreatic duct pathology. Surg. 58 (1965) 58

Troutman, R. C.: Interview in Highlights Ophthal. 7 (1964) 162

Troutman, R. C.: The operating microscope in ophthalmic surgery. Trans. amer. ophthal. Soc. 63 (1965) 335

Urschel, Jr., H. C., E. J. Roth: Small arterial anastomoses: I. Nonsuture. Ann. Surg. 153 (1961) 599

Urschel, Jr., H. C., E. J. Roth: Small arterial anastomoses: II. Suture. Ann. Surg. 153 (1961) 610

Villegas, L. D. de: Technique for end-to-end anastomoses between artificial grafts and arteries with minimal interruption of the circulation. Surg. 40 (1956) 1035

Voe A. G. De: Interview. Highlights Opthal. 7 (1964) 212

Weiss, E. W., C. R. Lam: Tantalum tubes in the nonsuture method of blood vessel anastomosis. Amer. J. Surg. 80 (1950) 452

Yaşargil, M. G.: Experimental small vessel surgery in the dog including patching and grafting of cerebral vessels and the formation of functional extra-intracranial shunts. Ed. by R. M. P. Donaghy, M. G. Yaşargil. Mosby. St. Louis, Thieme, Stuttgart 1967, pp. 87—126

CHAPTER 2

A. The Operating Microscope

The Operating Microscope and its Attachments

The operating microscope shown in Fig. 1 was developed in 1952. The microscope is supported on a stand which contains a counterbalancing weight. Recently, an electric motor was mounted to provide automatic up-and-down motion with foot pedal control. The microscope can be moved manually into any desired position. The vertical movement may be freely executed without use of the motor. When the microscope points directly downwards, the motorized vertical movement functions as a fine focus. In all other positions the microscope is focussed by adjusting the control knobs indicated in Fig. 2.

The straight binocular observer tube is detachable. Depending on the nature of the

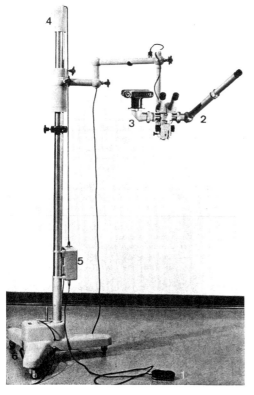

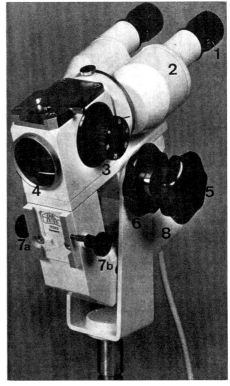

Fig. 1. The operating microscope: OPMi I on its stand with motorized head; 1, pedal for operating the electric motor; 2, observer tube; 3, adapter with camera; 4, motorized head; 5, power supply unit; 6, light switch.

Fig. 2. The operating microscope: 1, ocular; 2, straight ocular tube; 3, magnification changer; 4, objective; 5, focussing control; 6, clamping ring for adjusting tilt of head; 7a and 7b, daylight and red-free filter; 8, lamp.

operation, it can be inverted or replaced by an angled binocular tube. The field of operation is coaxially illuminated through the objective lens from a light source incorporated in the microscope. This is essential for operating on deep structures.

The focal length of the objective lens, which is indicated on the frame of the lens, must correspond to the operating space available, i. e., the distance between the patient's tissues and the lens. Objective lenses of varying focal lenght are available, and they are freely interchangeable. The objective lens is selected according to the operating space that is required. In neurosurgery the most useful lenses are those with focal lengths of 300—400 mm. These lenses are graduated in steps of 25 mm.: thus 300, 325, 350 mm., etc.

The optic system of the apparatus is shown diagrammatically in Fig. 3. The objective

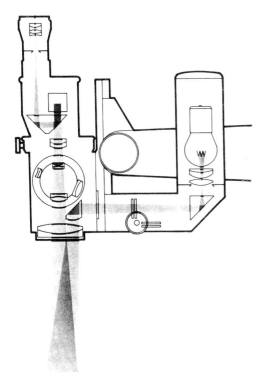

Fig. 3. Optical principles of OPMi I.

lens is on the left and behind it there is a rotating drum with two pairs of refractors that can be interposed in the beam; the one pair is for image enlargement and the other for reduction. In this way four grades of magnification are possible. Fig. 3 also shows the illumination system by which the light beam is coaxially directed through the objective lens of the microscope.

The magnification control knob is graduated, the various settings corresponding to the degree of enlargement through the microscope. However, they are indicated by mere numbers 6, 10, 16, 25 and 40 — and the actual magnification must be determined with the aid of a table (Table 1).

Microscope magnification depends on the following factors: the focal length of the objective, the magnification of the eyepiece, the focal length of the tube (fixed at 160 mm.) and the magnification setting used. By suitable combinations of these factors the microscope can be operated within a defined range over the operating space and magnification available. It is very useful, in the practical application of the microscope, to have the operating space, i. e., the distance between the objective and the field of operation, unaffected by changes in magnification brought about by adjustment of the magnification control knob. The diameter of the field of vision through the microscope depends simply on the magnification, so that this also can be controlled. The microscope magnification corresponds to the following equation:

$$V = f_t/f_o \cdot W/16 - V_{ok} \qquad (1)$$

where f_o = focal length of the objective lens in mm.

f_t = focal length of the tube. For both the long angled tube and the long straight tube — and only these are used here — this is 160 mm. Shorter tubes with f_t = 125 mm. are also available for this microscope.

W = setting on the magnification control knob.

V_{ok} = magnification of eyepiece. For this apparatus, lenses of $10\times$, $12.5\times$, $16\times$ and $20\times$ magnification are available.

Table I. Magnification with the OP Mi I Operation Microscope
(valid for long tubes, f = 160 mm.)

Objective Lens mm.	Control knob setting					Eyepiece
	6	10	16	25	40	
200	3	5	8	13	20	
300	2	3	5	8	13	10 ×
400	1.5	2.5	4	6	10	
200	4	6	10	16	25	
300	2.5	4	6	10	16	12.5 ×
400	2	3	5	8	13	
200	5	8	13	20	32	
300	3	5	8	13	20	16 ×
400	2.5	4	6	10	16	
200	6	10	16	25	40	20 ×
300	4	6	10	16	25	20 ×
400	3	5	8	13	20	

Microscope Magnification

Table I and Equation (1) reflect values that are valid for the three objective lenses and the eyepiece used in any of the five settings on the magnification control knob.

It is possible, with a fixed working distance, to vary the field of magnification by changing the eyepiece, e.g. with a working distance of 300 mm., a 2 to 13 × range of magnification is possible with the 10 × eyepiece and a 4 to 25 × with the 20 × eyepiece.

The optical parts of the microscope are so coordinated that the diameter of the field of vision in mm. is given by the following simple equation.

$$d = 200/V \qquad (2)$$

This equation is valid for all the microscopes described here, irrespective of the optical combination used to produce the magnification. For example, for the highest magnification shown in Table I, V = 40 ×, a field of vision of d = 5 mm. is obtained from the objective lens, while for the lowest magnification, V = 1.5 ×, the diameter of the field of vision is 133 mm.

Coaxial illumination provides a sharply defined, homogeneously illuminated field, with a diameter

$$d_L = 0.16, f_o \text{ mm.} \qquad (3)$$

This diameter depends only on the objective lens. For the 3 lenses listed in Table I, it amounts to the following: 32 mm. (objective lens 200 mm.); 48 mm. (objective lens 300 mm.); and 64 mm. (objective lens 400 mm.).

The working distance should be kept to a minimum at all times, consistent with surgical needs, because the brightness decreases progressively with increasing working distance.

If a beam divider is placed between the head of the microscope and the binocular tube, as is shown in Fig. 4, it is possible to attach still cine and television cameras as well as a second eyepiece to it. The beam divider has a mirror surface in the path of each of the two incident beams. It is semi-translucent, reflecting as much light as it allows to pass along the tube. Since the beam division occurs in parallel between the microscope and the tube, the optical picture of the

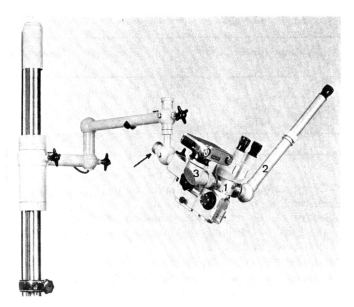

Fig. 4. OPMi I with 1, beam divider; 2, observer tube and 3, camera adapter, with the optical system tilted at an angle (arrow).

microscope is unaffected. The only effect observed by the operator is a diminution of brightness, and this can be overcome by using a stronger illumination source.

The beam divider serves a dual purpose, as is shown in Fig. 4. The beam from the right tube is used for a second eyepiece, while that from the left tube is passed through a photoadapter and used for 35 mm. photography. The view seen through the second eyepiece is the same as that seen by the right eye of the operator. By adjusting the tube to the most favorable position the observer has a wide range of movement around the horizontal axis and can rotate the image as well. He can change the axis, by rotating the ring around the middle of the tube. The photoadapter attachment can be used for a second observer tube instead of a camera, so that two observers may view the course of the operation in monocular vision at the same time. Conversely, the second tube can be replaced by a second photoadapter, so that stereophotography may be carried out (Fig. 8a).

The photoadapter contains a photographic objective lens with a 220 mm. focal length. It is principally intended for 35 mm. photo-

graphy. In theory, a 16 mm., cine camera or a television camera can also be linked to the photoadapter although the use of these devices is somewhat limited by the small size of the image obtained. A special cine and television adapter has been designed for this purpose (Fig. 9b).

The photoadapter produces an image, as is shown in Fig. 4, with the light controlled by the magnification knob. The photoadapter is so constructed that it portrays accurately, within an area of the 35 mm. negative, the picture seen by the observer with his left eye (Fig. 4), provided that a $12.5 \times$ eyepiece and a long tube ($f_t = 160$ mm.) are used. (With short tubes a $16\times$ eyepiece must be used, to gain the same effect.)

The photographic magnification V_p, produced on the film by the objective lens, depends on the magnification of the eyepiece and the length of the tube, since neither contributes to the origin of the image. V_p amounts to:

$$V_p = f_p \cdot W/16 - f_o \qquad (4)$$

where $f_p = 220$ mm. = the focal length of the photoadapter,

Table II. Photographic Magnification with the OPMi I Operating Microscope Photoadapter 220 mm.

Objective Lens	Control knob setting				
mm.	6	10	16	25	40
200	0.4	0.7	1.1	1.8	2.7
300	0.3	0.6	0.7	1.2	1.8
400	0.2	0.3	0.6	0.9	1.4
			Photographic magnification		

W = the setting of the magnification control knob, and f_o = the focal length of the objective of the microscope. Equation (4) is the basis for deriving the magnification values shown in Table II.

All the magnification values given in Table II are doubled when a $2 \times$ supplementary objective lens is placed between the adapter and the camera.

The photoadapter possesses an adjustable diaphragm to regulate the brightness and the sharpness of the image. In most cases these factors have to be determined empirically. The following specifications give approximate values:

With OPMi I it is possible with the use of a 300 mm. objective, the 220 mm. photoadapter, an electronic flash gun of 240 watt-seconds and color film of 160 ASA speed (Kodak Ektachrome High Speed) to obtain a photographic magnification of up to $V_p = 2$. Similar results may be achieved without the use of an electronic flash gun, by using a 6 volt 50 watt lamp and overloading it with 10 amps. With 125 ASA color film (Kodak Ektachrome High Speed), exposure times of 0.25–0.5 seconds are necessary.

It is possible to utilize the photoadapter in the same way to obtain 16 mm. cine magnifications of up to $V_p = 0.7$ with 16 frames/second or $V_p = 0.5$ with 24 frames/second, using color film, (e.g. Eastman Kodak Ektachrome EF Type B). It is to be noted here that the 16 mm. film, because of its small format, does not permit very great magnification of the image.

The OPMi I operating microscope described above can only be operated manually, in-cluding its focussing and magnification. With increasing sophistication of the operating technique, the need has become more urgent to free the operator, if possible, from manual contact with the microscope. This trend prompted the author and his colleagues to develop an automatic operating microscope*, which was first introduced in 1967. This instrument (Figs. 5a–b) comprises a flexible system of components, illumination attachments and adapters, from which various combinations can be selected and assembled. It incorporates many aspects of the OPMi I, including the objective, tubes, eyepiece and beam divider, with an attachment for additional observation or photographic, cine and television cameras as described above. Not only are all these parts interchangeable within the OPMi II system but they can be taken from an OPMi I and used in the construction of an OPMi II.

The microscope stand of the OPMi II contains a motorized zoom, i.e. a magnification control system which permits continuous adjustment of magnification — interrupting vision by means of a foot pedal contact — without focussing is also operated by a foot contact and, in fact, in any desired position in the direction of the optical axis. The microscope is attached to the stand by a system of brackets and the height is likewise controlled automatically by the foot pedal contact. The entire electrical circuit is incorporated within the brackets and the stand itself. This instrument has a Cardan suspension, i.e., it can be rotated on three axes.

---

* Operating Microscope OPMi II, manufactured by Carl Zeiss, Oberkochen, Germany.

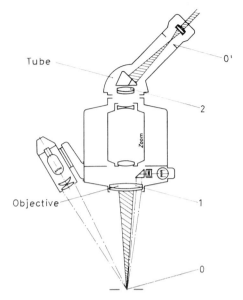

Fig. 6. Optical principles of OPMi II: 0, focal point; 1, objective lens; 2, objective lens of eyepiece tube; 0', intermediate picture.

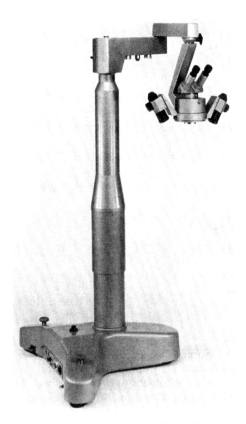

Fig. 5a. Operating microscope OPMi II.

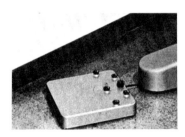

Fig. 5b. Foot pedal for operating the electric motor and for focussing and magnification.

The optical system of the instrument is generally similar to that of OPMi I, as shown in Fig. 6. The 5-stage magnification control knob may be substituted by the zoom system. In Fig. 6, a coaxial illumination lamp is shown on the right and the focus lamp on the left. Since the light beams are in the mi-croscope between the magnification knob and the binocular tubes, as in OPMi I, the same beam divider and all its adapters can be utilized. Figure 7 shows a combination consisting of photoadapter and second tube; Fig. 8a shows the arrangement for simultaneous stereophotography; and Fig. 8b shows the combination with a film camera. At present adapters are available for Bolex, Beaulieu or House-Urban* cine cameras. The House-Urban camera was specially designed for OPMi I and is, therefore, fully suited to OPMi II.

In view of the similarity between the optical systems of the two microscopes, the methods of determining the degrees of magnification and fields of vision in OPMi II are the same as those in OPMi I. Since the magnification V_z of the zoom system is directly indicated, the microscope magnification can be calculated according to Equation (5):

$$V - f_t \cdot V_z \cdot V_{ok/fo} \qquad (5)$$

* Manufacturer: Urban Engineering Company, Burbank, Calif., USA.

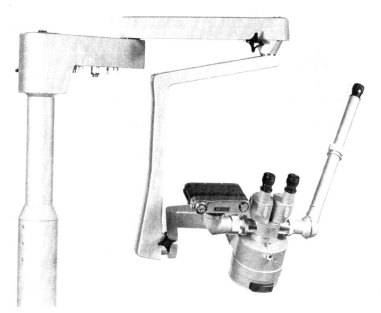

Fig. 7. OPMi II with elongated arm.

analogous to Equation (1). (The factor W/16 in (1) is identical with the respective degree of magnification indicated by the control knob settings in OPMi I).

The zoom system varies between $V_z = 0.5 \times$ and $V_z = 2.5 \times$. From this the degrees of magnification given in Table III can be estimated.

The diameter of the field of vision can be determined according to Equation (2). Since the same photoadapter is used for both microscopes, Equation (4) can be used for estimating the photographic magnification, except that W/16 is used for the zoom magnification V_z. Several important values are reviewed in Table IV.

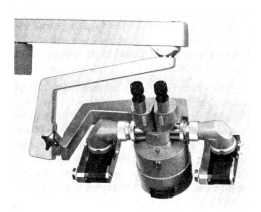

Fig. 8a. OPMi II with beam divider and two camera adapters for simultaneous stereophotography.

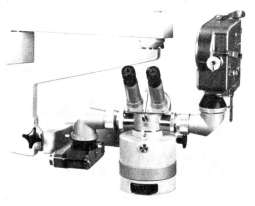

Fig. 8b. OPMi II with beam divider, and adapters for photographic and cine cameras (Bolex 16 mm.).

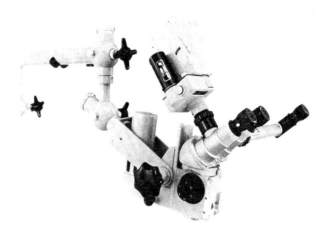

Fig. 9a. OPMi I with Urban 16 mm. cine camera mounted on ocular tube.

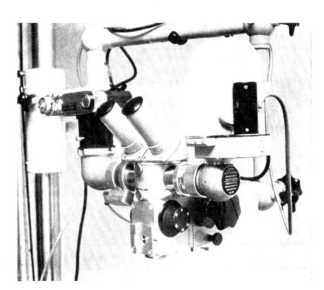

Fig. 9b. OPMi I with Urban camera attached on new adapter.

Fig. 9a shows the "House-Urban photo-tube" which has an attachment for a photographic camera and a fixed second eyepiece tube. A cine television camera, two photographic cameras or two observer eyepieces can also be attached. The same tube may also be used with the OPMi II operating microscope.

All the attachments and variations described here were originally developed for microsurgery of the ear and eye. This is particularly true of the stand and the ceiling mounted microscope which is not described here. It is evident that the use of the microscope in neurosurgery has placed new and completely different demands on the instrument. Following the brilliant results of preliminary application in this field, the time has come to develop specialized equipment exclusively for neurosurgery; a similar situation occurred some years ago in oto- and ophthalmo-microsurgery. The microscope and its attachments can be adapted with virtually no alteration but the stand and flexible arms require urgent modification.

*Table III. Magnification with the
OPMi II Operating Microscope*
(valid for long tubes ft = 160 mm.)

Objective Lens mm.	Zoom Magnification 0.5 × to 2.5 ×	Eyepiece
200	4 to 20	10 ×
300	2.5 to 13	
400	2 to 10	
200	5 to 25	12.5 ×
300	3 to 16	
400	2.5 to 13	
200	6 to 32	16 ×
300	4 to 20	
400	3 to 16	
200	8 to 40	20 ×
300	5 to 25	
400	4 to 20	

Microscope
Magnification

*Table IV. Photographic Magnification
with the OPMi II Operating Microscope*
(Photoadapter 220 mm.)

Objective Lens mm.	Zoom Magnification 0.5—2.5 ×
200	0.5—2.7
300	0.4—1.8
400	0.3—1.4

Photographic Magnification

Summary

Two operating microscopes and their attachments and adapters for photographic, cine and television cameras as well as for observer viewing in microsurgical operations are described. These apparatuses were originally devised for microsurgery of the ear and eye. Except for the stand and the flexible arms, these microscopes do meet requirements of neurosurgery. However, since this apparatus is the only one available at present and since further development of the flexible arms presents no major difficulties,

a description of their optical properties is justified. Of particular value are the details concerning visual and photographic magnification, fields of vision, exposure times, etc. which have already been tested in practical operations.

The Binocular Operating Microscope from the Surgical Standpoint

The Binocular Diploscope

In 1961 Littmann built the binocular diploscope out of two operating microscopes coupled rigidly in an axis of 180 degrees (Figs. 10a—b). Both microscopes function independently as regards focussing and magnification. Usually the surgeon's assistant employs a lower power of magnification than the surgeon, in order to observe a larger operating field. The diploscope, apart from its other advantages, allows the combined execution of subtle operative techniques, particularly the suturing of small-calibre vessels. In addition, it is invaluable for demonstration and teaching, in that the assistant obtains a stereoscopic view of the operation. In addition, it enables the teacher to supervise operations performed by trainees and to correct their mistakes. Difference in body build between the operator and his assistant may be corrected when using the diploscope by seats of different heights, or by various eyepieces (on one side straight, on the other side sloping). This instrument is suitable for operations on the surface (peripheral nerves and arteries, and skin, eye and ear operations) which entail no major changes in the axis of viewing. Of necessity, the paths of illumination and observation in the instrument lie very close together. For neurosurgical operations, in which the greatest possible mobility in all directions is desirable, the diploscope is unsuitable and cumbersome. The double microscope without internal illumination developed by Harms and Mackensen (1966) provides the

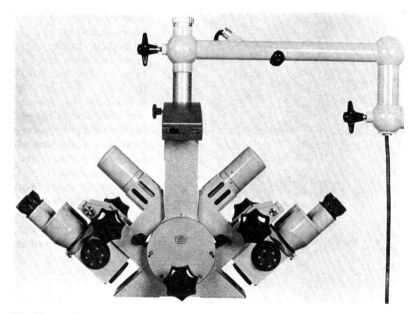

Fig. 10a. Diploscope with two straight binocular eyepiece tubes.

surgeon's assistant with a piece sloped at an angle of 20 degrees, freely mobile within 90–180° around the horizontal axis (Fig. 11).

This instrument is unsuitable for many intracranial procedures because diagonal movements are difficult to execute. It is, however, quite useful for spinal procedures.

The Electrically Driven Binocular Monoscope (Zeiss I)

The binocular monoscope is attached to a 2.2 m. stand by a double-jointed arm which makes it significantly more mobile and easier to handle. The use of a geared electric motor with magnetic brakes attached to the stand provides power-assisted vertical movements and automatic, noiseless focussing, by means of foot or finger contacts (see Fig. 1). The finger control knob is fixed to the observer eyepiece. The motor moves the microscope by a continous nylon strip and if this should break the microscope is pulled upward by a counterweight in the column.

A beam divider is inserted between the magnification control knob and the straight

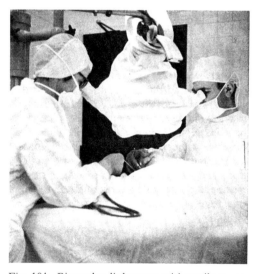

Fig. 10b. Binocular diploscope with sterile cover. Miss E. Roberts assisting the surgeon.

(or angled) binocular eyepiece in the parallel pathway of the rays. About half the light stream is beamed at right angles into each of the second eyepieces. An adapter can be fitted on the one side for a photographic, cine or television camera, and on the other

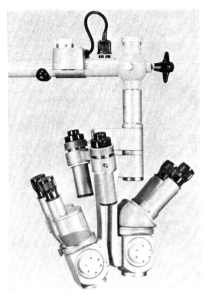

Fig. 11. Two binocular monoscopes linked together around an axis with independent movement. Constructed for ophthalmic surgery.

side around the horizontal axis for a second eyepiece (combinations such as bilateral second eyepieces, or a photographic camera on one side and a cine camera on the other side, are also possible). A correcting ring on the second eyepiece enables the picture to be rotated to any position. The use of an observer tube with a $20 \times$ eyepiece enables an assistant to follow all details of an operation and to assist the surgeon; although monocular, the color reproduction through this tube is perfect.

The Zoom Microscope (Zeiss II)

The zoom microscope, which was introduced at the end of 1967, has the same optical elements as the older binocular monoscope. The stand is solidly constructed, so much so that it supports the microscope on a bracket. The focussing adjustment, the magnification control knob (zoom) and the height of the microscope are automatically operated by foot controls

(seven buttons on a 50×50 cm. metal footplate) (see Fig. 5b). This extremely solid instrument fulfils the requirements of the opthalmologist, less so those of the neurosurgeon. The fact that the cranial vault and the brain are bullet-shaped structures makes it necessary for the neurosurgeon to carry out complicated diagonal movements with the operating microscope in order to examine structures at the base of the brain. In resecting basal tumors the movements are even more complicated in that the microscope needs to be manipulated over the cerebral hemisphere as well as the surface of the tumor, and the focussing adjusted as well. Operations on the central nervous system demand a highly mobile microscope. Ideally the surgeon should be freed of both manual and pedal controls.

The Automatic Microscope Stand

At the time of going to print, an advanced stage had been reached in the development of a mobile microscope stand for neurosurgeons. The feature of mobility causes the microscope to automatically follow all of the head movements of the operating surgeon. The new stand is *ceiling mounted* but it will be possible to provide a *floor mounting*. The principal design philosophy is to free the surgeon's hands during the displacement of the microscope to any new viewing position. Switches, actuated by the head, are attached to the microscope and trigger logic circuits. These, in turn, control a set of motors which serve to move the microscope. These movements are made extremely fine and precise, the speeds of rotation and translation being selected to assure comfortable zeroing-in on the desired new position.

One very attractive feature of the new stand is the principle governing rotational movements of the microscope. A change in the angular direction of viewing a given object can be performed with ease, the focal point of the microscope having been selected as the established center of rotation. It is possible, therefore, to practically eliminate changes of focus or maladjustments arising from a change in the viewing angle.

A single movement of the surgeon's head suffices to initiate displacement or rotation in the desired direction. The forces required to actuate the switches are kept small enough to obviate any motion of the eyes relative to the eyepiece.

Provision is made for a foot-switch which completes the logic circuits between head switches and driving motors. Without actuation of the foot switch, the head switches are ineffective in controlling the driving motors. The frame actuating the switches can then be used as a head support. Since there are no restraining attachments between the head and the head set, the surgeon is completely free to remove his head at any time.

Controlled translational movements can be performed over an area corresponding to that of a human head. The support is designed for a microscope having a focal length of 300 mm., but is adaptable to other focal lengths. Controlled rotational movements of approx. ± 90° in all planes can be carried out, with even greater angles being possible in one plane of rotation.

Photographic, movie, and television cameras may be mounted on the microscope, facilities having been provided on the support to counterbalance the weight of such equiment.

The prototype will be subjected to extensive testing in Summer 1969. After evaluation of experience gained with the microscope stand in the neurosurgical clinic, work will begin on a commercially available product in 1970.

Directions for Use of the Operating Microscope

As a preliminary each neurosurgeon must learn to carry out the movements of the microscope himself, which are the same with both the Zeiss I and the Zeiss II models. From personal experience it appears that the Zeiss I model is significantly easier to handle and more mobile for neurosurgical purposes. The automatic magnification chang-er (zoom) is not essential for neurosurgical operations because the specific magnifications (10- or 16-fold) once chosen are seldom altered.

The Objective

For superficial operations a 200 mm. objective can be used, which amounts to an object distance of 16 cm. For intracranial and spinal operations a 300 mm. objective is essential, ensuring an object distance of 26 cm., so that structures lying 10—15 cm. in tissue depth can be reached while maintaining a 10—15 cm. gap between the objective and the surface of the operating field. This distance is essential, otherwise long instruments cannot be used. Use of the 300 mm. objective with the angled second eyepiece does not restrict the surgeon's movements: on the contrary, it allows him to place his hands in a convenient position. The author is convinced that untoward incidents have occurred in many neurosurgical clinics through the use of the 200 mm. objectives. As alternatives, objective lenses of 250, 275, 325 or 350 mm. may be used.

The Eyepiece (ocular lens)

The 12.5-fold, 16-fold and the 20-fold ocular lens are used for operations with the 300 mm. objective (Fig. 12). An eyepiece lens marked with a cross on one side is necessary for precise focussing and centering on the operating field. Eyepieces for spectacle wearers with 10-, 12.5-, 16- and 20-fold magnification are available which have a wide aperture and are thus far more acceptable to surgeons than have been the lenses hitherto used (Fig. 13). The use of the eyepieces is greatly facilitated by two very practical points. One, the eyepiece should always be warmed to just above body temperature in an oven and placed in the microscope just prior to use. This prevents fogging of the lens. Secondly, once the focussing adjustments have been made the adjusting scale should be taped in position.

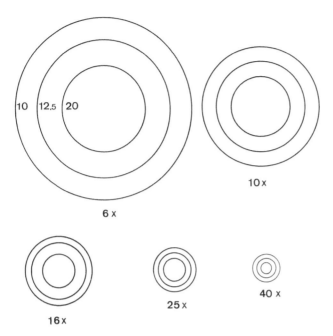

10 12.5 20

6 x

10 x

16 x

25 x

40 x

|||||||||||||||||||||||||||||||||||||||| cm.
  1   2   3   4   5

Fig. 12. The size of the field of vision, according to the magnification (6—40 ×) and the size of the ocular lens (10—20 ×).

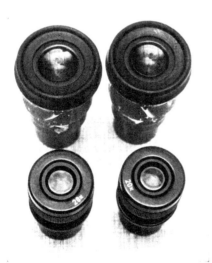

Fig. 13. Eyepiece (ocular lens) for spectacle wearers (wide opening) and normal ocular lens (below).

Positioning of the Microscope at the Start of the Operation

At the beginning of the operation the microscope is sharply focussed on the highest magnification (40-fold), so that later during the operation the object remains sharply focussed for each desired magnification between 6 to 40-fold. Both the requisite height changes and sharpness of the image may then be effected with the pedal (or digital) motor control; and the surgeon's hands are left free for manipulations in the operating field.

The Eyepiece Tube (ocular tube)

Straight or angled tubes are at present available (Figs. 1, 2, 4, 5a, 7, 8a—b, 9a—b). For operations performed in the direction of the axis of observation (e.g. exposure of Meckel's cave or angle tumors with the patient seated erect), the straight tube is best; for all other operations the angled one is used. Indeed, one of the principal advantages of the operating microscope lies in the fact that the optical axis can be rotated in all directions around 60—70 degrees and that the angled tube provides the surgeon with a convenient and well-illuminated binocular view.

Changing from the angled to the straight tube during the operation presents no difficulties if the microscope is used without a sterile cover: understandably, if the latter is used, the exchange is time-consuming and jeopardizes the sterility of the apparatus. For these reasons, the authors choose rather to dispense with an exchange of tubes than to remove the sterile covers from the microscope. It is extremely desirable that a mobile eyepiece tube should be built with a spherical prism so that the angle of the tube can be altered at will. This attachment has existed on ordinary microscopes for a long time.

Magnification

After opening the dura, it is advisable that a 6-fold magnification should be used, thereafter to adjust the degree of magnification according to the size of the object (Table V):

Table V

Object Size	Magnification
5 —10 mm.	6—fold
2 — 5 mm.	10—fold
1 — 2 mm.	16—fold
0.5— 1 mm.	25—40—fold

Sterile Covering of the Microscope

Sterile plastic caps are clipped onto the control knobs immediately before a Trikot cover is placed over the microscope (Figs. 14a—b). The sterility of the microscope makes greater demands on the skill of the operating room nurse, as is shown in Figs. 14c—h. To prevent contaminating the instruments on the objective lens during the operation, a 3×4—5 cm. sterilizable objective shell may be attached to the lens (Fig. 14h) through an opening in the cover. The stand is covered with a special sterile towel (Figs. 15a—b), secured by towel clips along its column. After the craniotomy or laminectomy has been performed, the stand is positioned just to the left of the surgeon alongside the operating table, so that his first assistant can stand or sit in front of or beside it. The optical system of the microscope is moved into the operating field from

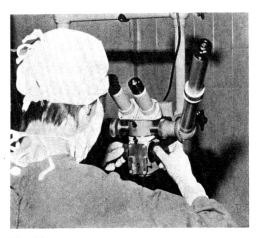
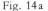
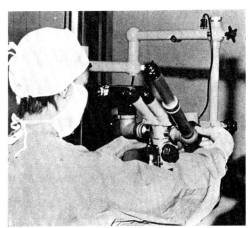

Fig. 14a

Fig. 14b

Fig. 14a and b. Sterile draping of the operating microscope by attaching the sterile caps over the 4 lateral knobs for magnification (a), and focussing (b).

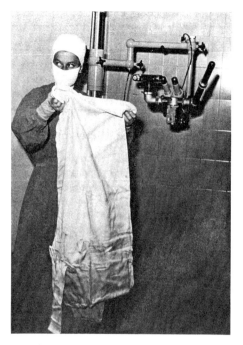

Fig. 14c. Sterile cover made of Tricot (double layer stockinet).

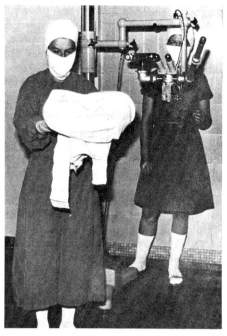

Fig. 14d. Method of drapping the Tricot over by rolling up the "stockings".

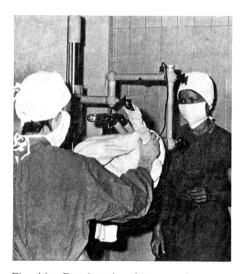

Fig. 14e. Draping the observer tube.

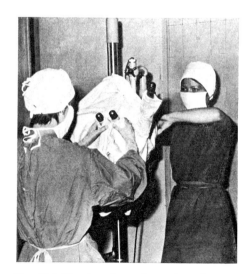

Fig. 14f. Draping the main ocular tubes.

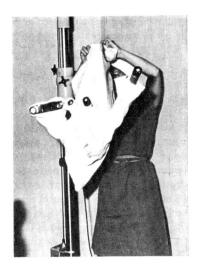

Fig. 14g. Covering the light source and attachment to stand.

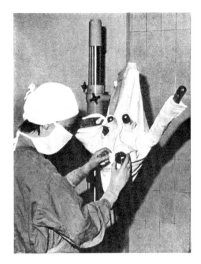

Fig. 14h. Attaching a sterile metal tube to the objective, to prevent contamination. This tube also prevents the sterile cover from sliding off.

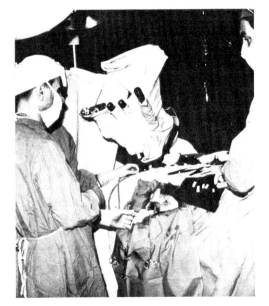

Fig. 15a. After covering the optical system with the sterile cover the stand is draped in a sterile sheet and the microscope is brought into the operating field from the left side.

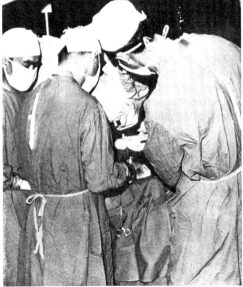

Fig. 15b. Use of the operating microscope during a craniotomy. Surgeon standing.

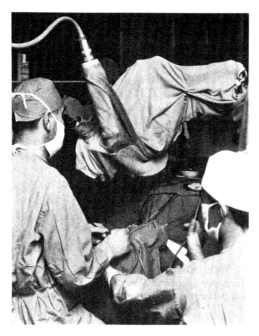

Fig. 15c. Using of the operating microscope during craniotomy. Surgeon seated.

the left side, in both craniotomies and laminectomies. The surgical nurse stands in front on the right (Fig. 15c), and dispenses her instruments from the right side. This sterile draping technique enables the surgeon to

move the microscope, alter the magnification or focus manually if desired.

Attachment for Still and Cine Cameras

The Zeiss-Ikon is used for still photography and the Bolex Paillard for cine studies. The latter camera is extremely heavy, and the attachment must be firmly fixed to the base stand to prevent its weight rotating the optical system of the microscope, or even capsizing it. This firm fixation is accomplished at the expense of the mobility of the microscope. Loading the cine film (30 m.) during the course of an operation is time-consuming and endangers the sterility of the apparatus. The adapter was originally designed for the still camera, not the cine, so that even high-speed film tends to be underexposed. Recently, however, the Zeiss-Company has perfected a new universal adapter for the cine camera (Bolex, Urban) and television camera. The cine camera of House and Urban (Los Angeles) possesses significant advantages on the grounds of camera weight, simplicity of cassette loading and improved film illumination. We now use this camera exclusively for cine photography. During still and cine photographic exposures, the aperture of the adapter is opened to its maximum (14), and good results can be obtained with an exposure time of 0.5

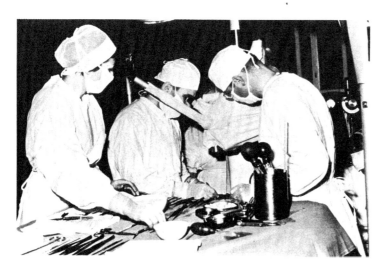

Fig. 15d. Use of the operating microscope during a thoracolumbar laminectomy. The observer tube is directed towards the surgical nurse.

seconds. Photographs made at 25- or 40-fold magnification are too dark and of little value.

Table VI lists the essential components of the operating microscope presently being used in Zürich.

Table VI

Microscope body with magnification changer objective f = 300 mm.
straight binocular tube f = 160
inclined binocular tube f = 160
eyepiece for spectacle wearers 20 × (2)
eyepiece for spectacle wearers 12.5 × (2)
bulb 6V 50W (5)
small sterilizable rubber cap (2)
large sterilizable rubber cap (2)
rollable stand 1.9 m. with built-in
transformer 80 VA 110—240 V, 50 cps
compensating weight
coupling K 90/260
coupling K 90/47
coupling K 120/76
protection cover, length 1.9 m.
long and short observation tubes
small beam splitter
eyepiece 20 ×
clamping device
spreader bolt
photo adapter
adapter for cine-camera and TV f = 137 mm.
camera housing
intermediate piece for camera housing
magnification attachment 2 ×
motorized head 24 V, 50—60 cps
power supply unit 5.5 VA with cable
holding clamp (2)
foot-switch
hand-switch
inset diaphragm 30 degrees for camera housing
sterilizable objective shell

Film Material

Color slides were made with Kodak High Speed Ektachrome (EHB 135 Type B) film, and the colored cine sequences with the Bolex camera and House-Urban camera with 16 mm. Kodak Ektachrome (Type 7242, EFB 449, Tungsten 3200 K). Ektachrome film may be developed by a special technique so as to give an ASA rating of 1000—1400. This provides adequate exposure with improved depth of field characteristics.

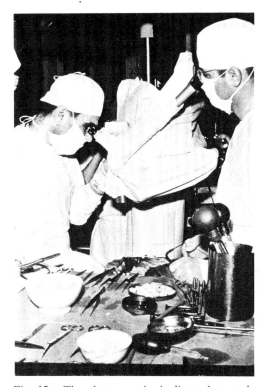

Fig. 15e. The observer tube is directed towards the surgeon's assistant.

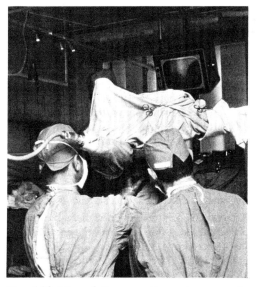

Fig. 15f. Use of the operating microscope in sitting position of the patient.

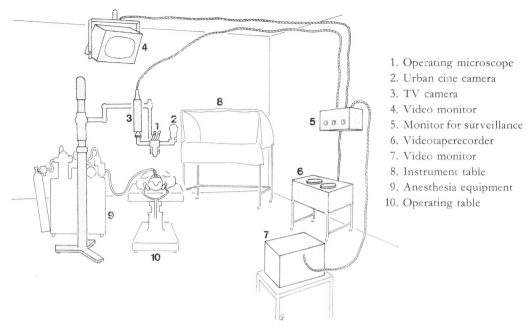

1. Operating microscope
2. Urban cine camera
3. TV camera
4. Video monitor
5. Monitor for surveillance
6. Videotaperecorder
7. Video monitor
8. Instrument table
9. Anesthesia equipment
10. Operating table

Fig. 16a. The layout of the operating theatre.

Television Camera

The attachment of a television camera to the operating microscope signifies a further advance in the field of micro-neurosurgery (Henderson, Holman 1964; Barraquer et al. 1966; Rand 1966; Hardy 1967 and Osterholm Pyneson 1967). By the use of monitors both within and outside the operating theater, an unlimited number of spectators can follow the course of the operation. It enables the surgical nurse and the surgeon's assistants as well as the anesthetists to follow the course and progress of the operation, and thereby to perform their tasks more intelligently.

Recording of the course of the operation on video tape provides, apart from precise documentation, the possibility of retrospective analysis of its various stages.

Attachment of a television camera by means of a cable does not influence the mobility of the microscope. Technical developments indicate that stereoscopic color television will soon be a possibility. It is to be hoped that cost of this development will remain within reasonable limits.

Technical Details of the Television Camera for Operating Microscopes

A TV equipment for application in the microsurgery consists of an industrial TV camera, a monitor for surveillance, a videotaperecorder as well as a videomonitor (Fig. 16).

The TV camera FA 30 with the control unit is particularly suited for the usage with the mobile operating microscope. The dimensions of this small camera are: length 10″, diameter 2.5″, weight 1700 g. The TV camera is connected with the control unit by means of a $^1/_2″$ cable. All connections as A. C. power, monitor for surveillance and video monitor are made by the control unit. The TV camera FA 30 is all transistored and adjusts itself to the objects illumination. It works automatically and can be adapted to any optical system.

The video monitor is mounted in a metal casing. The diagonal of the picture tube can be selected between 9″ and 26″ according to the view distance. The optimal view

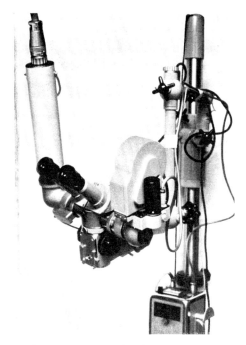

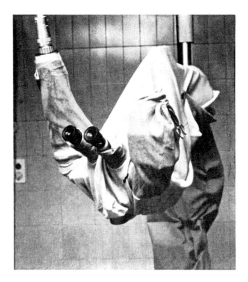

Fig. 16b. Microscope with television and Urban cameras.

Fig. 16c. Sterile covered microscope.

distance lies between four and eightfold's picture height.

It is possible to connect as many monitors as requested to one TV camera. However, attention has to be paid to the cable length between the camera and control unit on one side and between the latter and the last monitor on the other side which should not exceed 1.000 feet.

The combination of industrial TV equipment with microscopes has proven successful everywhere.

A camera adapter can be delivered to each microscope. The optic of the Zeiss operating microscope serves simultaneously as camera objective. The camera TV FA 30 can therefore be directly installed in place of a normal camera. If properly set up, no additional camera regulation at changing the enlargement rate is required.

In addition, it is possible to produce stereoscopical pictures using the TV cameras FA 30.

The AMPEX Videotaperecorder VR 7003 is specially built for the recording and the replay of operating procedures. This recorder is easy in handling and can be adapted for color. Each tape has a 60 minutes' play time and can be replayed, overplayed and erased as often as required like a normal taperecorder. On request the recording can be stopped everywhere in order to obtain a fixed picture. This recorder is equiped with two audio channels which can be recorded at the same time with the picture or later on. On the same tape two languages can be recorded. Each recorded tape can be replayed on any other AMPEX recorder. It is even possible to replay American tapes (American TV system) in Europe (European system) on the AMPEX videotaperecorder and *vice versa* without any adaptation on the machine.

Operating Microscope

References

Barraquer, S. I., J. Barraquer, H. Littmann: Nuevo microscopio para cirugia ocular. Arch. Soc. oftal. hisp. amer. 5 (1966) 271

Hardy, J.: L'exérèse des adénomes hypophysaires par voie transphénoidale. Un. méd. Canada 91 (1965) 933

Hardy, J., M. Wigser: Trans-sphenoidal surgery of pituitary fossa tumors with televised radiofluoroscopic control. J. Neurosurg. 23 (1965) 612

Harms, H., G. Mackensen: Augenoperationen unter dem Mikroskop. Thieme, Stuttgart 1966

Henderson, J. W., C. B. Holman: Closed circuit television in extraction of an intraocular foreign body. Proc. Mayo Clin. 39 (1964) 241

Jakubowski, H., H. Riedel: Der Motorkopf zur elektrischen Vertikalbewegung des Operationsmikroskopes. Zeiss-Informationen 63 (1967) 34

Littmann, H.: Ein neues Operationsmikroskop. Klin. Mbl. Augenheilk. 124 (1954 a) 473

Littmann, H.: Ein neues Operationsmikroskop mit Photoeinrichtung. Naturwissenschaftl. Rundschau 7 (1954 b) 391

Littmann, H.: Ein neues Photogerät. Photographie und Forschung 6 (1954 c) 2

Littmann, H.: Ein neues motorisiertes Operationsmikroskop für die Mikrochirurgie des Auges. Klin. Mbl. Augenheilk. (in press).

Osterholm, S. L., S. Pyneson: Television magnification in surgerey. J. Neurosurg. 26 (1967) 442

Rand, R. W.: Personal communication 1966

B. Instruments for Microsurgery

With the use of the operating microscope it is possible to undertake operations on mass lesions of varying size (cerebral and spinal tumors and aneurysms and arterio-venous malformations) as well as on small caliber blood vessels. Therefore, instruments are necessary that are broad, solid and heavy as well as thin, narrow and delicate. Existing instruments used in neurosurgery, otology, ophthalmology and vascular surgery have been modified and adapted to the requirements of neurosurgery. They should possess the following features.

The bayonet-shape is important so that the hand of the surgeon holding them remains outside the light beam of the microscope.

The blades should be slender and the tips, particularly the mouthpieces should be delicate so that they take up as little space as possible in the operating field and therefore not obstruct the surgeon's view.

The tips are available in various breadths (0.1—2.0 mm.), forms (straight and bent) and shapes (pointed, blunted, toothed, smooth or fluted inner surfaces).

Forceps

Powerful, long (18.5—22 cm.) and finely-sprung bayonet forceps are available for routine dissection under the microscope as follows:

Shape of blade	Inner surface		Tips	MM
straight	smooth		pointed	0.3—0.9
curved	diagonally	fluted	blunt	1.0—2.0
round	cross		toothed	$1 \times 2, 2 \times 3$, and
	longitudinally			more elaborate

They must be finely sprung, and the grip surface on their blades should be fluted for the thumb and index finger of the surgeon.

Some must be long (18.5—22 cm.), so that the deeper basal structures of the brain can be easily reached, although regular length instruments will be adequate for superficial structures.

The straight, very sharply pointed type of bayonet forceps may be used for micro-vascular operations on smallcaliber vessels of less than 3 mm. in diameter (see Fig. 18a—d).

Very deep structures can be reached by means of the straight spring-grip forceps (length 23 cm., mouthpiece 7 cm. and tips 3 mm.).

Length	Spring Grip	Blade	Cutting surface	Tip
18.5 cm.	straight bayonet	straight angled (15°, 30°, 90°)	1.3 cm. 0.5 cm.	0.1 mm.

Hunt-Forceps

This instrument is of great value in holding pathological tissue by virtue of its toothed circular tip. A similar forceps without teeth has been advocated by Dr. W. Hunt for holding vessels.

Scissors

All scissors have bayonet-shaped spring grips with a notched window or shell-closure mechanism.

Spring grips (length 18.5 cm.) are attached to the short-bladed ophthalmological Micro-Vanna scissors for microvascular work. Two types of blade, one straight and the other slightly angled, may be used (Figs. 17a—b, 18e—h). In order to protect these micro-instruments and facilitate their use, a metal case holder has been constructed (Figs. 19a and b).

Clamps

Dissecting Clamps

(Sylvian groove, basal cisterns)

Clamps 18.5 cm. in length with spring grips and a lock are available, angled either slightly (30°) or more (75°); the mouthparts are 22 mm. long, 1.0 mm. thick at their tips and fluted on their inner surface.

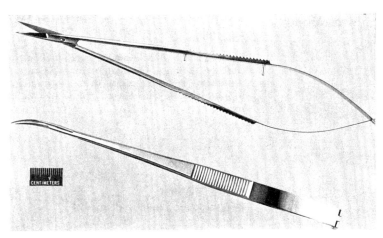

Fig. 17a   Fig. 17b

Fig. 17a. Jacobson scissors with straight or curved blades (Storz, St. Louis; V. Mueller, Chicago). Fig. 17b. Scissors with slightly curved tips and bayonet grips and serrated blades for cutting suture material (Aesculap, Tuttlingen, Germany).

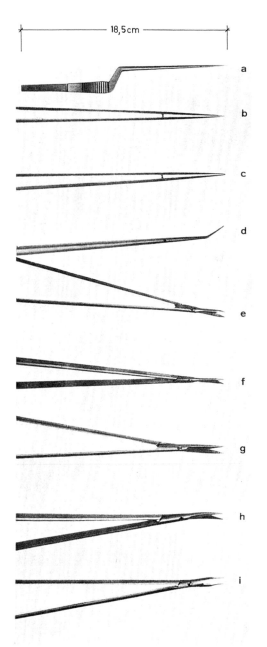

18,5 cm

a

b

c

d

e

f

g

h

i

Fig. 18a—i. Microforceps (a, b, c, d) micro-scissors (e, f, g, h) and needle holder (1) (Fischer, Freiburg, Germany).

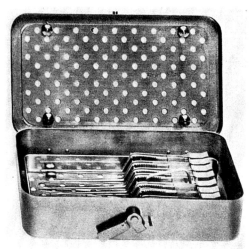

Fig. 19a

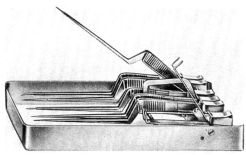

Fig. 19b

Fig. 19a and b. Metal case for micro-instruments (Fischer, Freiburg, Germany). a) double cassette for storage and sterilization of the instruments; b) inner cassette with hinged holder for the instruments.

Artery Clamps

(Vessels over 3 mm. in diameter)

The ordinary bulldog clamp with a straight, angled or simply inclined mouthpiece does not damage the tissues: it should possess effective Potts' teeth. The forceps are 15 cm. long.

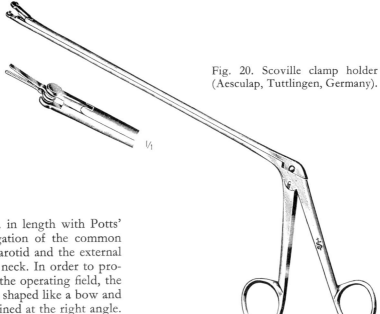

Fig. 20. Scoville clamp holder (Aesculap, Tuttlingen, Germany).

Carotid Clamps

(extracranial)

Bulldog clamps 8 cm. in length with Potts' teeth are used for ligation of the common carotid, the internal carotid and the external carotid arteries in the neck. In order to provide enough room in the operating field, the handle of the clamp is shaped like a bow and the mouthpiece is inclined at the right angle.

Jacobson Clamp

(intracranial)

Jacobson's pen-shaped clamp (length 15 cm.) with the parallel locking mouthpiece (7 mm.) has been modified, in that Pott's teeth have been added to it. The clamp was designed for temporary occlusion of the internal carotid in its intracranial part.

Scoville Clamp and Applicator

(1—3 mm. vessels)

This clamp with its smaller rounded head takes up significantly less room in the operating field than the Maxfield clamp with its broader end. Scoville clip applicators are available in 5 sizes: 0.6 and 1 cm. in length, either 0.5, 1.0 or 2.0 mm. in breadth. The inner surface of the mouthpiece is finely toothed to prevent sliding. They are either straight or angled and are available in two sizes (1.0 cm. in length, either 1.0 or 2.0 mm. in breadth). A clip holder 20 cm. long with a round mouth and a peg on the inside of one of the mouth surfaces has been developed for applying and releasing the clips with certainty at depths in the operating field (Fig. 20).

Micro-Clamp

(Vessels of 0.8—1.5 mm. in diameter)

These clips (0.5 cm. in length and 0.5—0.8 mm. in breadth, with smooth inner surfaces) are used for small-caliber vessels (Figs. 21a—b). For the clipping of saccular aneurysms we prefer the hemoclip (Edward Weck & Company, Inc., Long Island City, New York) with bajonet-shaped clip applicator (Aesculap, Tuttlingen, Germany).

Micro-Satinsky Clamp

This instrument, 1 cm. in length and 0.8 mm. in breadth, is developed from the mouthpiece of the Satinsky clamp and is intended for use during partial marginal occlusion of an opened vessel (Fig. 22).

Curettes and Dissectors

Slender instruments 18.5 cm. in length, bayonet-shaped and straight-tipped or angulated inwards or outwards, and with sharp endpieces of varying size (spoon, cutting edge) are available for the preparation of normal and pathological tissues. Double-

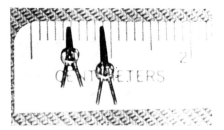

Fig. 21a. Microclamps of Stevenson for vessels with a diameter of 1.0 mm. (V. Mueller, Chicago).

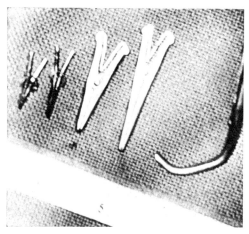

Fig. 21b. Straight and angled microclamps (Aesculap, Tuttlingen, Germany).

ended dissectors are also available, e. g. one with an oval curette at one end and a sharp pointed tip at the other.

Forceps and Punches

The otologist's microforceps mounted on a long thin tube (18 cm. in length, 1.0 mm. in diameter) is used for holding and resecting pathological tissues, as well as bone, cartilage

Fig. 22. Microclamp for tangential clamping of vessel (V. Mueller, Chicago).

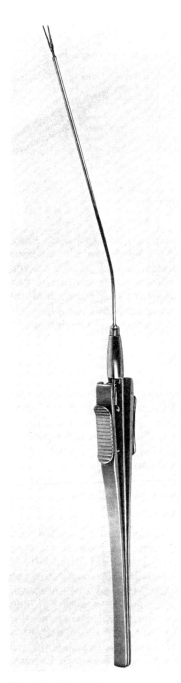

Fig. 23a. Hand formed microforceps (Fischer, Freiburg, Germany).

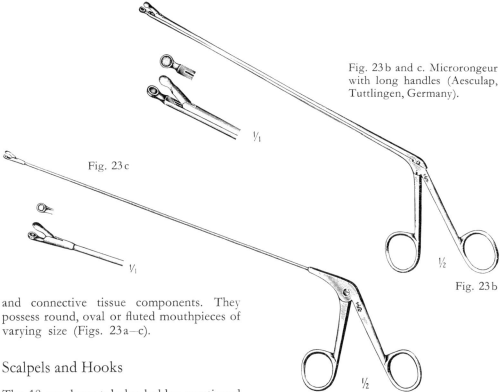

Fig. 23b and c. Microrongeur with long handles (Aesculap, Tuttlingen, Germany).

Fig. 23 c

¹/₁

½

Fig. 23 b

½

and connective tissue components. They possess round, oval or fluted mouthpieces of varying size (Figs. 23a–c).

Scalpels and Hooks

The 18 cm.-long tubular holder mentioned above serves many useful purposes, in that long thin pieces of razor blade fixed in the holder make extremely sharp knives. Personal experience has shown that no scalpel is quite as suitable for the incision of small-caliber vessels as pieces of razor blade.

Hooks are made from injection needles with their tip bent over and attached to the holder. Their size and sharpness can be altered at will. For operations on humans, hooks with blunt and round tips in two different sizes are used.

Needle Holder

Bayonet-shaped needle holders 18.5 cm. long with spring grips, with or without locks, are available. The mouthpiece possesses a smooth inner surface and a very fine tip (0.2 mm.) bent inwards, which does not obstruct the surgeon's view. Vessels with a diameter of less than 3 mm. can be sutured with the aid of

this microneedle holder (with 9.0–10.0 suture material) Figs. 24a–b).

Probes

After horizontal or longitudinal sectioning of a vessel and emptying of the blood from a segment between two clamps, the vessel walls immediately collapse and become adherent. In order to separate them without damaging the endothelium, Jacobson's one-headed microprobe is used. This probe is also useful as a dissector during embolectomy. The twin-headed Jacobson probe is used as a track during the insertion of a tube into small caliber vessels. The probe is passed through the incision for 2–3 mm. into the lumen, then the tube is pushed beyond the tip of the probe and the latter is withdrawn (Fig. 25).

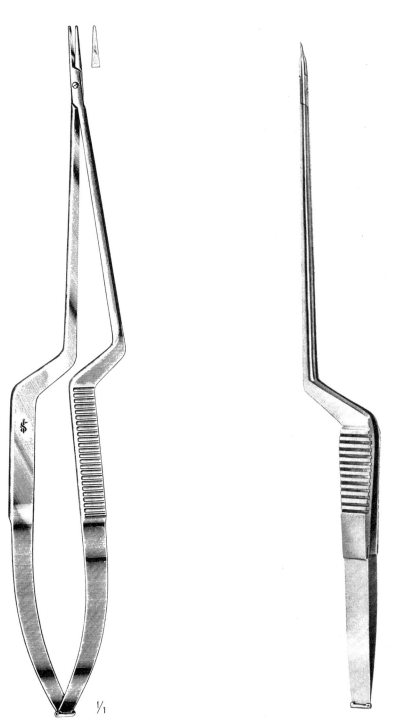

Fig. 24a. Needle holder with bayonet grips for 7.0 and 8.0 suture material (Aesculap, Tuttlingen, Germany).

Fig. 24b. Needle holder with bayonet grips for 9.0 and 10.0 suture material (Fischer, Freiburg, Germany).

Irrigator

A Silastic tube of the same dimensions as the vessel is used for irrigating the lumen. The tip of the tube inserted into the lumen is cut diagonally and the other end is attached to a syringe of saline solution.

Counterpressor ('Micro-fork')

With the aid of this instrument it is possible to suture arteries without gripping or damaging them. To prepare this instrument, the tip of an injection needle opposite to the bevelled surface is filed down under the microscope so as to produce a very fine two-pronged fork. By choosing needles of appropriate size, a series of microforks can be prepared, the prongs being used either straight or somewhat curved. When attached to a holder, this instrument serves a very valubale purpose during suturing: it is held against the needle tip during perforation of the wall, so that counterpressure is exerted against the pressure of the needle tip and the vessel wall is fixed between the prongs of the counterpressor and remains undamaged. After the vessel wall is pierced, the counterpressor lifted off and repositioned for the next suture. The counterpressor substitutes for the use of the forceps in a meaningful way; it fixes the vessel wall without gripping or damaging it. The tips of microforceps may also be utilized as a counterpressor: however, it is significantly easier and more reasonable to bend the prongs of the micro-fork, rather than the tips of the forceps, into the shape required by the course of the artery.

Retractors

Small automatic retractors (Adson and Beckman) should be used during transcervical clivectomy and temporal craniotomy in animals for spreading and fixing the musculature. Very long retractors are necessary for transcervical transoral clivectomy and transphenoidal hypophysectomy in humans. Our experiences for an ideal retraction of the brain with a newly developed selfretaining retractor have been very satisfactory (Fig. 26).

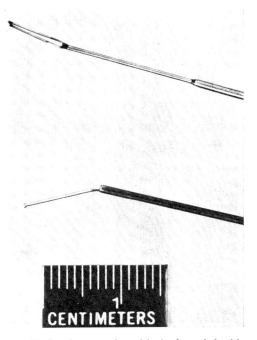

Fig. 25. Jacobson probe with single and double heads (Aesculap, Tuttlingen, Germany).

Suckers

Metal cannulae 16, 18 and 20 cm. in length and 1.0—3 mm. in caliber, angulated in varying degrees and consisting either of a single unit or of several pieces, are suitable for microsurgical operations.

A microsucker with a caliber of 0.1—0.2 mm. has been designed for operations on the base of the brain in the vicinity of the cranial nerves, which can be attached to the tips of other suckers. Cannulae are available for combined suction and irrigation of the operating field with saline. Their use is essential during bone drilling, both for keeping the drilling area clear and for protecting the adjacent structures from overheating. Simultaneous irrigation and suction is also useful in providing a better view of the operating field during diffuse capillary oozing from tumors.

A rugine with a hollow grip and a special tip can be attached to the tube of the sucker,

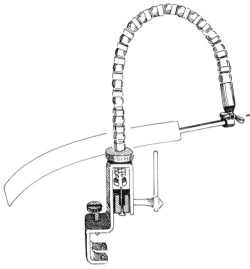

Fig. 26. Selfretaining retractor (Aesculap, Tuttlingen, Germany).

so that it can be used simultaneously as a sucker and a rugine.

The rotosucker (House-Urban, Los Angeles, USA), is intended for tumor excavation (acoustic neurinomas, pituitary tumors): by altering the speed of the rotating cutting blades and by regulating the strength of the sucker, it is possible to vary its action from one of predominant suction, on the one hand to one of predominant tissue resection, on the other.

Drills

For animal operations a hand drill or the simpler type of electric drill is quite adequate.

For transclival, transsphenoidal, transmastoid and transpetrosal craniotomies, a variety of electric dental drills is available, apart from those operated by gas.

Swab Material

Up to now small flat squares of cotton wool have been prepared, each attached to a silk thread. However, this material consists of many loose strands which may be a nuisance in the microscopic field during the operation.

Recently synthetic cotton wool squares have become available (American Silk Sutures Inc., Roslyn Heights, N. Y., USA) which can be cut into the sizes desired (2×2 mm., 3×3 mm., 4×4 mm., 5×5 mm. or larger) and each attached to a silk thread. These swabs are an essential aid in the indirect siphoning off of water, cerebrospinal fluid and blood, and in the exposure of blood vessels, nerves and brain substance.

Rubber Strips (Dam)

After preparation of the artery, a strip made from a rubber glove is placed under the mobilized segment to protect the underlying brain substance, nerves and other arteries during suturing. On completion and just before release of the artery forceps, the strip is wrapped around the sutured vessel and held lightly in place with a swab. The smooth surface of the rubber dam prevents it from adhering to the operating site, particularly the completed sutures, as is the case with cotton-wool squares. As many rubber dams as are necessary may be applied and light compression may be exerted upon them to ensure hemostasis. Instead of rubber, Silastic (Dow Corning Midland, Mich., USA) or Saran can be used and cut up into appropriate sizes to provide strips with a smooth surface.

Ligature Carrier

A right-angled or curved (semicircular or arc-shaped) hollow hook (diameter of 0.8 mm.) with a bullet-shaped head is used to carry the ligature around a vessel or around the neck of an aneurysm. First, a thin ligature (6.0 to 7.0) is pulled through, then a thicker one (2.0—4.0) attached to it.

Bipolar Coagulation in Microsurgery

In order to reconstruct a small vessel it is first necessary to have a meticulous exposure and isolation in a clear and bloodless field. The microsurgical bipolar coagulator can be of considerable aid in this procedure.

In 1940, Greenwood introduced the use of two point coagulation to neurosurgery. His first description of the technique included a specially designed forceps with two blades, insulated from each other. One blade was connected to the patient ground socket of the standard Bovie coagulation unit and the other blade was connected to the active electrode socket of the Bovie unit. A hand switch was used to disconnect the special forceps and to reconnect the ground plate and active electrode when the unipolar current was to be used. Greenwood demonstrated the advantages of the two point coagulation technique and proved its greater safety in critical areas of neurosurgical procedures.

Certain technical limitations prevented the full adoption of the method, however. The usual operating room unipolar coagulating machine is not designed to be isolated from ground. The indifferent or "patient" connection of these machines ordinarily has a fairly low impedence to ground even when disconnected from the patient. Also, in the modern operating room the patient generally has other connections (as to monitoring equipment) more or less adequately grounding his body. As a result the active electrode of the machine will still be a current source even when the ground plate is not connected. Therefore, when the bipolar forceps is connected to the unipolar type of coagulator, one blade tends to be active and may still produce a fair amount of current spread to the patient even if the other blade of the forceps is not in contact with the tissue.

In 1958, the present author built a new instrument specifically for bipolar coagulation. A damped wave spark unit was designed to provide a completely isolated output so that with the machine grounded there was negligibly low ground leakage from either electrode connection. The output wave form was shaped by matching transformer impedances with the rest of the circuitry so that

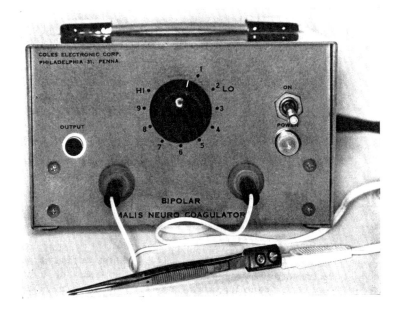

Fig. 27a. The complete bipolar coagulator unit, with miniature forceps attached.

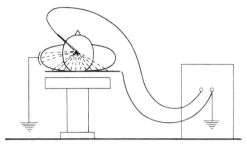

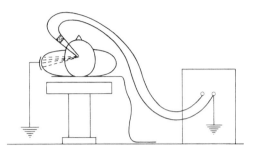

Fig. 27b. Unipolar coagulation technique. The current flows from the active electrode to the ground plate beneath the patient. From the point of active electrode contact where the highest energy level is released, the current decreases in strength to the area of the ground plate. Additional grounds which may be connected to the patient, such as electrocardiogram leads, or contacts to the operating table, or even intra-atrial catheters used for central venous pressure are also effective return points for the current.

a wave form was provided which caused minimal muscle stimulation for the amount of coagulation produced. The machine was designed for a continuous duty cycle, in order to provide a high degree of reliability. The units were then made available commercially with the most recent models utilizing a ten step switched control of intensity for reliable reproduction of the coagulation level (Figs. 27b–f).

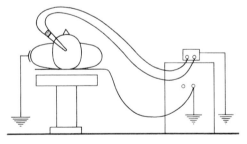

Fig. 27d. Bipolar forceps connected to an isolated source of coagulation current. Such a generator has no ground in its output circuit. Current flows only between the two forceps tips and no current flows to the ground regardless of how many are connected to the patient.

Fig. 27c. A bipolar forceps is connected to the ordinary unipolar coagulating generator with one side of the forceps connected to the ground connection, and the other side to the active electrode. While most of the current flows across the tips of the forceps as the nearest point to which a ground is applied, there is current leakage still from the active pole of the forceps to all other grounds attached to the patient. There is still a greater hazard if at the moment of coagulation, only the active side of the forceps touches the patient and the grounded side of the forceps does not make contact with the patient. In this case, all of the current flows as if there were a unipolar contact to the distant grounds and none across to the other pole. This would be particularly hazardous if the effective grounds were electrocardiogram leads or an intra-atrial catheter.

For general neurosurgical work the instrument is set at # 5 or # 6 and rarely used higher than # 6. In working around the spinal cord and brain system a setting of # 3 or # 4 is most often used with the standard forceps. If the fine forceps designed for work under the operating microscope are employed the usual setting is # 2. The # 1 setting is used only for very fine vessels under the microscope at powers above 15 diameters with very fine pointed forceps.

In the bipolar coagulation system, the current is restricted to the shortest path between the two electrode tips. There is no significant current flow from either electrode tip to ground or the patient in general. When the electrode tips touch each other the current is short circuited and no coagulation occurs. It is, therefore, essential that the vessel or tissue to be coagulated be held between the electrode tips and that the

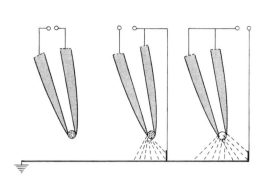

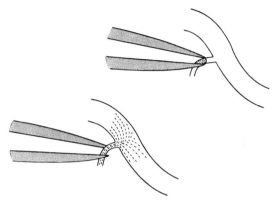

Fig. 27e. This figure recapitulates the various conditions. The diagram on the left shows bipolar coagulation from an isolated bipolar generator, and the current flows only across the vessel between the two tips of the forceps. The middle diagram of the figure shows the bipolar forceps connected to a unipolar generator with one leg active and the other leg grounded. Current flows across the blood vessel between the tips of the forceps but also flows from the active leg to ground. The diagram on the right of the illustration shows the situation when regular unipolar current is applied to an ordinary forceps. In this case the current flows incidently through the vessel while it is flowing from the forceps to ground.

Fig. 27f. The danger of thrombosis of a major vessel when a branch is coagulated is minimized with bipolar coagulation as shown in the right figure. Current flows only from one leg of the forceps to the other leg through the branch, thereby coagulating it. No current flows into the parent vessel. On the left side of the figure, the situation with unipolar coagulation is shown and the current takes the path to the best ground which is usually through the blood in the vessel and current is conducted from the small branch which is coagulated but return flow to ground is through the main vessel which may injure it and cause immediate or perhaps later thrombosis.

tips do not contact each other. Since the current flow is concentrated in the shortest path between the two electrode tips, it is not necessary to coat the blades of the forceps with insulation. In the experimental laboratory, for acute studies, the uninsulated forceps is often used barehanded without burning or shocking the experimenter. Coagulation may be carried out under a pool of saline solution as demonstrated in Figure 28 where the forceps is immersed in saline. For a more obvious photograph the power was turned up to ╫ 10 so that an actual spark would appear to show the area of current flow. The stream of bubbles comes from the tip as a result of local boiling of the saline at this very high power setting. Nevertheless, even in this situation significant passage of current takes place only between the tips of the forceps. Saline irrigation is used during the course of all coagulations with the bipolar

coagulator, thereby preventing any significant degree of tissue heating and minimizing shrinkage, drying and sticking to the forceps. If the forceps is used in a dry field without saline irrigation or under a layer of blood, there is a tendency for the forceps tips to be coated with a baked layer of charred blood which effectively insulates the points and prevents any further coagulation. This layer would be best scraped away with a scalpel blade. Even better, it should be prevented from occurring whenever possible by the use of saline irrigation.

In routine neurosurgery, major vessels, such as the middle meningeal, superficial temporal, or occipital arteries are readily closed with the bipolar unit. However, such vessels are readily occluded by ligature or clip or unipolar techniques. The most important advantage of the bipolar method in neurosurgery is its ability to handle vessels in areas where the use of the unipolar coagulating current would be hazardous. The dissection

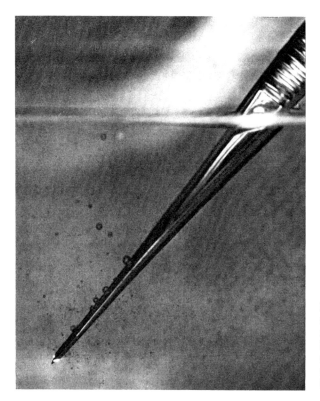

Fig. 28. The forceps is shown immersed in saline solution in order to demonstrate the current concentration between the forceps tips photographically, the power was set to maximum, causing a spark between the electrode tips and local boiling of the saline.

of an angle tumor from the pons can be handled bloodlessly without damaging the pons by current spread or heating, by picking up the individual vessels on the tumor capsule along the brain stem and coagulating while a small amount of saline is irrigated over the forceps. Ransohoff et al. (1961) have pointed out the improvement in angle tumor surgery that this technique allows. In cordotomy, vessels on the antero-lateral surface of the cord may be coagulated by stroking the cord with the forceps tips separated about a millimeter leaving a clearly demarcated thin line of coagulation through which the incision may be made. It is possible to do the actual separation of the anterior quadrant of the cord using the bipolar coagulator to coagulate the substance of the cord itself under direct vision. With the saline running on the field this is accomplished without danger of damage to the rest of the spinal cord by current spread or heating.

The ability to coagulate a very small tissue volume without current spread permits the application of the technique to meticulous hemostasis of skin flaps as in plastic surgery. The amount of devitalized tissue can readily be reduced to less than that of even precise use of fine ligatures, and postoperative reaction appears to be distinctly less marked. For microsurgical work a special bipolar forceps has been developed. This forceps is illustrated in Figure 29. A rather delicate forceps has been separated and then bolted back together with its blades insulated by fiber sleeves after the standard telephone relay technique. The rebuilt area is then potted in a high temperature epoxy for permanence. Two contacts are brought out, one from each blade of the forceps, to fit a standard type of electric razor cord which was selected for its lightness and the fact that its excellent quality of rubber would withstand repeated autoclaving. In addition, the limpness of these cords which are designed for repeated flexing minimizes the drag on the operator's hand. When necessary for work on extremely fine vessels under very high magnifications we have preferred to hand hone the tips of the forceps to even finer points than provided on the commercially available miniature bipolar.

With this forceps the isolation of small vessels becomes much more feasible since their tiny branches may be coagulated when necessary to permit the isolation of a sufficient segment to permit reparative or anastomotic surgery. Using very low currents under saline, it is possible to even seal tiny holes of vasa vasorum without appreciable shrinkage in the wall of the vessel being manipulated. Tiny bleeders may show up as very fine streams in a saline pool under the microscope. The source of such a bleeder may be difficult to see if the saline is removed from the field, but with the fine bipolar, the tiny bleeding point may be picked up under the saline and readily controlled. Subpial and subarachnoid diffusion of blood may thereby be prevented and prolonged waiting with the application of pressure on cottonoids to control such oozing may be avoided.

The use of the bipolar coagulation technique allows hemostasis to be made of almost any size vessel encountered in neurosurgical procedures, from vessels as large as the superficial temporal down to vessels too small to ligate or too small for the application of a silver clip. This may be done, as has been pointed out, in areas where ordinary unipolar coagulation with its attendant current spread would be dangerous or impossible.

The Author's Experience with the Bipolar Coagulator of Malis

The bipolar coagulator of Malis (1967) is essential for microsurgical procedures. The electric current flows only through the inner surface of the tips of the forceps and coagulates only the piece of tissue gripped by the forceps, without heating the surrounding

tissues. With the use of very sharply tipped forceps, microcoagulation may be effected of the vasa vasorum of small caliber vessels. It should be noted that homogeneous tissues are most effectively coaguletad because mixed tissues offer varying degrees of resistance. A variety of forceps of different size and tip sharpness is available for use with the Malis coagulator (Fig. 29), with which 6 graduations of current intensity are possible. Personal experience has shown that graduation 1 is best to use for the microcoagulation of vessels of 0.05—0.5 mm. in size; graduation 2 for vessels of 0.5—1.5 mm; and graduation 3 for vessels of 1.5—2.5 mm.

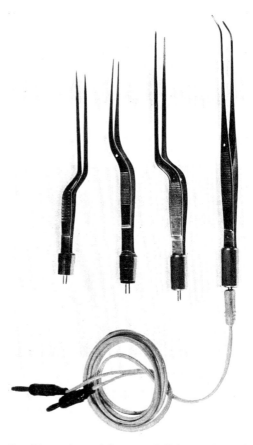

Fig. 29. Variety of forceps of different size and tip sharpness is available for use with the Malis coagulator (Mathys + Sohn, Zürich, Switzerland).

Instrumentation for Transsphenoidal Microsurgery of the Pituitary (Hardy)

The transsphenoidal approach to the pituitary requires special instrumentation such as the modified Cushing bivalve speculum, micro-enucleators, and forks with bayonet handles.

These instruments designed by Hardy are produced by Down Bros. (Mitcham, Surrey, G.B.) (Figs. 30a–d, 31a–e, 32a–c).

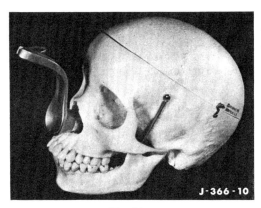

Fig. 30a

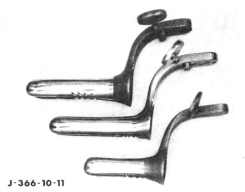

Fig. 30b

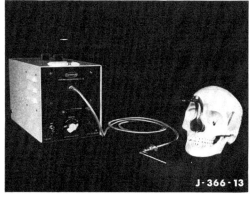

Fig. 30c

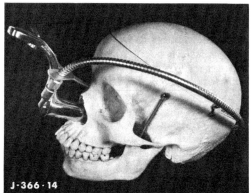

Fig. 30d

Fig. 30a. Hardy's modified Cushing bivalve speculum with 7 cm. blades for transsphenoidal hypophysectomy, toothed to engage superior edge of maxilla, non-illuminated for use in conjunction with surgical microscope.

Fig. 30b. The same as Fig. 30a, with 9 cm. blades.

Fig. 30c. Hardy's modified Cushing bivalve speculum with 7 cm. blades for transsphenoidal hypophysectomy, toothed to engage superior edge of maxilla, with fiber light illumination.

Fig. 30d. The same as Fig. 30c, with 9 cm. blades.

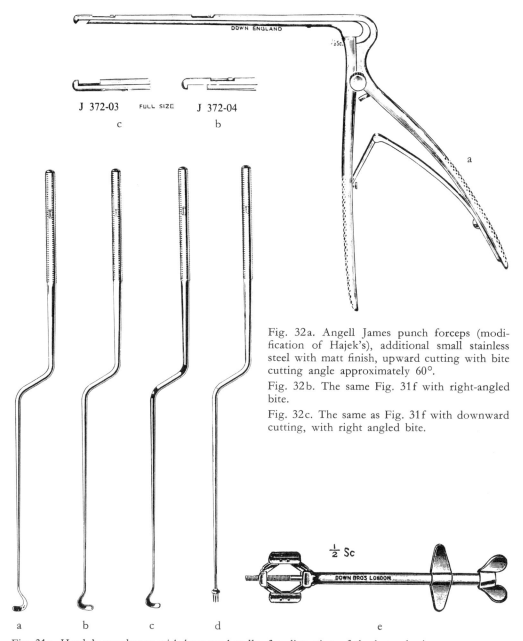

J 372-03   FULL SIZE   J 372-04

c   b

a

Fig. 32a. Angell James punch forceps (modification of Hajek's), additional small stainless steel with matt finish, upward cutting with bite cutting angle approximately 60°.

Fig. 32b. The same Fig. 31f with right-angled bite.

Fig. 32c. The same as Fig. 31f with downward cutting, with right angled bite.

½ Sc

a   b   c   d   e

Fig. 31a. Hardy's enucleator with bayonet handle, for dissection of the hypophysis.
Fig. 31b. Hardy's enucleator (left) with bayonet handle, for dissection of the hypophysis.
Fig. 31c. Hardy's sickle scalpel with the inner cutting edge and bayonet handle, for low stalk sectioning.
Fig. 31d. Hardy's fork with bayonet handle, for application of the sculptured portion of the nasal septum in the reconstruction of the pituitary floor.
Fig. 31e. Expanding device to assist in opening blades.

Instrumentation for Otoneurosurgery (Fisch)

A variety of retractors, excavators, neurotoms and scissors are necessary in otoneurosurgery. Some of these instruments modified by Fisch and produced by Fischer (Freiburg, Germany) are illustrated in Figs. 33, 34, 35, 36.

Fig. 33. Modified Urban-House mechanical dura-retractor. The retractor is fixed to the lateral edges of the craniotomy (Fischer, Freiburg, Germany).

Fig. 34a and b. a, neurotomy knife; b, neurotomy forceps (Fischer, Freiburg, Germany).

Fig. 35. Set of micro-dissectors (Fischer, Freiburg, Germany).

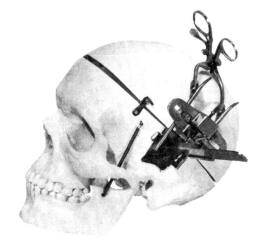

Fig. 33

Fig. 36. The irrigation suction device (Fischer, Freiburg, Germany).

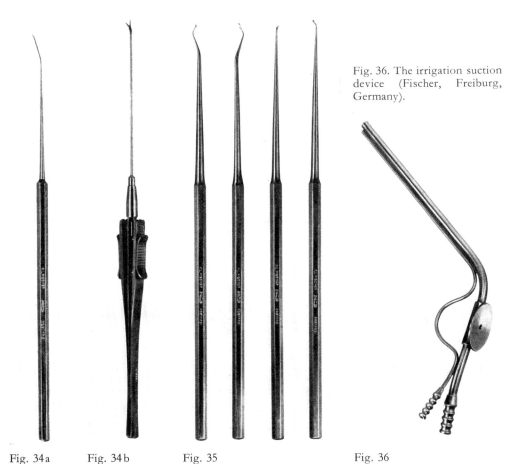

Fig. 34a   Fig. 34b   Fig. 35   Fig. 36

References

Bergi, G., L. M. Nyhus: A new vessel clamp for microsurgery. Med. Pharmacol. exp. 16 (1967) 45

Buncke Jr., H. J., W. P. Schulz: The suture repair of one millimeter vessels. In: Micro-Vascular Surgery. Ed. by R. M. P. Donaghy, M. G. Yaşargil. Thieme, Stuttgart 1967, pp. 24—35

Ferguson, D. A., D. E. Donald: A ligature carrier for experimental surgery. Proc. Mayo Clin. 36 (1961) 185

Gaertner, R. A.: A new principle in the design of vascular clamps. Surgery 59 (1966) 220

Greenwood, Jr., J.: Two point coagulation. A new principle and instrument for applying coagulation current in neurosurgery. Amer. J. Surg. 50 (1940) 267

Greenwood, Jr., J.: Two point coagulation. A follow-up report on a new technique and instrument for electrocoagulation in neurosurgery. Arch. phys. Ther. (Omaha) 23 (1942) 552

Greenwood, Jr., J.: Two point or interpolar coagulation. Review after a twelve year period with notes on addition of a sucker tip. J. Neurosurg. 12 (1955) 196

Jacobson, J. H.: The development of microsurgical technique. In Micro-Vascular Surgery. Ed. by R. M. P. Donaghy, M. G. Yaşargil. Thieme, Stuttgart 1967, pp. 4—14

Jacobson, J. H.: The large chamber for hyperbaric oxygenation: Instrumentation and monitoring problems. Trans. N. Y. Acad. Sci. 26 (1964) 474

Jacobson, J. H.: Arterial patency showed by implantable detector. Med. Tribune, 28, March, 1966

Jacobson, J. H., M. C. H. Wang, T. Yamaki, H. J. Kline, A. E. Kark, L. A. Kuhn: Hyperbaric oxygenation: diffuse myocardial infarction. Arch. Surg. 89 (1964) 905

Lougheed, W. M., G. Khodadad: A new clip for surgery of intracranial and small blood vessels. J. Neurosurg. 22 (1965) 397

Malis, L. I.: Bipolar coagulation in microsurgery. In: Micro-Vascular Surgery. Ed. by. R. M. P. Donaghy, M. G. Yaşargil. Thieme, Stuttgart 1967, pp. 126—130

Pearlman, D. M.: The immobilization of small vessels to be sutured. Surg. Gynec. Obstet. 121 (1965) 1343

Polin, S. G., F. B. Hershey: Technic of shunt removal from the carotid artery without interruption of blood flow. Amer. J. Surg. 111 (1966) 296

Rand, R. W.: Personal communication 1966

Ransohoff, J., J. Potanos, F. Boschenstein, J. L. Pool: Total removal of recurrent acoustic tumors. J. Neurosurg. 18 (1961) 804

Roe, B. B., P. B. Kelly Jr.: Heat fusion of synthetic suture knots during prosthetic valve implantation. Ann. thorac. Surg. 1 (1965) 775

Salmon, P. A., C. Assimocoupolas: Pneumatic needle holders for vascular and microvascular procedures. Angiology 16 (1965) 690

Sharp, W. V.: Incisional drape of microsurgery. Amer. J. Surg. 110 (1965) 1006

Trusler, G. A.: A vascular clamp for use in infants. J. thorac. cardiovasc. Surg. 50 (1965) 603

Yaşargil, M. G.: Experimental intracranial-extracranial shunts and patching and grafting on brain arteries of the dog. In: Micro-Vascular Surgery. Ed. by R. M. P. Donaghy, M. G. Yaşargil. Thieme, Stuttgart 1967, pp. 87—137

Plastic Tubes and Plastic T-Tubes

The tube serves three functions in vascular surgery:

1. Maintenance of the continuity of blood flow (bypass) around the segment of vessel that is interrupted.

2. Provision of a method by which the vessel, when fixed to the T-tube, may be rotated (Donaghy, 1967).

3. Protection of the vessel by the tube from within, in the sense of a plug.

Absorbable tubes have been made in various sizes from gelatin and sugar, all of which have proved unsatisfactory in respect of softness, elasticity and smooth surface. Moreover, pieces of these tubes tend to break off and form emboli. Silastic tubes (Holter Company, Bridgeport, Penna., USA, and Dow Corning, Midland, Mich., USA) are very supple and elastic, possess no toxic properties and are useful as intra- and extravasal bypass. The simple silastic tube is available in sizes from 0.305 mm. inner diameter and 0.635 outer diameter to 15.050 inner diameter and 25.400 outer diameter in 20 different lengths (Dow Corning, Midland, Mich., USA).

The simple tube is used as a vessel support and as an internal and external bypass (Donovan 1954, Diaz de Villegas 1956, Keirle et al. 1960, Ballinger et al. 1963, Nasbeth et al. 1965, Polin, Hershey 1966, Som et al. 1966). When utilized as an internal bypass, the passage of a thread through the tube is advised, in order to simplify the removal from the lumen later on.

When utilized as an external bypass, needles can be applied to both ends of the tube and passed through the proximal and distal ends of the respected artery and fixed with thread ligatures.

The T-tube possesses the following advantages:

1. Various substances (saline, heparin, etc.) may be injected through the third opening of the tube, which protrudes from the lumen of the vessel.

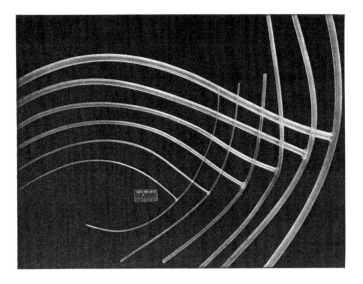

Fig. 37a. Various sizes of T-tube (Holter Company, Bridgeport).

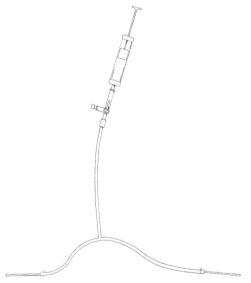

Fig. 37b. T-tube for bypass preparation.

2. The pulsating column of blood in the third limb of the tube enables a permanent check to be made on the circulation, e. g. by brief occlusion of the distal and proximal limbs, the direction and force of the blood flow can be tested at will.

3. The third limb can be used for rotating the vessel so that sutures can be applied to the posterior wall of the artery. Figs. 37a—b.

The ends of the T-tube are cut diagonally to the desired lengths, since diagonal tips are most easily inserted into the lumen of the vessel.

References

Ballinger, W. F., C. Fineberg, D. Figlio: Repair of small vessels with minimal interruption of flow. J. surg. Res. 3 (1963) 475

Diaz de Villegas, L.: Technique for end-to-end anastomoses between arterial grafts and arteries with minimal interruption of the circulation. Surgery 40 (1956) 1035.

Donaghy, R. M. P.: Patch and by-pass in microangeional surgery. In: Micro-Vascular Surgery. Ed. by R. M. P. Donaghy, M. G. Yaşargil. Thieme, Stuttgart 1967, pp. 75—86

Donovan, T. J.: The uses of plastic tubes in the reparative surgery of battle injuries to arteries with and without intra-arterial heparin administration. Ann. Surg. 130 (1954) 1024

Keirle, A. M., W. A. Altemeier: Resection of the carotid arteries for neoplastic invasion with maintenance of circulation. Amer. J. Surg. 26 (1960) 588

Nasbeth, D. C., O. Eiken, B. Kekis: Arterial patch grafts with minimal interruption of blood flow: a new method. J. cardiovasc. Surg. 6 (1965) 199

Polin S. G., F. B. Hershey: Technic of shunt removal from the carotid artery without interruption of blood flow. Amer. J. Surg. 111 (1966) 296

Som, M. L., C. E. Silver, B. Seidenberg: Excision of carotid body tumors using an internal vascular shunt. Surg. Gynec. Obstet. 122 (1966) 41

C. Suturing Techniques

Five different techniques are available at present for constructive and reconstructive vascular surgery.

1. Stapler

The precursors of the stapler were the tube-shaped intra- and extraluminal prostheses first used seventy to eighty years ago, made either of non-absorbable material (glass, goose-quill, iron, magnesium, gold, silver, steel, tantalum, Teflon, nylon) or of absorbable material (sugar, gelatin, fibrin and collodion), and applied to vascular surgery (for detailed references, see Khodadad and Lougheed 1964).

Several stapling machines have been developed for facilitating and speeding up organ transplant surgery (Androsov 1956, Inokuchi 1958, 1961, Vogelfanger et al. 1958, 1961, 1962, 1967, Sterling 1959, Carton et al. 1960, Rohman et al. 1960, Goetz et al. 1961, Mallina et al. 1962, Mallina 1963, Healey et al. 1962, 1965, Nakayama et al. 1962, Miller 1963, Gonzalez, Nathan 1963, Williams, Takaro 1963, Zingg, Khodadeh 1964, Carroll 1964, 1965, Brunius et al. 1966, Irvine et al. 1966, Bellman et al. 1967). The microstapler developed by Vogelfanger and Beattie 1967 enables anastomoses to be performed on vessels with a diameter as small as 1 mm. However, this apparatus is *unsuitable* for present microneurosurgical practice. During end-to-end anastomoses the end of the artery tends to curl around the attachments of the apparatus shortening it by 2—3 mm., increasing the frequency with which the vessel is handled and adding considerably to the time necessary for anastomosis. As well, the designs presently available do not permit end-to-side anastomoses and are too large to be used on the basal vessels of the brain. Because they are manufactured singly, these prototypes of the microstapler are difficult to obtain and are prohibitive in price.

Nonetheless, it is possible that the finished product will in the future serve a useful purpose in bridge transplants between the common carotid artery and the intracranial arteries.

References

Androsov, P. I.: New method of surgical treatment of blood vessel lesions. Arch. Surg. 73 (1956) 902

Bellman, S., A. Kövamees, K. A. Rietz: Reconstruction of small arteries: Androsov's and Nakayama's apparatuses and microangiography. In: Micro-Vascular Surgery. Ed. by R. M. Donaghy, M. G. Yaşargil. Thieme, Stuttgart 1967, pp. 67—74

Brunius, U., G. L. Helander, C. M. Rudenstam, B. Zederfeldt: Experience with staplers in anastomosing small blood vessels in dogs. Acta chir. scand. 131 (1966) 30

Carroll, S. E.: Experimental anastomosis of the left internal mammary artery to the divided circumflex coronary artery using the NRC-Vogelfanger stapling device. Canad. J. Surg. 7 (1964) 463

Carroll, S. E.: Aanastomosis of small arteries with the NRC-Vogelfanger stapling device. Med. Serv. J. Can. 21 (1965) 711

Carton, C. A. et al. (see Adhesives) 1960

Goetz, R. H., M. Rohman, J. D. Haller, R. Dee, S. S. Rosenak: Internal mammary-coronary artery anastomosis. A nonsuture method employing tantalum rings. J. thorac. cardiovasc. Surg. 41 (1961) 378

Gonzalez, E. E., P. Nathan: A new method for anastomosing blood vessels by manual applied clips. Angiology 14 (1963) 178

Healey, Jr., J. E., E. B. Moore, B. F. Brooks, K. S. Sheena: Vascular clamps for circumferential repair of blood vessels. Surgery, 51 (1962) 452

Healey, J. E., E. B. Moore: An anastomosing instrument for ductal repairs. Amer. J. Surg. 109 (1965) 689

Inokuchi, K.: A new type of blood vessel suturing apparatus. Arch. Surg. 77 (1958) 954

Inokuchi, K.: Stapling device for end-to-side anastomosis of blood vessels. Arch. Surg. 82 (1961) 337

Irvine, A. H., W. E. Collins, P. Murphy, J. V. Berry, A. C. Scott, I. J. Vogelfanger: The problem of ureteral anastomosis. Brit. J. Urolo 38 (1966) 44

Khodadad, G., W. M. Lougheed: Repair of small arteries with contact cement and teflon graft. J. Neurosurg. 21 (1964) 552

Mallina, R. F., T. R. Miller, P. Cooper, S. G. Christie: Surgical stapling. Sci. Amer. 207 (1962) 48

Mallina, R. F.: The technical aspect of the vascular stapler. Trans. N. Y. Acad. Sci. 25 (1963) 353

Miller, T. R.: The Russian stapling device. N. Y. Acad. Sci. 25 (1963) 378

Nakayama, K., T. Tamiya, K. Yamamoto, S. Akimoto: A simple new apparatus for small vessel anastomosis (free autograft of the sigmoid included). Surgery 52 (1962) 918

Nakayama, K., K. Yamamoto, T. Tamiya: A new simple apparatus for anastomosis of small vessels. Preliminary report. J. int. Coll. Surg. 38 (1962) 12

Rohman, M., R. H. Goetz, R. Dee: Double coronary artery-internal mammary artery anastomosis, tantalum ring technique. Surg. Forum 11 (1960) 236

Selker, R. G., P. M. Carney: A non-suture small vessel prosthetic connector. In: Micro-Vascular Surgery. Ed. by R. M. P. Donaghy, M. G. Yaşargil. Thieme, Stuttgart 1967, pp. 50—52

Sterling, J. A.: Experimental use of an apparatus for stapling small blood vessels. J. A. Einstein med. Cent. 7 (1959) 192

Vogelfanger, I. J., W. G. Beattie: A concept of automation in vascular surgery. Canad. J. Surg. 1 (1958) 262

Vogelfanger, I. J., W. G. Beattie: A concept of automation in vascular surgery: a preliminary report on a mechanical instrument for arterial anastomosis. Canad. J. Surg. 4 (1961) 22

Vogelfanger, I. J., W. G. Beattie: Microvascular stapling. In: Micro-Vascular Surgery. Ed. by R. M. P. Donaghy, M. G. Yaşargil. Thieme, Stuttgart 1967, pp. 39—50

Vogelfanger, I. J., W. G. Beattie, F. N. Brown, J. E. Devitt, T. K. Scobie, D. H. Scobie: The problem of small vessels anastomosis. Surgery, 52 (1962) 354

Williams, C. L., T. Takaro: The Russian stapler in small artery anastomoses and grafts. Angiology 14 (1963) 470

Zingg, W., M. Khodadeh: Vascular anastomosis, sutures, staples or gene. Canad. med. Ass. J. 91 (1964) 791

2. Adhesives

Since 1952 the well-known adhesives of the alkylcyanoacrylate series have found numerous applications in experimental and clinical surgery, particularly in the field of blood vessel anastomosis.

Eastman 910 Adhesive contains ninety per cent methyl-2-cyanoacrylate as the active agent, ten per cent methylacrylate as the thickening substance, ferrous sulphate as an inhibitor and sebasate as the plastic agent. This polymer adhesive possesses ideal qualities, i. e. appropriate thickness, and elastic and uninterrupted spread over the surface of the vessel opening to be repaired. The clinical use of Eeastman 910 adhesive has recently been banned in the U.S.A. because of the carcinogenic properties of the methylacrylates (Laskin et al. 1954, Oppenheimer et al. 1955, Bering et al. 1955, Healey et al. 1965).

Eastman 910 Monomer contains only methyl-2-cyanoacrylate and is dispensed in 5 ml. ampules, also in 1 ml. ampules under the title M2C-1. M2C-2 contains ferrous sulphate in addition to methyl-2-cyanoacrylate. While this adhesive is not carcinogenic, it possesses thrombogenic and histotoxic side effects and leads to necrosis of the vessel wall (Fassett et al. 1961, Weissberg, Goetz 1964, Hoppenstein et al. 1965, Sachs et al. 1966, Tsuchiya et al. 1968). Gottlob and Bluemel (1967) tested methyl-2-cyanoacrylate (Eastman 910 Monomer), butyl-cyanoacrylate (Histocoll T 100 B, Braun, Melsungen, Germany) and aron alpha-ethyl-cyanoacrylate (Sankyo, Tokyo, Japan), on the rabbit aorta: they found that butyl-cyanoacrylate showed the least tissue toxicity, while Japanese researchers (Inou et al. 1965, Ota et al. 1965) regard ethyl-cyanoacrylate as the ideal adhesive. Gottlob and Bluemel attach the vessels with adhesive to the inside of conical rings, which hold the vessels in a stretched position and thereby prevent any shrinkage at the side of anastomosis. Both rings are inserted into a Teflon tube and joined together. Tsuchiya et al. (1968) tested the effects of various adhesives on the cerebral meninges, the femoral artery and the extracranial part of the carotid artery in rabbits. The following substances may be used:

Table VII

Eastman 910 Monomer (Selverstone mixture)	Methyl-2-cyanoacrylate Polyvinyl polyvinyledene chloride Epoxy polyamide resin
(Pudenz mixture)	Silastic RTV-502
(Aneuroplastin)	Methyl-metacrylate
(AD/Here)	Methyl-alpha-cyano-acrylate
Biobond "EDH-Adhesive"	(Nitrile rubber + polyisocyanate + a small amount of methyl-2-cyanoacrylate monomer in a nitromethane solution).

All the above-mentioned substances have been shown to produce an inflammatory reaction of the leptomeninges, destroying the adventitia and media. The histotoxic effect was maximal in the 30th day, thereafter it diminished. An unusually severe reaction was observed with methyl-2-cyanoacrylate, the least severe with Biobond.

The principal use of the various adhesives is in the reinforcement of the walls of inoperable aneurysms and the sealing of suture lines. They are of little use in the end-to-end anastomosis of small vessels without sutures and impossible to use in end-to-side anastomosis. At present there is no ideal adhesive and it remains for the chemical industry to develop substances to meet all the requirements.

References

Agnew, W. F., E. M. Todd, H. Richmond, W. S. Chronister: Biological evaluation of silicone rubber for surgical prosthesis. J. surg. Rrs. 2 (1962) 357

Albin, M. S., A. N. D'Agnostino, R. J. White, J. H. Grindlay: Nonsuture sealing of a dural substitute utilizing a plastic adhesive, methyl-2-cyanoacrylate. J. Neurosurg. 19 (1962) 545

Araki, C., H. Handa, T. Ohta: Coating and reinforcement of intracranial aneurysm with synthetic resin and rubbers. Neurochirurgia (Stuttg.) 6 (1963) 123

Bering, Jr., E. A., L. R. McLaurin, J. B. Lloyd, F. D. Ingraham: The production of tumors in rats by the implantation of pure polyethylene. Cancer Res. 15 (1955) 300

Bernhard, W. F., A. S. Cummin, G. F. Vawter, J. G. Carr, Jr.: Closure of vascular incisions utilizing a new flexible adhesive. Surg. Forum 13 (1962) 231

Bernhard, W. F., A. S. Cummin, P. D. Harris, E. W. Kent: New flexible vascular adhesive for use in cardiovascular surgery. Circulation 27 (1963) 739

Carter, E. L., E. J. Roth: Direct nonsuture coronary artery anastomosis in the dog. Ann. Surg. 148 (1958) 212

Carton, C. A., L. A. Kessler, B. Seidenberg, E. S. Hurwitt: Experimental studies in the surgery of small blood vessels. IV. Nonsuture anastomoses of arteries and veins, using flanged ring prosthesis and plastic adhesive. Surg. Forum 11 (1960) 238

Carton, C. A., L. A. Kessler, B. Seidenberg, E. S. Hurwitt: Experimental studies in the surgery of small blood vessels. II. Patching of arteriotomy using a plastic adhesive. J. Neurosurg. 18 (1961) 188

Carton, C. A., M. D. Heifetz, L. A. Kessler: Patching of intracranial internal carotid artery in man using a plastic adhesive (Eastman 910 adhesive). J. Neurosurg. 19 (1962) 887

Carton, C. A., J. C. Kennedy, M. D. Heifetz, J. K. Ross-Duggan: The use of the plastic adhesive (methyl 2-cyanoacrylate monomer) in the management of intracranial aneurysms and leaking cerebral vessels. A report of 15 cases. In: Intracranial Aneurysms and Subarachnoid Hemorrhage. Ed. by W. S. Fields, A. L. Sahs. Thomas, Springfield, Ill. 1965, pp. 372—443

Coe, J. E., C. E. Bondurant, Jr.: Late thrombosis following the use of autogenous fascia and cyanoacrylate (Eastman 910 monomer) for the wrapping of an intracranial aneurysm. J. Neurosurg. 21 (1964) 884

Coover, Jr., H. V., F. B. Joyner, N. H. Shearer, Jr., T. H. Wicker Jr.: Chemistry and performance of cyanoacrylate adhesives. Soc. Plastic. Engrs. S. 15 (1959) 413

Dutton, J. E. M.: Intracranial aneurysm. A new method of surgical treatment. Brit. med. J. 2 (1956) 585

Dutton, J. E. M.: Acrylic investment of intracranial aneurysms. Brit. med. J. 2 (1959) 597

Egdahl, R. H., D. M. Hume: Non-suture blood vessel anastomosis. Arch. Surg. 72 (1956) 232

Fassett, D. W., R. L. Rondabush, I. C. Emley, L. B. Graulich: Microbiological growth from Eastman 910 Monomer and adhesive. Cohesive News 1 (1961) 5

Faul, P.: Untersuchungen zum Ersatz der chirurgischen Naht durch Klebstoff. (Methyl Cyanocrylat). Med. Diss. München 1966

Ganett, H. E., S. W. Law: Control of vascular anastomosis hemorrhage in heparinized dog with a rapidly polymerizing adhesive. Surg. Forum 12 (1961) 254

Genest, A. S.: Experimental use of intraluminal plastics in the treatment of carotid aneurysms. Preliminary report. J. Neurosurg. 22 (1965) 136

Goetz, R. H., D. Weissberg, R. Hoppenstein: Vascular necrosis by application of Methyl-2-Cyanoacrylate (Eastman 910 Monomer) Ann. Surg. 163 (1966) 242

Gott, V. L., D. A. Koepke, R. L. Dagett, W. P. Young: The coating of intravascular plastic prostheses with colloidal graphite. Surgery 50 (1961) 382

Gottlob, R., G. Bluemel: Über Gefäßwandveränderungen nach Einwirken von Alkylcyanocrylat-Klebern. Langenbecks Arch. clin. Chir. 317 (1967) 160

Hafner, G. D., T. J. Fogarty, J. J. Cranley: Non-suture anastomosis of small arteries. Surg. Forum 11 (1963) 417

Handa, H.: The neurosurgical treatment of intracranial vascular malformation, particularly with the use of plastics and polarographic measurements. Clin. Neurosurg. 9 (1963) 223

Harrison, J. H.: Synthetic materials as vascular prostheses. Long-term studies on grafts of Nylon, Dacron, Orlon and Teflon, replacing large blood vessels. Surg. Gynec. Obstet. 108 (1959) 433

Hayes, G. J., R. C. Leaver: Methyl methacrylate investment of intracranial aneurysms. A report of seven years experience. J. Neurosurg. 25 (1966) 79

Healey, Jr., J. E., B. J. Brooks, H. S. Gallager, E. B. Moore, K. S. Sheena: A technique for nonsuture repair of veins. J. surg. Res. (1961) 267

Healey, Jr., J. E., R. L. Clark, H. S. Gallager, P. O'Neill, K. S. Sheena: Nonsuture repair of blood vessels. Ann. Surg. 155 (1962) 817

Healey, J. E., H. S. Gallager, E. B. Moore, R. L. Clark, K. S. Sheena, C. M. McBride: Experiences with plastic adhesive in the nonsuture repair of body tissues. Amer. J. Surg. 109 (1965) 416

Healey, Jr., J. E.: The use of liquid plastic adhesives in vascular repairs. In: Micro-Vascular Surgery. Ed. by R. M. P. Donaghy, M. G. Yaşargil. Thieme, Stuttgart 1967, pp. 63—67

Hoppenstein, R., D. Weissberg, R. H. Goetz: Fusiform dilatation and thrombosis of arteries following the application of Methyl-2-Cyanoacrylate (Eastman 910 Monomer). J. Neurosurg. 23 (1965) 556

Hoppenstein, R.: Surgeons cautioned on use of plastic adhesive. Med. World News, 11 February, 1966, p. 40

Hosbein, D. J., D. A. Blumenstock: Anastomosis of small arteries using a tissue adhesive. Surg. Gynec. Obstet. 118 (1964) 112

Jacobson, J. H., R. A. Moody, B. K. Kusserow, T. Reich, M. C. H. Wang: The tissue response to a plastic adhesive used in combination with microsurgical technique in reconstruction of small arteries. Surgery 60 (1966) 379

Inou, R., S. Mori, K. Mizuno, K. Ota: A new adhesive for vascular surgery. J. cardiovasc. Surg. (Toronto) 44 (1965) 241

Khodadad, G., W. M. Lougheed: Repair of small arteries with contact cement and Teflon graft. J. Neurosurg. 21 (1964) 552

Khodadeh, M., H. M. Ross, C. C. Ferguson, W. Zingg: Investigations on a plastic bonding agent in vascular surgery. Canad. J. Surg. 8 (1965) 106

Kline, D. G., G. J. Hayes: An experimental evaluation of the effect of plastic adhesive, methyl-2-cyanoacrylate, on neural tissue. J. Neurosurg. 20 (1963) 647

Krayenbühl, H.: Behandlung intrakranieller Aneurysmen mit synthetischem Klebstoff. Münch. med. Wschr. 106 (1964) 1370

Laskin, D. M., I. B. Robinson, J. P. Weinmann: Experimental production of sarcoma by methyl methacrylate implants. Proc. Soc. exp. Biol. (N. Y.) 87 (1954) 329

Leonhard, F.: The in vivo and in vitro fate of alkyl alpha cyanoacrylate. In monograph: A Symposium on Physiological Adhesives. University of Texas Press (in press)

Manax, W. G., J. H. Bloch, J. K. Longerbean, R. C. Lillehei: Plastic adhesive as an adjunct in suture anastomoses of small blood vessels. Surgery, 54 (1963) 663

Messer, H. D., L. Strenger, H. J. McVeety: Use of plastic adhesive for reinforcement of ruptured intracranial aneurysm. J. Neurosurg. 20 (1963) 360

Nathan, H. S., M. M. Nachlas, R. D. Solomon, B. D. Halpern, A. M. Seligman: Nonsuture closure of arterial incisions using a rapidly-polymerizing adhesive. Ann. Surg. 152 (1960) 648

Oppenheimer, B. S., E. T. Oppenheimer, A. P. Stout: Sarcomas induced in rodents by imbedding various plastic films. Proc. Soc. exp. Biol. (N. Y.) 70 (1952) 366

Oppenheimer, B. S., E. T. Oppenheimer, I. Danis-Hefsky, A. P. Stout, F. R. Eirich: Further studies of polymers as carcinogenic agents in animals. Cancer Res. 15 (1955) 333

Ota, K., S. Mori: Nonsuture anastomoses of vascular prosthesis utilizing plastic adhesives. Angiology. 16 (1965) 521

Ota, K., S. Mori, T. Koike, T. Inou: Blood vessels repair a new plastic adhesive. J. Surg. Res. 5 (1965) 453

Sachs, E., A. Erbengi, G. Margolis, D. H. Wilson: Fatality from ruptured intracranial aneurysm after coating with methyl-2-cyanoacrylate (Eastman 910 Monomer, M2C-1). Case report. J. Neurosurg. 24 (1966) 889

Seidenberg, B., E. S. Hurwitt: Non-suture technique for vascular anastomosis. Dis. Chest. 44 (1963) 229

Seidenberg, B., E. S. Hurwitt, C. A. Carton: The technique of anastomosing small arteries. Surg. Gynec. Obstet. 106 (1958) 743

Selverstone, B.: Aneurysms at middle cerebral „trifurcation": treatment with adherent plastic. J. Neurosurg. 19 (1962) 884

Selverstone, B.: Treatment of intracranial aneurysms with adherent plastic. Clin. Neurosurg. 9 (1963) 201

Selverstone, B., R. Deghan, N. Ronis, R. A. Deterling, Jr., A. D. Callow: Adherent synthetic resins in experimental arterial surgery. Arch. Surg. (Chic.) 84 (1962) 80

Selverstone, B., N. Ronis: Coating and reinforcement of intracranial aneurysms with synthetic resins. Bull. Tufts-New Engl. med. Cent. 4 (1958) 8

Simeone, F. A.: The anastomosis of several arteries by a nonsuture method. Surg. Clin. N. Amer. 27 (1947) 1088

Smith, R. F., D. E. Szilagyi: Healing complication with plastic arterial implants. Arch. Surg. (Chic.) 82 (1961) 14

Sugar, O., G. Tsuchiya: Plastic coating of intracranial aneurysms with "EDH-adhesive". J. Neurosurg. 21 (1964) 114

Todd, E. M., B. L. Crue, Jr.: The coating of aneurysms with plastic materials. In: Intracranial Aneurysms and Subarachnoid Hemorrhage. Ed. W. S. Fields, A. L. Sahs. Thomas, Springfield, Ill. 1965, pp. 357—371

Todd, E. M., C. H. Shelden, B. L. Crue Jr., W. F. Agnew: Plastic jackets for certain intracranial aneurysms. J. Amer. med. Ass. 179 (1962) 935

Troupp, H.. T. Rinne: Methyl-2-cyanoacrylate (Eastman 910) in experimental vascular surgery. With a note on experimental arterial aneurysms. J. Neurosurg. 21 (1964) 1067

Tsuchiya, G., O. Sugar, D. Yashon, J. Hubbard: Reactions of rabbit brain and peripheral vessels to plastic used in coating arterial aneurysms. J. Neurosurg. 28 (1968) 409

Urschel, Jr., H. C., E. J. Roth: Small arterial anastomosis: I. non-suture. Ann. Surg. 153 (1961) 599

Weissberg, D., R. H. Goetz: Necrosis of arterial wall following application of methyl-2-cyanoacrylate. Surg. Gynec. Obstet. 119 (1964) 1248

Woodward, S. C., J. B. Herrmann, J. L. Cameron, G. Brandes, E. J. Pulaski, F. Leonard: Histotoxicity of cyanoacrylate tissue adhesive in the rat. Ann. Surg. 162 (1965) 113

Yashon, D., J. A. Jane, M. C. Gordon, J. L. Hubbard, O. Sugar: Effects of methyl-2-cyanoacrylate adhesives of the somatic vessels and in central nervous system of animals. J. Neurosurg. 24 (1966) 883

3. & 4. Microlaser and Micro-Electrocoaptation

At present the notion of uniting or reuniting vessel walls by means of focussed, modulated laser beams or by electrocoagulation remains a pipedream. Concerning the problems of laser irradiation, the reader is referred to the works of Beaz and Kochen (1965), Stellar (1965), Brown et al. (1966), Strully and Yahr (1967), Yahr and Strully (1967). The problems of electrocoaptation are dealt with in the papers of Schwartz (1962) and Sigel et al. (1965 and 1967). Observing that tissues being coagulated at surgery adhered to the coagulating instrument, Sigel and Acevedo wondered if this tendency could be exploited to make one tissue adhere to another. In 1962 they published a paper in which they indicated this was possible and practical for closure of veins and venous anastomosis. The following year they published their experience with arteries. In 1963 their conclusions were: "In veins linear closure can be accomplished with relative safety and in less time than in suture closure. End-to-side porto-caval shunts have also been constructed in dogs. However, we have been unable to achieve consistent satisfactory closure of arteries".

References (Laser)

Baez, S., J. A. Kochen: Laser-induced microagglutination in isolated vascular model system. Ann. N. Y. Acad. Sci. 122 (1965) 738

Brown, T. E., C. True, R. L. McLaurin, P. Homby, R. J. Rockwell: Laser radiation. Acute effects on cerebral cortex. Neurology (Minneap.) 16 (1966) 730

Stellar, S.: Effects of laser energy on brain and nervous tissue. Laser Fows I, 15 (1965) 3

Strully, K. J., W. Z. Yahr: The effect of laser on blood vessel wall: a method of non-occlusive vascular anastomosis. In: Micro-Vascular Surgery. Ed. by R. M. P. Donaghy, M. G. Yaşargil, Thieme, Stuttgart 1967, pp. 135—138

Yahr, W. Z., K. J. Strully: Laser theory and biomedical application. In: Micro-Vascular Surgery. Ed. by R. M. P. Donaghy, M. G. Yaşargil. Thieme, Stuttgart 1967, pp. 130—135

References (Electrocoaptation)

Engler, H. S., C. I. Hancock, C. B. Thomas: Use of a negative electric current at small artery anastomosis. Abstr. Circul. 26 (1962) 713

Kendall, K. L., A. Richard, B. Sigel: Electrocoaptive closure of linear incisions in the ureter. J. Urol. 99 (1968) 401

Schwartz, S. I.: Effects of electric environment on thrombosis. Clin. Neurosurg. 10 (1962) 291

Sigel, B., F. J. Acevedo: Vein anastomosis by electrocoaptive union. Surg. Forum 13 (1962) 233

Sigel, B., F. J. Acevedo: Electrocoaptive union of blood vessels. J. surg. Res. 3 (1963) 90

Sigel, B., M. R. Dunn: The mechanism of blood vessel closure by high-frequency electrocoagulation. Surg. Gynec. Obstet. 121 (1965) 823

Sigel, B., F. L. Hatke, M. R. Dunn: Electrocoaptation of small blood vessels. In: Micro-Vascular Surgery. Ed. by R. M. P. Donaghy, M. G. Yaşargil. Thieme, Stuttgart 1967, pp. 53—57

5. Suture Material

The suturing of tissues with a thread remains, now as always, a wholly surgical method. Metals, silk and nylon have been used for this purpose. Silicone-treated suture material has been recommended by Pollack and Devick (1960), negatively-charged nylon by Winfrey and Foster (1962), and elastic nylon (Lycra) by Wagner et al. (1966) and steel wire by Dormandy and Goetz (1966). In 1953 Sawyer and Pate notet that the normally negative charge at the level of the intima was reversed following trauma. They subsequently found that one could induce thrombus formation by creating a positive charge in the vessel wall, but also one could prevent or diminish such formation by creating a negative charge in an injured wall.

Winfrey and Foster in 1962 demonstrated that negatively charged wire used as a suture material could diminish thrombosis and Schwartz and Muyshondt developed a small

(dime-sized) inlying battery which could maintain a negative charge at the suture line for up to 30 days (Donaghy).

Size of Thread

In the microsurgery of nerves and vessels, untwisted i. e. monofilament nylon thread of 7.0—10.0 sizes has been found to be particularly suitable. It is sufficiently strong and elastic, can be easily knotted, and provokes only a mild tissue reaction. The following sizes of thread with the corresponding size of needle should be used, depending on the diameter of the vessel being operated upon:

Table VIII

Thread Size	Diameter of Vessel		Examples of Blood-Vessel Size
6.0	5—6	mm.	Common carotid artery
7.0	4—5	mm.	Internal carotid or vertebral artery
8.0	3—4	mm.	Basilar or middle cerebral artery
9.0	2—3	mm.	Anterior or posterior cerebral arteries
10.0	0.8—1.5	mm.	Sylvian arteries, cortical arteries

In operations on experimental animals, the following thread sizes should be used: 9.0—10.0 for the cerebral arteries of the dog; 8.0 for the common carotid artery of the rabbit or cat; and 10.0 for the femoral artery. Thread sizes of 8.0—10.0 are recommended for nerve sutures (Fig. 38).

Needles

Until 1968 8.0 Davis-Geck and 8.0 Ethicon atraumatic needles with a 3/8 curve and 8—10 mm. length were available, while 10.0 Ethicon atraumatic needles (BV-3; 3/8 curve 6,35 mm. length, 2.778 mm. radius and 0.127 mm. diameter) could be supplied by the firm on a special order. Atraumatic round 1/2 or 3/8 curved needles of 3, 5, 7 and 10 mm. lengths, 0.100 mm. diameter are necessary for microsurgery and are now available (Spingler, Tritt, Jestetten, Germany).

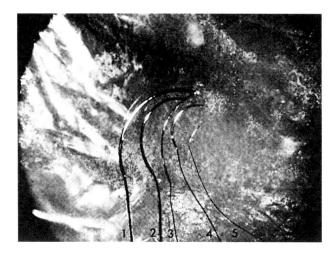

Fig. 38. Various types of suture material: 1, 7.0 silk; 2, 7.0 nylon (Ethicon); 3, 8.0 nylon (Davis & Geck); 4, 10.0 nylon (Ethicon); 5, 17.5 μ nylon (Buncke).

In superficial vessels and nerves the length of the needle is less important than its diameter and the strength of the thread attached to it. In operations on deeply-situated structures (basal vessels of the brain, nerves, Sylvian arteries) exceptionally short needles are essential, in order to prevent damage to the surrounding tissues during their use in the restricted operation field. The width of the clivectomy exposure in the dog is 6 mm., that in the cat and rabbit 4.5 mm., so that a needle of no greater length than 3 mm. can be used in this situation.

Thread and needle sizes are given in the following table:

Table IX

	Thread (μ)	Needle (μ)
6.0 Silk	63	406
6.0 Dacron	70	330
6.0 Nylon	94	559
7.0 Silk	32	236
7.0 Dacron	25	229
8.0 Silk	32	247
8.0 Nylon	43	155
9.0 Nylon	40	150
10.0 Nylon	26	120

Attempts to harden the one end of the thinnest possible nylon thread (2–10 μ) by means of metal coating for use as a needle have not been an unqualified success. The suture material of Buncke and Schulz (1967) has not yet been marketed. With the increasing trend in microsurgery to operate on smaller arteries and nerves, the need to produce still finer suture material will be accentuated.

Suture Technique

Standard vascular surgical suture techniques, modified for microsurgery form the basis for small vessel anastomoses. Attention to the following points has proven to be of value.

The surgeon himself should open the pack of microsuture material, unroll the thread, cut up the double thread material into appropriate lengths, then place the needle on the ball of his left index finger and grip it at the junction of its anterior and middle thirds with the needle holder. The microneedle should not be gripped in its posterior third because it will bend and a bent needle unnecessarily widens the hole made in the wall of the artery. The tip of the needle should be inserted at regular intervals from the artery (or nerve) edge; the regularity of the distance between individual holes may be viewed as a measure of the skill of the surgeon. Because of the cramped space in a deep field, the thread can only be pulled through tangentially to the surface of the vessel, while it is guided to and from the

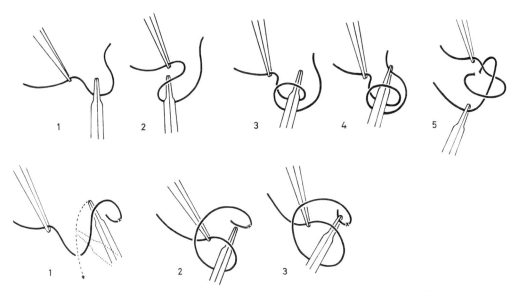

Fig. 39. Techniques of tying knots with instruments: top row the knot is tied from the front; bottom row the knot is tied from behind.

entrance and exit holes respectively over the splayed ends of a forceps (see Fig. 42a—c). If the thread is directed in an oblique or vertical direction, it may tear the thin wall of the artery and enlarge the hole; which should be avoided. Everted vertical sutures (Donati) and oversewn single sutures are applied to end-to-end and end-to-side anastomoses, the latter (simple oversewn continuous or continuous everted mattress sutures) are used with patches. In vessels with a diameter of less than 2 mm., the suture passes through all three layers, while in larger arteries only the adventitia and media are secured. The knots are tied with the use of instruments (Fig. 39). With a pair of forceps in the left hand, a 1.5—2 cm. length of thread is held close to the vessel and a second pair of forceps in the right hand is used to make a loop. The short end of the thread (3—5 mm.) is then passed back through the loop with the aid of the right-hand forceps, and returned. Three knots are always made. Instead of the right-hand forceps, a needle holder with a fine mouthpiece may be used. With practice it is possible to learn to tie knots instrumentally at speed, so that this procedure which is essential for microsurgery can be carried out deep in a narrow field with the least possible movements.

Roe and Kelly (1965) applied the technique of electrothermal fusion of Dacron threads (No. 2) to heart-valve surgery. A 6-volt soldering iron with a pencil-sized gold tip sterilizable in gas is used to melt the Dacron thread at 482° F. (250° C).. This may represent an improved tying technique. It remains to be shown whether this technique is suitable for 8.0—10.0 nylon threads.

In connection with suturing techniques, reference should be made to the method of Kunlin et al. (1963), who apply a ring around the site of the anastomosis and attach the sutures to this ring, in order to prevent narrowing at the suture site. This method, however, has attracted no followers. While narrowing of the suture line is in fact prevented, a relative narrowing can be expected of the segments immediately adjacent to it.

References

Buncke, Jr., H. J., P. Schulz: The suture repair of one millimeter vessels. In: Micro-Vascular Surgery. Ed. by R. M. P. Donaghy, M. G. Yaşargil. Thieme, Stuttgart 1967

Donaghy, R. M. P.: Personal communication.

Dormandy, S. A., R. H. Goetz: Wire suture short-circuit thrombi. Med. World News 85, 4 Nov., 1966

Kunlin, J., F. Lengua, S. Richard: Anastomoses et greffes d'artères de petit calibre (entre 1 et 2 milimètres) par la technique de la suspension de la suture dans un anneau. C. R. Soc. Biol. (Paris) 156 (1962) 228

Pollack, H. S., J. R. Devick: Silicone treated sutures in small artery anastomosis. Tex. Rep. Biol. Med. 18 (1960) 271

Roe, B. B., P. B. Kelly, Jr.: Heat fusion of synthetic suture knots during prosthetic valve implantation. J. thorac. Surg. 1 (1965) 775

Sawyer, P. N., J. W. Pate: Bio-electric phenomena as etiologic agents in intravascular thrombosis. Surgery 34 (1953) 491

Sawyer, P. N., J. W. Pate: Bio-electric phenomenon as etiologic factor in intravascular thrombosis. Amer. J. Physiol. 175 (1953) 103

Schwartz, Muyshondt: Quoted by R. M. P. Donaghy

Wagner, M., G. Reul, J. Teresi, K. L. Kayser: Experimental observations on a new and inherently elastic material for suture and vascular prostheses. Lycra. Amer. J. Surg. 111 (1966) 838

Winfrey, E. W., J. H. Foster: Prevention of arterial thrombosis with a negatively charged wire suture. Surg Forum 13 (1962) 229

D. Future Developments

The Microscope

An automatically adjustable microscope will become a reality in the near future. However, the problem of the surgical cooperation of two or three surgeons in the simultaneous use of the microscope remains unsolved, because the use of two or even three microscopes in a given narrow space over the operating field cannot be solved in practice. Apart from this, the exposed area in neurosurgical operations is so small and narrow that only rarely there is room in it for more than two hands. Of course there are situations in which the use of additional instruments (sucker, forceps, scalpel, etc.) by a second operator can be extremely valuable. Indeed, through a second eyepiece an experienced assistant can follow the course of the operation monoscopically and in color, and provide the help required. Through the use of two additional eyepieces, two assistants can observe the operation. By attaching a television monitor, its course can be followed by still more in the operating theater and by a unlimited number outside it. Stereoscopic color television monitors would enable the combined work of several operators, the surgical nurse and the anesthetist to be followed under ideal and equivalent viewing circumstances. The use of non-stereoscopic color television monitors has already considerably facilitated the work of the operating team (surgeon, assistants, surgical nurse, neuroanesthetist). The psychological significance alone of this method is not to be underestimated, by which each participant can follow the course of the operation himself, instead of experiencing the monotony of merely standing about and marking time.

Technical development presages the development in the near future of two color television cameras linked to the microscope, one on each side, by means of a disk on the monitor revolving through 60—70 turns a second. By alternating coupling with the pictures of both television cameras, a stereoscopic effect can be achieved. A monitor placed outside the operating field enables the surgeon to operate not only through the narrow opening of the eyepiece, which is very tiring, but also indirectly with the aid of the monitor. Current technical development makes it possible, with the aid of laser beams of varying height, position and size, to project planes of perspective through the air. The future may well, therefore, see the replacement of the operating microscope by a television camera with improved resolution characteristics at 10—20 times magnification. Becoming accustomed to the technique of indirect operating appears to be solely a question of practice.

Combination of Microscope, Television and X-ray Image Amplifiers

In basal craniotomies as well as in operations on related structures in animals, and in intraventricular or mesencephalic tumors, the use of X-ray image amplification increases the precision of operation. From time to time the surgeon can orientate himself regarding the true position of the operating field. Hardy and Wigser (1965) made use of these facilities for transsphenoidal hypophysectomy (see Fig. 114). Recording can be made from both monitors on video tape, so that the course of the operation is precisely recorded and documented. Since 1965 an organization in the U.S.A. (NCME — Network for Continuing Medical Education) has concerned itself with the provisioning, cataloging and distribution of video-tape recordings. In this way it is possible for qualified specialists, as well as medical students and assistants to obtain prompt, relevant and useful information. This development will significantly enrich, rather than completely supercede, existing methods of teaching and the exchange of information, but will require standardisation of recording equipment by international agreement.

Instruments

Pneumatic (Salmon, Assimocoupolas 1965) or hydraulic (Buncke, Schulz 1967) instruments (forceps, needle holders and scalpels) are already available. They will probably undergo refinement in the near future, and their mechanism be perfected. Various models of micromanipulators are used in laboratories in the isolation of microstructures. The modification and application of these instruments to neurosurgical requirements is only a matter of time. Laser beams that can be better modulated and focussed, without side effects, will probably also one day be linked to the operating microscope (L'Esperance, 1968) and find their application in neurosurgery in microcoagulation and microcoaptation.

References

Assimacopoulos, C. A., P. A. Salmon: A modified pneumatic needle holder suitable for fine suture techniques. Surg. Gynec. Obstet. 119 (1964) 356

Buncke, Jr., H. J., W. P. Schulz: The suture repair of one millimeter vessels. In: Micro-Vascular Surgery. Ed. by R. M. P. Donaghy, M. G. Yaşargil. Thieme, Stuttgart 1967, pp. 24—35

L'Esperance, Fr. A. Jr.: An ophthalmic argon photocoagulation: design, construction and laboratory investigation. Trans. Amer. Ophthal. Soc. 66 (1968) 827

Hardy, J., S. M. Wigser: Trans-sphenodial surgery of pituitary fossa tumors with televised radiofluoroscopic control. J. Neurosurg. 23 (1965) 612

Salmon, P. A., C. Assimocoupolas: Pneumatic needle holders for vascular and microvascular procedures. Angiology 16 (1965) 690

CHAPTER 3

Experimental Microsurgical Operations in Animals*

Special Remarks

In order to master the technique of using an operating microscope many months of preliminary practice on animals is essential. Only by this means can the surgeon accustom himself to the altered circumstances of microsurgery. One must learn to accept the need for maintaining the head and body in new positions for prolonged periods (four to five hours or longer) become accustomed to the indirect view provided by the angled optical system of the microscope, and acquire the coordination of eyes and hands necessary with indirect viewing of the object.

Complete familiarity with the potentials and limitations of the microscope (magnification, axial adjustments and operation of various pedals) and microinstruments should first be gained in the animal laboratory. Similarly, perfection of an atraumatic microtechnique is essential and may be acquired by operating on blood vessels of small caliber (0.8–1.5 mm.) in animals. When one achieves the necessary manual dexterity required for these difficult manipulations, one gains the confidence and ability necessary to carry out similar procedures (usually on larger vessels) in human operations.

A purposeful, calm and disciplined work method in the operating room is essential. The procedure should be planned and rehearsed with the surgical nurse and other members of the operating team so that positioning of the patient, draping, auxillary lighting and instrument exchange may be carried out smoothly and efficiently.

The microsurgical technique can only be acquired by daily practice for at least six months. The training program should be planned as follows:

1. Two weeks are spent at the laboratory bench in handling blood vessels (arteries and veins) removed at autopsy, in order to become completely familiar with the microinstruments, and also with dissection and suture technique.

2. The following four weeks are occupied in practical experiments on the common carotid and femoral arteries of animals (rabbits, cats, guinea pigs and rats). Rats are an ideal animal to operate on at first because their vessels are relatively easy to handle, show little spasm and the animals are readily available and inexpensive.

3. After the introduction, the next six to eight weeks are occupied in carrying out a series of precisely-planned operations. The animals are then sacrified weeks or months later, and the operative results followed up by angiography and post mortem examination and the mistakes corrected whenever necessary.

4. In the succeeding three months the techniques of basal and posterior-fossa craniotomy are learnt, as well as exposure of the basilar, internal carotid and middle cerebral arteries in animals (dogs and monkeys).

* The experimental work at the laboratory of the neurosurgical department of Zürich has been supported by Swiss National Funds No. 4921.3.

Surgical Exercises on Rats

Carotid Artery

The animals are anesthetized with Hypnorm (0.5 ml./kg. body weight intramuscularly) and anesthesia is maintained with Numal (Roche) (0.3—0.4 ml. intramuscularly) a dose being given as soon as any movement is noted, and then they are fastened to a dissecting stand in the supine position. After removal of the hair of the neck a 4 cm. midline skin incision is made extending from the hyoid to the sternum. The skin flaps are retracted and fixed to the stand with sutures. After incision of the superficial fascia the prominent thyroid gland is mobilized and displaced either upwards or laterally. The external jugular vein, the main venous drainage in the rat, is now prominently exposed and should be preserved. A muscular triangle is now visible formed by the pretracheal strap muscles medially, the sternocleidomastoid laterally and inferiorly and the omohyoid laterally and superiorly. The strap muscles should now be separated in the midline and after opening a small window in the anterior wall of the trachea a 2—2.5 mm. diameter, and 4 cm. long polyethylene tube inserted. This tracheal intubation is most important if one wishes to maintain normal respiratory function with the animal in the supine position for more than one hour.

Using retraction sutures in the sternocleidomastoid the muscular triangle is opened and by dividing the thin remnants of muscle lying within the investing layer of fascia the common carotid artery and its accompanying vagal nerves and small veins are exposed. The preparation of the carotid artery over a length of 2—3 cm. should be carried out under the microscope and with microtechnique so that small vascular branches are not divided, coagulation is not required and the carotid artery is never directly handled with forceps. It is essential that all dissection be sharp and performed with direct incision of the tissues with microscissors. Blunt or spreading techniques of dissection are to be condemned; not only do these methods result in unnecessary damage to vascular structures they cannot be applied to the central nervous system and are therefore of no value to the neurosurgeon.

With the carotid artery mobilized, it is isolated from surrounding tissues with a rubber dam and temporarily occluded with a microclip as proximal as possible and a second just proximal to the bifurcation so that a 1.5 to 2 cm. length of common carotid artery about 1.0 mm. diameter is excluded from the circulation.

Half-ring bypass graft

A useful exercise in the technique of end-to-side anastomosis may be carried out on the carotid artery and aorta of the rat and on the carotid and femoral arteries or the aorta of the rabbit and cat. After preparation of the vessel a second length of artery of slightly smaller or similar diameter and 1.0—1.5 cm. in length is obtained from the same or another animal. After bevelling the ends of this donor graft artery to an angle of 45° they may be sutured to the margins of small elliptical arteriotomies in the recipient artery. During the fashioning of the anastomosis a small polyethylene or silastic tube should be inserted in the recipient vessel to support the wall. Interrupted or continuous sutures may be used. This exercise is useful as one can readily test the function of the prepared bypass by varying the position of the graft and the occluding clamps.

Aorta and Vena Cava

The intimate association of the abdominal aorta and vena cava provides an exceptional opportunity for the neurosurgeon to perfect microtechniques. The abdominal wall is opened in the midline and the bowel displaced to the left and covered with a moist sponge. At the root of the mesentary the posterior peritoneum is opened exposing the great vessels. The vena cava is remarkably thin-walled and adherent to the adventitia of the aorta. Using sharp microdissection it is possible to prepare a length of aorta and vena cava without damage to the wall. The technical expertise necessary for this maneuver is in many ways similar to that required in the preparation of a cerebral aneurysm prior to ligation. On the prepared aorta and carotid artery the various microvascular procedures (incision and suture, patch, grafts etc.) may be carried out with ease.

Operations on the Femoral Artery (Rabbit, Cat)

The femoral artery in rabbits possesses an outer diameter of 1.0–1.2 mm.; it is unusually sensitive to external stimuli, reacting to rough handling by severe spasm — so much so that it is a measure of a surgeon's dexterity if he is able to lay bare this artery without producing spasm.

A 5–6 cm. incision is made in the anterior surface of the thigh from the inguinal region downwards, and the skin reflected laterally and fixed with sutures. The course of the artery between the rectus and vastus femoris muscles and the adductor group is carefully exposed under the microscope, the fascial planes being dissected with microscissors. During the dissection it is particularly important that the artery, which is obscured by veins and nerves, is not itself gripped or held with the forceps. Care should also be taken with the connective tissue fibers which surround the artery in a meshwork and are closely bound to the adventitia. The small branches of the artery passing to the femoral nerve and femoral vein should be individually coagulated, and then divided 3–4 mm. from their origins. All bleeding should be avoided in the vicinity of the artery to prevent spasm. The connective tissue covering the anterior surface of the artery is purposely left intact; a microforceps is used delicately to grasp these tissues and to lift the artery somewhat from its bed, and also to dissect free the surrounding meshwork of connective tissue and the remaining arterioles. The femoral artery gives off no major branches between the inguinal ligament and the adductor canal, so that it can be exposed, untethered by large branches, for 3–4 cm. of its length. A piece of rubber 4×3 cm. (fashioned from an old operating glove) is pulled through under the artery so as to isolate it and to cover over the muscles, vein and femoral nerve. During the next stage, the operating field, especially the artery, is kept constantly moist with a saline solution from an infusion set, the plastic connection being directed to the edge of the operation field (Crowell, 1969).

After this mobilization, the remaining intact connective tissue fibers and the adventitial fibers are gradually dissected free with a microscissors under 25-fold magnification, care being taken not to damage the artery. The artery itself is then occluded with two microclamps applied 2–2.5 cm. apart. All the blood within this segment is siphoned off with a small-bore needle. The lumen is then carefully irrigated with a saline solution so that no blood remains within it or comes in contact with its outer wall.

Longitudinal Arteriotomy

The anterior wall of the artery is incised with a broken-off razor blade for the desired length (8–10 mm.); if the walls collapse, an artery probe is first inserted, and then a Silastic tube. Throughout this procedure, handling of the arterial walls should be completely avoided, in order to prevent damage to the 4–5 μ-thick endothelial cells.

Introduction of the Tube

The delicate technique of inserting an ordinary tube or T-tube can only be perfected by experience. The tube should be inserted smoothly, i. e. without using force or pressure. It should be of the correct caliber, neither too thin nor too thick. The wall of the tube is molded so that the tip passes easily into the lumen of the artery. The tube is advanced 3—4 mm. or more beyond the site of the incision to within a few mm. of the clamp. In this way, the tip lies far enough removed from the incision opening, yet the tube remains sufficiently loose to permit intraluminal movements (upwards or downwards) when it is removed. A silk thread of appropriate strength is used for fixation, e. g. 7.0 twisted thread for blood vessels 1—3 mm. in diameter, and 6.0 thread for those 3—5 mm. in diameter.

The ligature should be tied neither too tightly nor too loosely around the artery: if too loose, the isolated segment will refill with blood; if too tight, the endothelial cells in the wall will be damaged. After correct positioning of the T-tube, the third limb is used for instilling heparin, saline solution, etc.

Suture Technique

Closure of the adjacent opening in the vessel demands a delicate suture technique if an 'hour-glass' stenosis of the orifice is to be prevented (Fig. 40). After performing a 3—4 mm. arteriotomy in arteries 2.0—2.5 mm. in caliber, the vessel may be closed with single sutures. In arteries with an outer diameter of less than 2.5 mm., it is worthwhile to use a patch, not so much to increase the normal caliber of the artery as to ensure that the lumen has an equivalent diameter throughout. In this regard, the following papers are relevant: Senning (1959), Crawford et al. (1959), Ellis, Cooley (1961), De-Leon et al. (1961), Chatterjee et al. (1962), Schamaun (1964), Vogt (1965), and Dale, Lewis (1965). The patch may be obtained from an artery or vein in another limb.

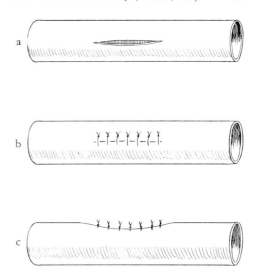

Fig. 40a—c. Incision and single sutures of a small-caliber vessel causing narrowing of the lumen.

The vessel chosen for this purpose is dissected no less carefully than the recipient artery. The adventitia must be handled with especial care: its resection requires a great deal of time and patience to avoid damaging the endothelial cells during fixation into a flat surface. From this transplant preparation, a spindle-shaped graft is fashioned, corresponding in size to the length of the incision, and this is then applied to the site of the incision (Fig. 41a—d). The patch is attached to the adventitia, not to the inner surface. It is then fixed by sutures to the upper and lower ends, and care is taken to ensure that the third limb of the T-tube protrudes from the anterior wall. The suture is applied in the direction: patch-arterial wall, in order to ensure that neither the patch nor the arterial wall is gripped by the forceps. During piercing, first the patch then the arterial wall is lightly supported by a counterpressor ('micro-fork') so that only the needle pierces the arterial wall (Fig. 42a—b). In order to keep the entry and exit needle wounds as small as possible, a round atraumatic micro-needle is used which after passage through the wall is carefully pulled away in a horizontal direction to avoid tearing or enlarging

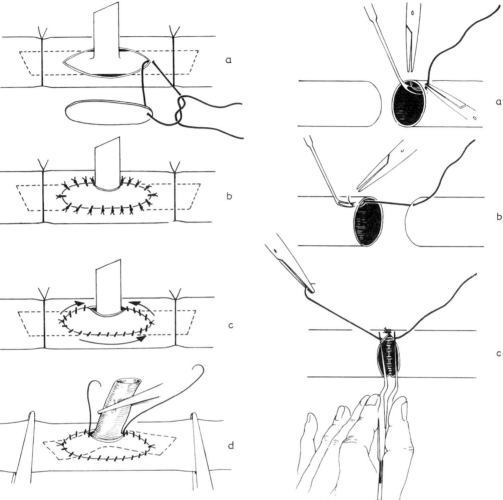

Fig. 41a—d. Closure of an incision in a small-caliber vessel. Insertion of a T-tube and application of a patch.

Fig. 42a—c. End-to-end anastomosis. Technique: a, facilitating the passage of the needle through the wall of the vessel by compression over the puncture site with the microfork; b, position of the microfork on the outer wall of the vessel; c, pulling through the thread under the slightly opened tips of a pair of forceps. This maneuver prevents tearing of the arterial wall at the site of puncture.

the hole. Then the thread is handled in the same way (Fig. 42c). The suture which is held between the tips of one pair of forceps, is knotted around the tips of a second pair — a procedure demanding the minimum of movement. Mastery of this instrumental suturing technique is essential (especially in operations on the arteries at the base of the brain, the approaches to which are always narrow and deep). In cases in which the patch is only 3—4 mm. in length, several

U-sutures are sufficient; with larger patches continuous suturing (U- or horizontal mattress suturing) is used. The posterior wall is first sutured, then the anterior wall, and in the case of continuous suturing from both

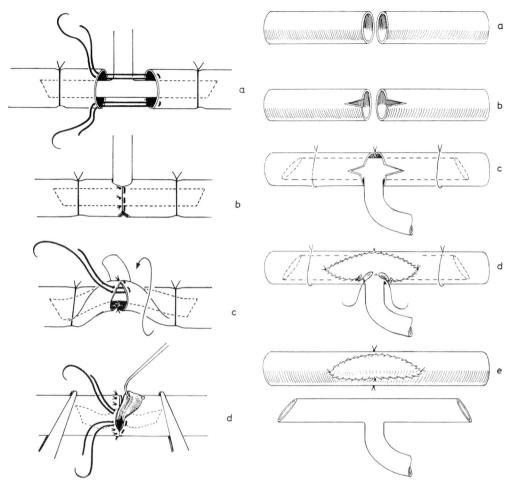

Fig. 43a—d. End-to-end anastomosis of vessels over 2 mm. in diameter: a, insertion of the T-tube and fixation by means of two ligatures wrapped around the vessel wall; b, tightening of two U-sutures inserted 120° apart into the anterior wall, and insertion of additional U-suture lengthwise along the artery; c, rotation of the artery around its own axis and insertion of U-sutures into the posterior wall; d, removal of the T-tube prior to tying the final sutures.

Fig. 44a—e. End-to-end anastomosis of vessels under 2 mm. in diameter with T-tube and patch; a, the vessels to be anastomosed; b, shaping of the open end; c, insertion and fixation of T-tube; d, application of patch; e, removal of the T-tube prior to tying the final sutures.

ends towards the middle against the T-tube (Fig. 41 d). For the final suture, two artery forceps are again applied, the sling suture placed around the T-tube and the tube carefully extracted. Then the final sutures are applied and knotted. Before releasing

the artery clamps a rubber dam or saran is placed around the artery in the region of the patch and light compression applied with a cotton-wool pledget. Direct application of the pledget to the patch results in strands of the wool becoming adherent to the edges of the wound (fresh coagulum, thread ends) so that when it is removed the wound edge may be pulled upon and torn; undesirable oozing then follows. The rubber

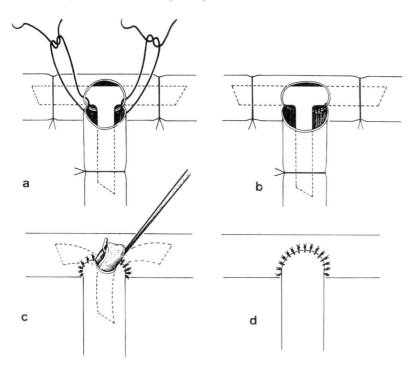

Fig. 45a—d. End-to-side anastomosis with T-Tube: a, application of two fixing sutures; b, interrupted sutures into far wall of anastomosis; c, removal of the T-tube before completion of the final sutures, and closure of the opening with two additional sutures; and d, complete closure of the end-to-side anastomosis.

dam possesses a smooth surface which is ideal for compression and appears to enhance hemostasis. It is important when removing the clamps to detach the distal one first and then the proximal one. With minor oozing hemostasis can usually be achieved by soaking up the blood for 2–3 minutes with a cotton-wool pledget applying light pressure on the suture line. If the oozing continues, the bleeding point must be found (rinsing the patch site with a saline solution and lightly dabbing with a cotton-wool pledget) and closed with further sutures. Reapplication of the clamps should be avoided if possible at this stage, because of the risk of thrombus formation in the occluded segments. When the forceps are then again removed these thrombi are swept into the peripheral circulation or the fresh thrombi adherent to the inner surface of the wound

edge may become a nidus for occlusive thrombus formation. If brisk bleeding occurs from the patch site, the spurting blood should be diverted with a microsucker while additional sutures are applied.

The future will show whether adhesive substances can be developed which, when applied to the sutured graft, cover it in an elastic envelope. From the experience obtained to date, no other method appears to equal manual suturing in its results. The more precisely and patiently it is carried out, the more successful will be the results. Respect for anatomical boundaries and physiological parameters is rewarded immediately following the procedure, when the reconstructed artery, without stenosis or aneurysmal dilatation and without spasm, commences again to pulsate.

End-to-End Anastomosis
(Termino-terminal Anastomosis)

The femoral artery is exposed and severed crosswise or diagonally. To prevent retraction, it may be grasped by means of a special U-clamp but we have not found this very satisfactory. Alternatively, after the occlusive clamps have been applied at the appropriate levels, the anterior wall of the artery is divided, and a tube or T-tube inserted and fixed with encircling silk ligatures 4—5 mm. above and below the incision; then the posterior wall is incised. In this way, retraction of the artery is kept to a minimum, so that when the ends are joined they do not pull apart and tear out the sutures (Fig. 43a—d). To prevent stenosis at the site of the anastomosis, an oblique incision across the artery is advised. In arteries of small caliber (less than 1 mm.) direct end-to-end anastomosis can result in stenosis at the suture line. To overcome this difficulty the anterior wall is incised in the long axis of the vessel for 2—3 mm. and after conventional suturing of the posterior wall the diamond-shaped defect of the anterior wall is now closed with a patch graft wrapped around the T-tube (Fig. 44a—e). This technique was developed by *Donaghy*. In the reconstruction of larger arteries (diameter 2 mm. and over) without patch or tube, two fixing sutures are placed at either end of the artery at 120-degree angles. Either by rotation of the thread ends or the T-tube, 4—5 simple or U-shaped separate sutures can be placed at regular intervals in the posterior wall of the artery; the anterior wall can then be closed with 6 to 8 single sutures. The arterial wall is punctured without touching it, only the two-pronged counterpressor being used.

End-to-Side Anastomosis
(Termino-lateral Anastomosis)

For end-to-side junction, e. g. when a branch artery is resutured to its main trunk, the vessel to be sutured is prepared with a

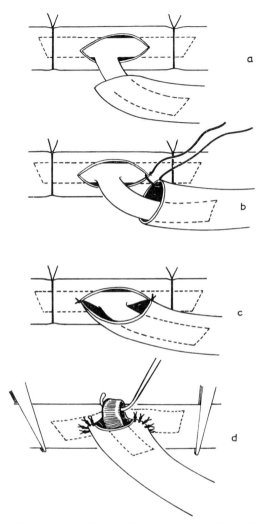

Fig. 46a—d. End-to-side anastomosis of small-caliber vessels, with oblique insertion of the anastomosed vessels.

blunt rounded tip for joining to an oval defect. After fixation of the branch artery with stay sutures at the obtuse and acute angles of the junction, the anastomosis is completed by interrupted or continuous sutures which are first placed on the wall furthest from the surgeon. The smaller the trunk artery, the longer and more acutely should the junction be shaped, and then secured with single sutures (Figs. 45a—d, 46a—d).

Duplication (after *Donaghy*)

The artery is exposed and separated from the adventitia and 5–6 mm. long parallel incisions made in the anterior and posterior walls. The 3–4 mm. transplant is then taken from a vein (diameter 3 mm.). After careful separation from its adventitia it is slipped over the end of a forceps and turned inside out. A tube is passed through the transplant and the two ends inserted into the open ends of the artery, so that the segment of vein lies precisely across the gap in the artery (Fig. 47a). The vein is first attached to the anterior wall, then after rotation of the tube to the posterior wall, by continuous mattress or simple sutures. In this way, the lumen of the artery is divided into two compartments. The surgeon may gauge the precision of his technique by the symmetry of the two resulting arteries (Fig. 47b). An unexpected hemorrhage that cannot be arrested may occur from the wall of the vein if the transplant contains a very small tributary which has been inadvertently cut and then dilates under the arterial pressure and begins to bleed. For this reason, the vein transplant should be taken from a segment that contains no tributaries. An artery may be used instead of a vein for the transplant. The duplication technique provides a good exercise in all the technical aspects of microvascular surgery. In the future, this technique may be applied to cerebral aneurysms hitherto classified as inoperable (fusiform dilatations, e. g. at the Sylvian trifurcation) as soon as a suitable bypass technique has been developed for this purpose (Donaghy 1966, personal communication).

Bridge Transplantation (Interposition)

A vein or artery transplant of any length is linked by end-to-end anastomosis between the two ends of a sectioned artery. A tube is inserted with the transplant, and the two ends then inserted into the open ends of the artery and secured by encircling silk ligatures. This procedure enables the blood flow to be maintained during the suturing, providing

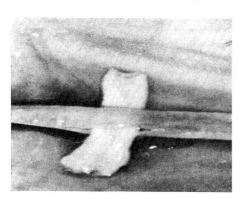

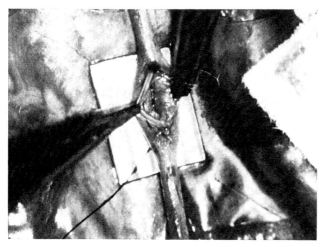

Fig. 47a and b. Arterial duplication: a, passage of a vein through the incised artery; and b, following bilateral suturing of the vein to the arterial wall at the incision site.

the surgeon with more time for his delicate work. After clamps are again applied in the final stage of the anastomosis, the tube withdrawn, the last two sutures tied and the clamps removed (Crowell, 1969).

With practice these manipulations can be carried out within 1—2 minutes. If a vein is used as a transplant, care must be taken to ensure that the direction of the valves does not impede the blood flow.

Operations on the Common Carotid Artery (Rabbit, Cat)

All the operations on the femoral artery described above may be carried out in the same way on the common carotid artery. The artery is exposed by a paramedian longitudinal skin incision over the sterno-mastoid muscle. The common carotid artery of the cat, rabbit and dog has an outer diameter of 2—3 mm. It is better to begin with the rat, however, whose carotid artery has a diameter of 0.8—1.1 mm. as mentioned previously.

Elaboration of Work Conditions

In order to prepare for operations on the cerebral arteries at the base of the skull and the brain, the above-mentioned operations on the femoral and common carotid arteries should be performed through a metal cone (Donaghy). This cone (6—7 cm. long, a 6 cm. diameter upper rim and a 4 cm. diameter lower rim) is fixed to the edge of the operating table and then, after exposure of the artery, placed in position over the operation wound. Thereafter the surgeon performs all manipulations on the artery through the cone. This elaboration of actual operative conditions has proved invaluable in teaching the surgeon to handle his instruments in a gentle and purposeful manner in a restricted space. The impossibility of executing wide free movements obliges him, after patient practice, to acquire the essential work discipline for this new dimension. One of the main advantages of the discipline of microsurgery is that it increases the surgeon's respect for the tissues of the nervous system because often for the first time he is able to see the essential detail and thereby spare the adjacent structures.

Transcervical-transclival Exploration of the Basilar Artery on Rabbit, Cat and Dog

In animals dorsal craniotomy is easier and quicker to perform than the transclival operation. For the beginner, however, the difficult basal approach is recommended, because the basilar artery presents significantly better relations in regard to its position, caliber and the thickness of its wall than the small-caliber and thin-walled cortical arteries.

The animal to be operated upon (rabbit, cat, dog or monkey) is placed on its back on the operating table under intravenous

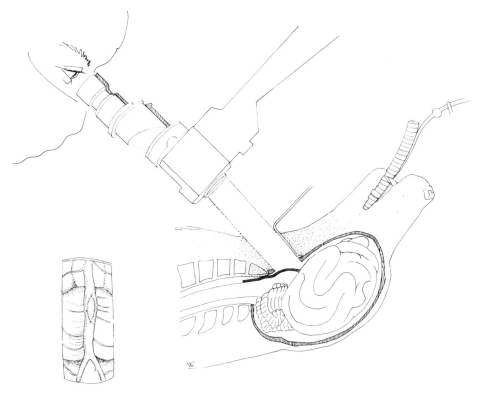

Fig. 48. The position for transcervical, transclival approach to the basilar artery.

pentothal anesthesia. In *acute* experiments (cats or rabbits) an oblique incision is made in the neck (anterior paramedian incision) on the right side alongside the trachea, and a plastic tube inserted (White, Donald 1962, White, Albin 1962). In *chronic* experiments (dog, rabbit or monkey) the animal is intubated perorally (Fig. 48). A paramedian incision is then made, extending from the level of the hyoid bone to 2—3 cm. below the lower margin of the thyroid cartilage. After opening the fascia, the sternomastoid muscle, the cervical vessels (common carotid artery and jugular vein) and the vagus nerve are retracted laterally and the trachea and esophagus medially, and held apart with a retractor. For the next step, the height of the hyoid bone should be noted, because the lingual artery and the hypoglossal nerve

run beneath it. These structures need not be sacrificed since the clivus lies more caudally than is generally believed by sectioning provided the head is extended. The groove between the inferior border of the clivus and the anterior arch of the atlas can be palpated in the midline under the hyoid bone. Above this groove the median rim of the clivus can be felt. These structures are covered by two paramedian pads of prevertebral muscles, attached from the tip of the clivus to the occipital condyles along the skull base and lateral edges of the clivus. In rabbits two veins 1—2 mm. in diameter run caudally alongside the clivus between the two prevertebral muscles and anastomose in the groove between the clivus and the arch of the atlas with the infratentorial sinuses and vertebral plexus of veins. These veins must be coagulated before the prevertebral muscles can be loosened and retracted. In the dog there are no extracranial veins at this site, so that the prevertebral muscles can be displaced laterally and fixed by a retractor. In this way the clivus can be well exposed in its whole length; its width in the rabbit is 3—4 mm. in the cat 4—5 mm. and in the dog 6—7 mm. A tough membrane covers the groove between the inferior margin of the clivus and the arch of the atlas, which exudes fluid when opened, and this may lead to the impression that the dura and arachnoid have been opened and cerebrospinal fluid is leaking out. However, this is only the shiny synovial fluid present in the extradural space. A burrhole is placed in the lower third of the clivus (drill diameter 3 mm.) and the hole then enlarged cranially and laterally with microrongeurs until an opening 1½— 2 cm. in length and 4—8 mm. in breadth has been fashioned. The clivus of the rabbit and cat possesses two thin lamellae including surprisingly thick diploe; in the dog it is 2—3 mm. thick in the midline and somewhat thinner laterally. The inferior margin of the clivus is exceptionally strong in the dog: the dura beneath it containing the circular sinus is exceptionally firmly attached to the inner surface of the bone so that great care is advised when resecting it. The electric microdrill enables extensive craniotomies to be performed and markedly simplifies the operation.

No venous plexus are encountered in the extradural space beneath the clivus, although the dura itself possesses a delicate plexus of veins. In the dog one or two arteries arise direct from the basilar artery and pass downwards in the midline to enter the dura: with a longitudinal incision into the dura these branches are exposed and must be dealt with. If they are damaged, profuse bleeding results with a loss of clear vision in the operating field. Moreover, the basilar artery reacts to any arterial hemorrhage by a narrowing of its lumen. It is advisable to perform the clivectomy and dural splitting under 8—10-fold magnification of the operating microscope. The dura, split vertically in

the operating field, is secured laterally over the edges of the bones and muscles by 2 or 3 single sutures. The vertebral and basilar arteries and their bulbar, pontine and cerebellar branches are now completely exposed and vulnerable in the operating field, framed in the background by the anterior surface of the pons and medulla oblongata — an unusual and breath-taking view for the neurosurgeon, who is suddenly confronted with the fact that these vessels are surgically accessible.

The arachnoid is opened under 16-fold magnification off-center from the basilar artery, so that the layer remains over the anterior surface of the artery. A 1-cm. segment of the basilar artery between its two large branches (circumflex brevis and circumflex longus) is now prepared for various micro-operations. The animals survive the operation without neurological deficit provided no large branches, other than 2—3 paramedian arterioles necessary for the mobilization of the basilar artery, are sacrificed. The arachnoid covering the anterior surface of the basilar artery serves as a grip surface for the forceps in order to grasp the basilar artery and lift it slightly. Between the artery and its bed there are numerous delicate but tough arachnoid fibres accompanied by small arterioles, which should be coagulated and sectioned. A 1×1 cm. rubber dam is inserted under the artery to prevent the underlying structures from being directly touched or damaged by further manipulation during the operation. The basilar artery in the cat and rabbit has a diameter of 0.4—0.5 mm., so that suture material of a finer grade than 10.0 is necessary for microvascular operations on it. The cat and rabbit are used to gain practice in the transcervical-transclival approach and to perform pharmacological tests on the basilar artery. In dogs and monkeys the basilar artery has an outer diameter of 1.0—1.3 mm. so that the desired vascular operations can be carried out in these animals.

Two microclamps are applied to the exposed area of the basilar artery, sparing its larger branches and providing a 7—8 mm. length of the artery for the implant operation. The anterior wall of the artery is now incised for 4—5 mm. with a very sharp knife (razor blade), and the lumen of the artery rinsed with saline. A T-tube is inserted with the aid of arterial probes and fixed with two circular silk threads (7.0 silk), and the artery clamps removed. As only healthy animals are used and as numerous collateral pathways substitute for the occluded segment it is possible to occlude the artery for 1—2 hours. The same suture technique as was described on page 63 is used in the repair of the incision with a patch (from a vein or artery). Since the width of the exposed clivus in ideal cases is at most 7—8 mm. and usually 5—6 mm., the suture needle must be no larger than 4—5 mm. Patch, graft or bypass operations may be carried out on the basilar artery of dogs. The dura is left open after the operation. The defect in the clivus is packed with 2—3 layers of Oxycel

(Tampotamp), and then the prevertebral neck muscles are carefully closed in two layers with continuous sutures. No respiratory disturbances, pulse irregularities or cardiac arrest, nor any postoperative cerebrospinal-fluid leakage, have been observed in any of the 55 such operations performed on the basilar artery. If the circular sinus below the rim of the clivus is damaged, profuse hemorrhage will result, and after severe blood loss the animal will undergo respiratory arrest. It is possible to keep the animal alive by means of artificial respiration (Bird apparatus), and glucose-saline replacement therapy.

The animal begins to drink 2—4 hours later: it is wise first to moisten the animal's parched pharynx and tongue manually and then gently rince it. During the first week the animal is fed on finely minced meat or meat extract.

Follow-up Angiography

After several weeks or months the animal is reexamined on the operating table on its back under intravenous pentothal anesthesia, and a transverse incision made in the supraclavicular region. The vertebral artery is identified and temporarily occluded between two

artery clamps. It is sectioned longitudinally, and a catheter inserted into it for 3—4 cm. in a cranial direction and fixed with a circular thread ligature. The injection of 4—5 ml. of contrast medium is adequate for visualizing the cerebral arteries and veins.

Autopsy

If the reconstructed basilar artery is to be examined histologically, it is wise to remove the whole brain, including the scar tissue

surrounding the basilar artery and the clivus, through a dorsal craniotomy.

Operations on Rhesus Monkeys: Transoral (Transmesopharyngeal) Clivectomy

Extensive clivectomy by the transcervical approach, is not possible in rhesus monkeys because of their prominent mandible. Echlin (1965) split the mandible in his acute operations on rhesus monkeys in order to perform a 2×1.5 cm. clivectomy and to expose the

basilar artery in its entire course. This technique is not practical in long-term investigations. No facilities for monkey experiments were available to the author in the Neurosurgical Laboratories either in Burlington or Zürich, but recently the opportunity did present itself at the Brain Research Institute, Zürich (Chief: Professor K. Akert). The following technique for demonstrating the basilar artery has been developed.

Following intubation anesthesia the animal is tied to the operating table. The mandible is fixed in an open position without undue force by a blunt retractor. The soft palate is incised laterally as far as the rim of the hard palate, is folded back and fixed with interrupted sutures. The mucus membrane and underlying soft tissues of the mesopharynx on the ventral surface of the clivus are divided with electrocautery and reflected caudally. A cavity is then made in the clivus under microscopical control with an electric drill, extending from the level of attachment of the vomer to 2—3 mm. above the anterior rim of the foramen magnum, 1.5—1.8 cm. in length and 0.8—1 cm. in breadth. Continuous rinsing of the drill apparatus with cold water is essential to avoid overheating of the adjacent structures of the brain. The dura is incised longitudinally and fixed laterally with check sutures. The basilar artery of rhesus monkeys has an outer diameter of 1.3—1.4 mm., so that microvascular operations can be performed upon it.

Operations on the Middle Cerebral Artery (Dog)

The head of the animal (dog) is positioned on the operating table for frontotemporal craniotomy. An oval skin incision is made along the superior margin of the zygomatic arch, around the glabella and then backwards along the median frontoparietal osseous ridge. The skin flap is reflected backwards over the ear. The powerfully developed temporal muscle (3—5 cm.). is then divided along the same line as the skin with the electrocautery; the muscle is separated from the processus muscularis in the temporal fossa and reflected backwards over the ear. Muscle remnants are displaced downwards with a swab. Since there are no bony walls between the lateral margin of the orbit and the temporal fossa in the dog, the soft tissues in the anterior part of the temporal fossa should be exposed with great care in order to prevent damage to the orbital contents. The bone is opened in the spheno-frontoparietal area with a hand or electric drill and the cavity enlarged in the vertical as well as in the anteroposterior direction to a diameter of 3—4 cm. A star-shaped incision is made in the dura, which is reflected and sutured along the bone edges to the muscles. The operating microscope is now brought into use. In the dog the insula lies on the surface, thus the middle cerebral artery (1.0—1.2 mm.) and its branches (0.8—1 mm.) are easy to locate. The arachnoid is next incised on one side of the insular arteries, then lifted up with forceps, so that the small arachnoid fibers and arterioles on its undersurface can be exposed and divided. Mobilization of the middle cerebral artery itself calls for an experienced and subtle technique, in order to avoid damaging the lenticulostriate arteries; injury to these fine vessels results in immediate contralateral paralysis. A rubber strip is placed under the mobilized artery. Two microclamps are applied to obtain temporary arterial occlusion 1—1.5 cm. apart, either simply or combined with a T-tube (see page 63 for method of insertion and fixation), and various experimental procedures can then be performed, e.g. incision and fixation of a patch, end-to-end anastomosis, end-to-side anastomosis, a graft joining two insular arteries, a bypass between the middle cerebral and superficial temporal arteries and the insertion of an autograft (page 76) between the common carotid in the neck and the middle cerebral artery.

Extracranial-Intracranial Anastomoses: Anastomosis between the Superficial Temporal Artery and the Middle Cerebral Artery (Dog) (Fig. 49)

The superficial temporal artery is covered with the thin layer of platysma over the temporalis muscle. The artery runs from the upper rim of attachment of the ear to the lateral margin of the orbit 5 mm. above the zygomatic arch, accompanied in its course by two veins and giving off six to eight thin muscular branches which run downwards. These branches must be identified, coagulated, and divided. A thin, protective covering of muscle and connective tissue is wrapped around the whole length (5—6 cm.) of the mobilized artery and its two veins. This vascular bundle with its thin muscle covering is displaced slightly downwards over the zygomatic arch and then wrapped with temporalis muscle, resected from the temporal fossa and reflected backwards, as described above. Fronto-temporo-basal craniotomy gives access to the middle cerebral artery. This artery is exposed proximal to its trifurcation to a depth of up to 6—5 mm., and mobilized. A rubber patch is then inserted under it. At this stage of the operation the superficial temporal artery is freed in its distal part (adjacent to the lateral orbital margin) from the surrounding muscle and connective tissues as well as its adventitia for a length of 5—6 mm., and two microclamps applied.

The anterior wall of the artery is incised and a Silastic tube inserted for 1—2 cm. in a retrograde direction, and fixed externally with a circular thread ligature. A heparinized saline solution is injected through the distal end of the tube and a microclamp then applied. The superficial temporal artery is now incised around the tube at its mouth and sectioned somewhat obliquely. This intubation technique is advisable because it is significantly more difficult to insert a tube into a sectioned artery, and the vessel wall may be mechanically damaged. After this preparation the superficial temporal artery is pulled through a gap in the temporalis muscle and its end positioned in the vicinity of the middle cerebral artery. The superficial temporal artery must be sufficiently long to ensure that it does not retract during or following the anastomosis and produce spasm. Under ideal circumstances, the middle cerebral artery is ligated between two microclamps before this, and then sectioned obliquely immediately adjacent to the proximal clamp. The tube protruding from the superficial temporal artery, which has previously been prepared, is inserted into the distal stump of the middle cerebral artery for a distance of 3—4 mm. and then externally fixed with a circular

→

Fig. 49 (1—5). End-to-end anastomosis between the superficial temporal artery and the middle cerebral artery in the dog: 1, position of the dog on the operating table; 2, operative incision with exposure of the superficial temporal artery and veins; 3, Isolation and mobilization of the superficial temporal artery with the veins and a muscle pedicle, as well as preparation of the middle cerebral artery; 4, end-to-end anastomosis between the superficial temporal artery and the middle cerebral artery; and 5, end-to-end anastomosis with application of a patch. Details of the end-to-end anastomosis with the T-tube are given in the line drawings (a—c).

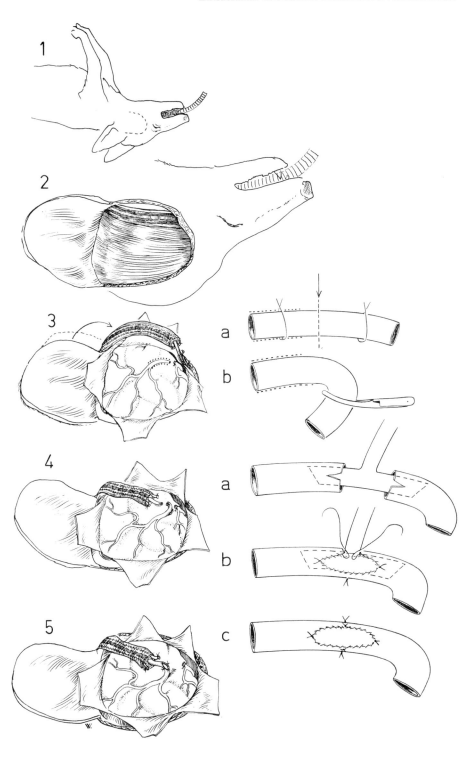

sling ligature. The microclamps on the superficial temporal artery are removed, thereby ensuring a flow of blood from the superficial temporal artery to the middle cerebral artery and its branches. The anastomosis between the sectioned arteries is secured by ten to twelve simple everted or single U-sutures. The middle cerebral artery at this level possesses an outer diameter of 1.0–1.2 mm., and the superficial temporal one of 1.0–1.4 mm. Nylon 10.0 is recommended as the suture material. A microclamp should be applied to the superficial temporal artery before the final two sutures are tied, and the simple or T-tube carefully removed from the artery. Upon completion of the sutures the microclamps are finally removed, and blood then flows along the new vascular channel to the middle cerebral

territory. With practice, ligation of the artery and the insertion, fixation and removal of the tube should take no longer than two to three minutes. The stump of the middle cerebral artery is ligated with 7.0 nylon thread. Particular care must be taken to protect the lenticulostriate arteries. The dura is closed with several sutures, and Oxycel is placed in the gap in the temporalis muscle through which the superficial temporal artery is passed. The scalp muscles are re-sutured in two layers to the processus muscularis of the mandible and then carefully re-attached along the rim of the zygomatic bone. The skin flaps are closed with subcutaneous and cutaneous sutures. The skin is sprayed with a plastic film (Nobecutane), which seals it satisfactory.

Extracranial-Intracranial Anastomoses: Bypass between the Common Carotid Artery and the Middle Cerebral Artery (Dog)

The superficial femoral artery is used as an autograft. It is exposed under the operating microscope for a length of 12–14 cm. from its origin from the femoral artery to the middle of the shank. All branches are ligated very close to their origin, to prevent blood accumulating within them and later becoming the sites of thrombus formation. After removal, the artery is rinsed with a heparinized saline solution and then preserved in ice saline. The second stage of the operation is a frontotemporal craniotomy, as described above. The middle cerebral artery is prepared and mobilized for anastomosis but it is not ligated. Next, the common carotid artery is exposed at the level of the bifurcation in the neck. After ligation of the external carotid, the proximal end of the superficial femoral artery is anastomosed end-to-end to the origin of the internal

carotid artery with single U-sutures. It is important to ensure that no stumps of branch arteries remain behind on the internal and common carotid arteries. The distal end of the superficial femoral artery is then passed through the subcutaneous tissues in the submandibular region and temporal fossa with an artery forceps, and anastomosed end-to-end or end-to-side to the middle cerebral artery. The superficial femoral artery is sutured to the common carotid artery with 8.0 monofilament nylon and to the middle cerebral artery with 10.0 monofilament nylon.

During the operation heparin is used for irrigating the T-tube (1 ml.: 5000 i.e. 50 mg. in 100 ml. physiological saline), otherwise no anticoagulants are used during or after the operation.

Pre- and Postoperative Management and Anesthesia in Laboratory Animals

Rabbits:

The animal is starved from the night before the operation. Three-quarters of an hour before the operation commences the animal is weighed, given Hypnorm 0.5 ml./kg. body weight intramuscularly, and put in a cage. As soon as the animal falls asleep, it is placed supine on the operating table and the extremities tied down. The operating area on the thigh or the neck of the animal is shaved, the remaining hairs epilated with an aluminium acetate applied to the skin. After preparation of the area, 0.5 ml. Numal (Roche) is injected into an ear vein; 0.3 to 0.5 ml. may be added. According to the wound is sprinkled superficially with Nobecutane to produce a protective covering. For the first 3 days the animals are given antibiotics intramuscularly.

Dogs:

Water and food are withheld from the animals from the night before the operation. The anesthetic is commenced one hour prior to operation with two ampules of 0.02 g. morphine hydrochloride given subcutane-ously into the skin of the dog's back. The dogs are then encouraged to walk about, since this helps to empty the bowel and bladder. Immediately before the operation the following are injected slowly intravenously: 2 ml. Combelen (Bayer) and 4 ml. Polamivet (Hoechst) and 3 ml. Pentothal (Abbott), until the animal is asleep. After intubation the dog is positioned and secured on the operating table. A mixed glucose-saline infusion is then commenced through a three-way system. The hair is now shaved and epilated, and desinfected with benzine and Merfen. Additional injections of 2—3 ml. Pentothal may be necessary, depending on the duration of the operation.

At the end of the operation and after closure of the incision, the wound area is sprayed with Nobecutane and the animals given antibiotics. Thereafter the rectal temperature is measured daily, bladder function is carefully controlled — if necessary by catheterization, and the animal observed during eating and drinking. It is removed from the cage and allowed freedom of movement as soon as possible. The sutures are removed on the tenth day.

Follow-up Angiography

After anastomosis between the superficial temporal artery and middle cerebral artery, the pulsation of the superficial temporal artery which can be palpated immediately above the superior rim of attachment of the ear is a good sign that the artery is intact. In order to perform arteriography, the artery is exposed in the subcutaneous tissues in front of the ear and incised through its anterior wall between two forceps. A Silastic tube is then inserted and advanced cranially for 1.5—2 cm., and fixed in position. Radiological contrast medium is injected through this tube and radiographs are made during the injection. By this means it can be shown that the contrast medium reaches the middle cerebral artery directly *via* the superficial temporal artery and not through the collateral channels.

In bypass operations between the common carotid and middle cerebral arteries, follow-up angiography is performed as follows: after weeks or months of postoperative survival, the common carotid is exposed in the neck proximal to the site of the operation, and a tube is inserted *via* the common carotid into the bypass for the contrast injection.

Summary of the Surgical and Physiological Problems of Vascular Surgery

Review exploration.

Atraumatic microinstruments.

During exposure of the blood vessels, isotonic saline should be constantly dripped into the operating field, to save the artery from dessication.

Longitudinal and oblique incisions should be undertaken with the sharpest scalpels available. Oblique sectioning of an artery is not advisable in embolectomy, because the arteriotomy cannot be extended if this procedure becomes necessary.

(Prior to the incision the contents should be aspirated and the lumen rinsed with saline.)

In arteries with a diameter of under 1 mm., the longitudinal incision should be closed with a patch. The latter should not be too wide since this leads to aneurysmal bulging of the artery, with all its ill-effects (turbulence of blood flow, the formation of mural thrombi, peripheral embolization).

The finest possible suture material should always be used.

The sutures should be spaced at very precise distances around the arterial wall and also at regular intervals from each other.

It is vitally important that the suture material does not come in contact with the blood or tissue fluids in the operating area for any length of time, in order to prevent microclots from becoming attached and being introduced into the lumen of the artery during further suturing. The sutures should be short, and should be wiped with a pledget and rinsed carefully in a saline solution each time they are inserted.

The edges of the artery are everted so that no adventitial tissue remains in the lumen of the artery.

It is advisable to use three square knots with nylon suture.

Very small arteries may be dilated by the insertion of a blunt forceps which is carefully released, to enable a small tube to be inserted (mechanical dilatation).

It is advisable to insert a rubber dam under the artery in order to protect the neighboring structures. After the initial fixing sutures, the sutures are cut to a length of 1—1.5 cm. and used for rotating the artery, in order to facilitate insertion of the sutures in the posterior wall.

The efforts of surgeons to operate on the blood vessels may be traced to previous centuries (Hallowell 1759, Asman 1785, Jassinowsky 1889), but the actual pioneer in the field was Carrel (1908). The monographs of Vogt (1965), Vollmar (1967) and the paper of Khodadad and Lougheed (1966) provide comprehensive reviews of the guidelines laid down by Carrel. The principles of macrovascular surgery are broadly applied to the circumstances of microvascular surgery. A bibliography of microvascular surgery, including a list of the papers dealing with the problems of autografts, homografts, allografts and heterografts, is appended to this chapter.

While technical perfection is a prerequisite for the success of any operation, it alone does not ensure satisfactory results. Narrowing of the arterial lumen (edema of the artery walls or spasm, or both) and thrombus formation as a reaction to mechanical physical, chemical and biological stimuli present a huge field for research. Even a brief discussion of recent investigations is beyond the scope of this monograph. The most important papers in this field are mentioned in the bibliography.

Some research workers and clinicians advocate antispasm medication — either alone or in combination with anticoagulants before, during, and after the operation. Contrary views can be found which deprecate these pharmacological measures and report equally good operative results. Similarly, the value of the hyperbaric chamber for operations also remains unclear. It is to be hoped that any application of physiological pharmacological and biochemical research to the problems of microsurgery will yield significant facts about the function of the blood vessels as an organ.

A very important, as yet unsolved problem is the fact that, apart from follow-up angiography and re-exploration, no simple, non-operative and non-taxing method is available for checking the immediate functional state of the repaired artery. The monitoring of blood flow utilizing an implanted detector in the arterial wall (Jacobson 1964), radioactive phosphorus (Kiehn et al. 1952) or the Doppler technique are methods that remain in the experimental stage.

References

Abbe, R.: The surgery of the hand. N. Y. med. J. 59 (1894) 33

Asman, C.: The aneurysmate. In: Scriptorum latinorum de aneurysmatibus collectio. T. Lauth, Ed. Argentorati: A. König, 18 (1785) pp. 564—583

Ayala, G. F., W. A. Himwich: Subtemporal approach to the basilar artery in the dog. J. appl. physiol. 15 (1960) 1150

Brown, R. B., C. E. Huggins, D. R. Koth: An experimental revaluation of the problem of smal vessel replacement. Surgery 43 (1958) 63

Buncke, H. J., W. P. Schulz: Experimental digital amputation. Plast. reconstr. Surg. 36 (1965) 62

Buncke, Jr., H. J., W. P. Schulz: Total ear reimplantation in the rabbit utilizing microminiature vascular anastomoses. Brit. J. plast. Surg. 10 (1966) 15

Buncke, Jr., H. J., C. M. Buncke, W. P. Schulz: Immediate Nicoladoni procedure in the Rhesus monkey, or hallux-to-hand transplantation utilizing microminiature vascular anastomoses. Brit. J. plast. Surg. 19 (1966) 332

Buncke, Jr., H. J., A. I. Daniller, W. P. Schulz, R. A. Chase: The fate of autogenous whole points transplanted by microvascular anastomosis. Plast. reconstr. Surg. 39 (1967) 333

Carrel, A.: Results of the transplantation of blood vessels, organs and limbs. J. amer. med. Ass. 51 (1908) 1662

Carrel, A.: The surgery of the blood vessels. Johns Hopkins, Hosp. 18 (1909) 18

Carter, P. D.: Suture and nonsuture methods of small vein anastomoses. Arch. Surg. (Chic.) 84 (1962) 350

Chase, M. D., S. I. Schwartz: Consistent patency of 1.5 milimeter arterial anastomoses. Surg. Forum 13 (1962) 220

Chase, M. D., S. I. Schwartz: Suture anastomosis of small arteries. Surg. Gynec. Obstet. 117 (1963) 44

Chi'en Yun Ch'ing, Ch'en Chung-Wei, Lin Eh'ing-Tien, Pao Yüeh-Se: Some problems concerning small vessel anastomosis in the reattachment of complete traumatic amputation. Chin. med. J. 85 (1966) 79

Cobbett, J. R.: Microvascular Surgery. Surg. Clin. N. Amer. 47 (1967a) 521

Cobbett, J. R.: Diameter changes in small vessel anastomoses. In: Micro-Vascular Surgery. Ed. by R. M. P. Donaghy, M. G. Yaşargil. Thieme, Stuttgart 1967b, pp. 35—38

Collins, R. E., F. M. Douglass: Small vein anastomosis with and without operative microscope. A comparative study Arch. Surg. (Chic.) 88 (1964) 740

Crawford, E. S., A. C. Beall, P. R. Ellis, Jr., M. E. De Bakey: A technic permitting operation upon small arteries. Surg. Forum 10 (1959) 671

Crowell, R. N., M. G. Yaşargil: Experimental microvascular autografting. Technical note. J. Neurosurg. 31 (1969) 101

Cullen, M. L., A. J. Silvestri, N. J. Skvevsky: Small artery anastomosis — an experimental study. J. A. Einstein Med. Cent. 10 (1962) 14

DeLeon, A. R., P. S. Crane, F. C. Spencer: Use of autogenous vein patch in the performance of end-to-end anastomoses in small arteries. Surg. Forum 12 (1961) 258

Donaghy, R. M. P.: Patch and by-pass in microangeional surgery. In: Micro-Vascular Surgery. Ed. by R. M. P. Donaghy, M. G. Yaşargil. Thieme, Stuttgart 1967, pp. 75—86

Donaghy, R. M. P., M. G. Yaşargil: Micro-Vascular Surgery. Report of First Conference, 6—7 Oct., 1966, Mary Fletcher Hospital, Burlington, Vermont. Thieme, Stuttgart and Mosby, St. Louis, Mo. 1967

Dormandy, S. A., R. H. Goetz: Wire suture short circuit thrombi. Med. World News, Nov. 4, 85 (1966)

Dorrance, G. M.: An experimental study of suture of arteries with a description of a new suture. Ann. Surg. 44, (1906) 409

Echlin, Fr. A.: Spasm af basilar and vertebral arteries caused by experimental subarachnoid hemorrhage. J. Neurosurg. 23 (1965) 1

Ellis, Jr. P. R., D. A. Cooley: The patch technique, an adjunct to coronary endarterectomy. J. thorac. cardiovasc. Surg. 42 (1961) 236

Ellis, F. H., I. V. Doumaniau, G. R. Plum: Methods of coronary arteriotomy closure in the dog. Arch. Surg. 84 (1962) 132

Fisher, B. Lee Sun: Microvascular surgical techniques in research with special reference to renal transplantation in the rat. Surgery 58 (1965) 904

Gaetano, L. De.: Sutura delle arterie; recerche sperimentali sul processo di guarigione delle fechite delle arterie, in rapporto alla rigenerazione delle fibre elstiche. Giorn. Intern. Sci. Med. 25 (1903) 289

Green, G. E. M. L. Som, W. I. Wolff: Experimental microvascular suture anastomosis. Circulation, Suppl. I, 33—34 (1966) 199

Goldwyn, R. M., P. M. Beach, D. Feldman, R. E. Wilson: Canine limb homotransplantation. Plast. reconstr. Surg. 37 (1966) 184

Hallowell: quoted by Khodadad, G., W. M. Lougheed

Holt, G. P., F. J. Lewis: A new technique for end-to-end anastomosis of small arteries. Surg. Forum 11 (1960) 242

Höpfner, E.: Über Gefäßnaht, Gefäßtransplantationen und Replantation von amputierten Extremitäten. Arch. klin. Chir. 70 (1903) 417

Isenberger, R. M., D. C. Carroll: Muscle flap repair of perforation in the larger arteries of dogs. Surgery 6 (1939) 265

Jacobson, J. H., E. L. Suarez: Microsurgery in the anastomosis of small vessels. Surg. Forum 11 (1960) 243

Jacobson, J. H., D. B. Miller, E. L. Suarez: Microvascular surgery: a new horizon in coronary artery surgery. Circulation 22 (1960) 767

Jacobson, J. H., T. Katsumura: Small vein reconstruction. J. cardiovasc. Surg. 6 (1965) 157

Jacobson, J. H.: Microsurgical technique. In: Craft of Surgery, Ed. by P. Cooper, Little, Brown & Co., Boston, Mass. (1964), pp. 799—819

Jacobson, J. H.: Arterial patency shown by implantable detector. Med. Trib. 28 March, 1966

Jassinowsky, A.: Die Arteriennaht. Med. Diss. Dorpat 1889

Jensen, G.: Über zirkuläre Gefäßsutur. Arch. klin. Chir. 69 (1903) 938

Kabat, H.: A new method of arterial anastomosis for acute experiments without use of an anticoagulant. Proc. Soc. exp. Biol. (N. Y.) 37 (1938) 698

Khodadad, G.: Repair and replacement of small arteries. M. S. thesis, Toronto, 1965

Khodadad, G., W. M. Lougheed: Repair and replacement of small arteries. Microsuture technique. J. Neurosurg. 25 (1966) 61

Khodadad, G., W. M. Lougheed: Stapling technique in segmental vein autografts and end-to-end anastomosis of small vessels in dogs. Utilization of the operating microscope. J. Neurosurg. 24 (1966) 855

Kiehn, C. L., L. Benson, D. M. Glover, M. Berg: Study of revacularization of blood vessel graft by means of radioactive phosphorus. Arch. Surg. 65 (1952) 477

Klotz, O., H. W. Permar, E. C. Guthrie: End results of arterial transplants. Ann. Surg. 78 (1923) 305

Krizek, T. J., T. Tasaburo, J. D. Desprez, C. L. Kiehn: Experimental transplantation of composite grafts by microsurgical vascular anastomoses. Plast. reconstr. Surg. 36 (1965) 538

Leon, A. R. De, P. S. Crane, F. C. Spencer: Use of autogenous vein patch in the performance of end-to-end anastomoses in small arteries. Surg. Forum 12 (1961) 258

Lindstrom, B. L., G. de Takats: Bifurcational anastomosis of small arteries with pedicled grafts. Surgery, 53 (1963) 340

Littler, J. W.: Neurovascular skin island transfer in reconstructive hand surgery. Transactions of the International Society of Plastic Surgeons, 2nd Congress: Livingstone, Edinburgh, 6 (1960) 175

Man, B., Z. Kohn: Experiments on the anastomosis of small vessels. J. cardiovasc. Surg. 3 (1962) 195

McCune, W. S., J. R. Thistlethwaite, J. M. Keshiskian, S. B. Blade: Nutrition of blood vessel grafts: India ink injection study of their vascularization. Surg. Gynec. Obstet. 94 (1952) 311

Mozes, M., B. Man, M. Agmon, R. Adar: Small vessel anastomoses. Surgery 54 (1963) 609

Murphy, J. B.: Resection of arteries and veins injured in continuity; end-to-end suture. Med. Rec. (N. Y.) 51 (1897) 73

Pearlman, D. M.: The immobilization of small vessels to be sutured. Surg. Gynec. Obstet. 121 (1965) 1343

Phelan, J. T., W. P. Young, J. W. Gale: The effects of suture material on small artery anastomoses. Surg. Gynec. Obstet. 107 (1958) 79

Reeves, M. M.: Microsurgical technic in patch-graft closure of coronary arterectomy. Dis. Chest. 47 (1965) 304

Sadd, J. R., J. T. Mendenhall, R. C. Hickey: Value of microsurgical techniques in small vessel anastomosis in grafting. Circulation, Suppl. I, 33—34 (1966) 196

Salmon, P. A. and Assimacopoulos, C. A.: Microsurgery. Minn. Med. 47 (1964) 679

Sauvage, L. R., S. J. Wood, K. M. Eyer, A. H. Bill Jr.: Experimental coronary artery surgery. J. thorac. cardiovasc.. Surg. 46 (1963) 826

Schamaun, M.: Internal mammary annd coronar artery suture-anastomosis with use of patch grafting. Angiology 15 (1964) 322

Schumacker, Jr. H. B., R. J. Lowenberg: Experimental studies in vascular repair. Comparison of reliability of various methods of end-to-end arterial sutures. Surgery 24 (1948) 79

Senning, A.: Stript-graft technique. Acta chir. scand. 118 (1959) 81

Smith, J. W.: Microsurgery and vasa vasorum. In: Micro-Vascular Surgery. Ed. by R. M. P. Donaghy, M. G. Yaşargil, Thieme, Stuttgart, pp. (1967) 57—62

Sobin, S. S., W. G. Frasher, H. M. Tremer: Vasa vasorum of the pulmonary artery of the rabbit. Circulat. Res. 11 (1962) 257

Stahl, W. M., T. Katsumura: Reconstruction of small arteries. Arch. Surg. 88 (1964) 384

Stahl, W. M.: Coronary endarterectomy in calves. Angiology 16 (1965) 303

Stich, R., H. Zoeppritz: Zur Histologie der Gefäßnaht der Gefäß- und Organtransplantationen. Beitr. path. Anat. 46 (1909) 337

Sundt, T. M., J. D. Nofzinger, F. Murphey: Arteriotomy patching by means of intraluminar pressure sealing venous autografts. J. Neurosurg. 23 (1965) 452

Urschel, Jr., H. C., E. J. Roth: Small arterial anastomosis. I. Suture. Ann. Surg. 153 (1961) 611

Vogt, B.: Die rekonstruktive Gefäßchirurgie bei Behandlung chronischer Arterienverschlüsse der unteren Extremität. Thieme, Stuttgart (1965) p. 83

Vollmar, J.: Rekonstruktive Chirurgie der Arterien. Thieme, Stuttgart (1967) p. 416

White, R. J., M. S. Albin: The technique and results of ligation of the basilar artery in monkeys. J. surg. Res. 2 (1962) 15

White, R. J., D. E. Donald: Basilar artery ligation and cerebral ischemia in dogs. Arch. Surg. 84 (1962) 470

Wolma, F. J.: The wire suture of blood vessels: an experimental study. Arch. Surg. 78 (1959) 490

Yamanoüchi, H.: Über die zirkulären Gefäßnähte und Arterien-Venenanastomosen, sowie über die Gefäßtransplantationen. Dtsch. Z. Chir. 112 (1911) 141

Yaşargil, M. G.: Experimental small vessel surgery in the dog including patching and grafting of cerebral vessels and the formation of functional extra-intracranial shunts. In: Micro-Vascular Surgery. Ed. by R. M. P. Donaghy, M. G. Yaşargil, Thieme, Stuttgart, 1967, pp. 87—126

Zwaveling, A.: Anastomoses in small-calibre arteries. Arch. chir. neerl. 15 (1963) 237

Allograft

Belcher, H. V., F. D. Roller: The use of Teflon felt in vascular anastomoses. J. surg. Res. 6 (1966) 498

Blakemore, A. H., A. B. Voorhees, Jr.: The use of tubes constructed from Vinyon »N« cloth in bridging arterial defects, experimental and clinical. Ann. Surg 140 (1954) 324

Bradham, R. R., D. B. Nunn: Autogenous vein grafts and Teflon grafts as small vessel prostheses. Ach. Surg. 81 (1960) 136

Contzen, H., F. Straumann, E. Paschke, R. Geissendörfer: Grundlagen der Alloplastik mit Metallen und Kunststoffen. Thieme, Stuttgart 1967

Eiken, O.: Combined Teflon-autologous vein grafts for small artery replacement in dogs. Acta chir. scand. 121 (1961) 200

Eiken, O.: Small artery replacement by autologous vein, homologous arteries and Teflon tubes in dogs. Acta chir. scand. 121 ((1961) 183

Gott, V. L.: The causes and prevention of thrombosis on prosthetic materials. J. surg. Res. 6 (1966) 274

Holman, E., R. Hahn: The application of the Z-plasty technic to hollow cylinder anastomosis. Ann. Surg. 138 (1953) 344

Hufnagel, C. A.: The use of rigid and flexible plastic prosthesis for arterial replacement. Surgery 37 (1955) 165

Massel, T. B.: Woven Dacron and woven Teflon prostheses. Arch. Surg. 84 (1962) 73

Murray, G., J. M. Jones: Prevention of failure of circulation following injuries to large arteries. Experiments with glass cannulae kept patent by administration of heparin. Brit. med. J. 2 (1940) 6

Payr, E.: Beiträge zur Technik der Blutgefäß- und Nervennaht nebst Mitteilungen über die Verwendung eines resorbierenden Metalles in der Chirurgie. Arch. klin. Chir. 62 (1900) 67

Poth, E., J. K. Johnson, J. H. Childer: The use of inert, plastic fabrics as arterial prostheses. Tex. Rep. Biol. Med. 13 (1955) 124

Smith, S. A.: A soluble rod as an aid to vascular anastomosis an experimental study. Arch. Surg. 41 (1940) 1004

Voorhees, A. B., A. Jaretzki III, A. H. Blakemore: The use of tubes constructed from Vinyon „N" cloth in bridging arterial defects. A preliminary report. Ann. Surg. 135 (1952) 332

Weiss, E., C. R. Lam: Tantalum tubes in the non-suture method of blood vessel anastomosis. Amer. J. Surg. 80 (1950) 452

Wesolowski, S. A., C. C. Fries, W. J. Liebig, P. N. Sawyer, R. A. Deterling Jr.: The synthetic vascular graft. New concepts, new materials. Arch. Surg. 84 (1962) 56

Autograft

Bellman, S.: Experimental reconstruction of small arteries using autogenous vascular grafts. Acta chir. scand. 128 (1964) 509

Chatterjee, K. N., R. Warren, I. Gore: Autogenous arterial patch graft for arteriotomy closure. Surgery 52 (1962) 890

Dale, W. A., M. R. Lewis: Lateral vascular patch grafts. Surgery 57 (1965) 36

Edwards, W. S.: Autogenous vein patch reconstruction of small leg arteries after endarterectomy. J. cardiovasc. Surg. (Torino) 3 (1962) 161

Eiken, O.: Autogenous connective tissue tubes for replacement of small artery defects. A preliminary report of an experimental study in dogs. Acta chir. scand. 120 (1960) 47

Eiken, O.: Bridging small defects in the dog with in situ performed autologous connective tissue tubes. Acta chir. scand. 121 (1961) 90

Horton, C., F. Campbell, R. Connar, A. Smith, K. Pickerell: The use of autogenous skin grafts to repair arterial defects. Surgery 39 (1956) 926

Scobie, D., T. Scobie, I. Vogelfanger: Venous autografts. Canad. J. Surg. 5 (1962) 471

Sparks, C. H., M. A. Melgard, J. Raaf: Carotid artery replacement with reinforced autogenous vein grafts. Angiology 14 (1962) 542

Wylie, E. J.: Vascular replacement with arterial autografts. Surgery 57 (1965) 14

Heterograft

Copley, A. L., P. L. Stefko: Arterial anastomosis in dogs, employing vein grafts from chickens and turkeys. Science 102 (1945) 338

Greco, F. Del: The use of immunosuppressive drugs in organ transplantation. New Physician (1966) 162

Rosenberg, N., J. Henderson, G. H. Lord, J. W. Bothwell: An arterial prosthesis of heterologous vascular origin. J. amer. med. Ass. 187 (1964) 165

Rosenberg, N., A. Martinez, N. P. Sawyer, S. A. Wesolowski, P. W. Postlethwait, M. L. Dillion: Tanned collagen arterial prosthesis of bovine carotid origin in man. Ann. Surg. 164 (1966) 247

Vickery, C. M., H. L. Combs, R. Warren: Experimental small artery grafts in dogs treated with immuno-suppressive drugs. New. Engl. J. Med. 272 (1965) 325

Homograft

Bellman, S., B. Gothman: Vascularization of one year old homologous aortic grafts. Ann. Surg. 139 (1954) 447

Goldwyn, R. M., M. Beach, D. Feldman, R. E. Wilson: Canine limb homotransplantation. Plast. reconstr. Surg. 37 (1966) 184

Moore, F. C., A. Ribiri, H. Kajikuri: Freeze-dried and alcohol preserved homografts for replacement of small arteries. Surg. Gynec. Obstet. 103 (1956) 155

Myers, R. N., E. W. Shearburn: Long-term follow-up on alcohol preserved homografts for small artery replacement. J. cardiovasc. Surg. (Torino) 3 (1962) 151

CHAPTER 4

Reconstructive and Constructive Surgery of the Cerebral Arteries in Man

A. Cerebral Vasculature

Blood vessels, arteries in particular comprise a highly variable, vital organ system. They vary in structure, age at different rates and have distinctive susceptibilities to disease. Furthermore, although it is known that arteries are metabolically active organs containing a number of enzyme systems there is little understanding of the regional variations in metabolism suggested by the striking regional differences in function and susceptibility to disease (Lansing 1959, Comèl, Laszt 1966). The absence of atherosclerosis in intraspinal arteries and the presence in the same individual of destroyed coronary or cerebral vessels of similar size is but one example.

In general all arteries contain the same basic components; namely, endothelium, elastic and collagen fibers, fibroblasts, ground substance and smooth muscle. Each of these components vary quantitatively in different arteries while maintaining a constant structure of three layers; the tunica intima, tunica media and tunica adventitia. The innermost layer, the tunica intima, consists mainly of endothelium supported by collagen, fibroblasts and ground substance generally orientated in a longitudinal fashion. The endothelial layer forms a tight, smooth, semipermeable membrane which is capable of complete regeneration within 3 weeks. The new endothelial cells arise from fibroblasts. The tunica media comprises the thickest part of the wall and the predominant type of tissue element contained in this layer is used to classify the artery. Thus, in conducting arteries (aorta, inominant, subclavian and the proximal common carotid) the media contains a predominance of elastic fibers whereas

in distributing or muscular arteries (from the elastic type to the arterioles) this layer is primarily composed of smooth muscle. The tunica adventitia forms the outermost layer and consists of a loose arrangement of collagen, fibroblasts, bundles of axons, Schwann cells and vasa vasorum, generally running parallel to the long axis of the vessel and blending with the surrounding connective tissue which accompanies every blood vessel. Between the tunica intima and media, and between the tunica media and adventitia there is a dense accumulation of elastic tissue forming almost complete circular membranes. The internal elastic membrane is particularly noticeable in muscular arteries and cerebral vessels; the external elastic membrane being absent in the latter. The change from an elastic to muscular type of artery takes place gradually with intermediate regions often designated as arteries of mixed types. In mixed arteries such as the carotid and vertebral arteries the tunica media consists of two layers for a varying distance; the internal layer predominantly muscular and the external layer mainly elastic.

Of the peripheral muscular arteries, the arteries of the central nervous system are unique. Depending upon their location (extracranial, intraosseous, intracavernous, subarachnoid and intracerebral) the vessels supplying the brain show an unusually varied structure. According to the morphology and thickness of the wall and the nature of accompanying structures, nine segments can be differentiated in the carotid and four in the vertebral arteries (Figs. 50, 51) (Platzer 1956). Within the carotid canal the adventitia and media of the internal carotid artery become gradually thinned by the loss of smooth muscle cells and collagen fibers. Although this change in vessel wall is gradual and progressive between the entrance of the canal and the exit from the cavernous sinus, abrupt changes in structure occur at the petrous curvature and the first knee of the carotid siphon (Platzer 1957). Certainly, at the

knee of the carotid siphon, the loss of three fourths of the thickness of the tunica media and tunica adventitia, the disappearance of the characteristic external limiting membrane of elastica and the condensation of elastic fibers into the dense internal elastic layer mark the transformation of a conventional peripheral muscular artery into an intra-

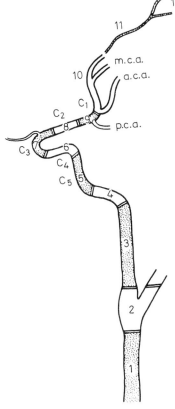

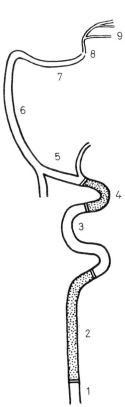

Fig. 50. Diagrammatic representation of the various sections of the internal carotid artery, subdivided according to structural differences of the wall: 1, common carotid artery; 2, carotid bulb; 3, internal carotid artery, extracranial part; 4, internal carotid artery, at the entrance to the carotid canal; 5, internal carotid artery, in the carotid canal; 6, internal carotid artery, in the cavernous sinus; 7, internal carotid artery, exit from the cavernous sinus; 8, internal carotid artery, in the subarachnoid space; 9, internal carotid bifurcation; 10, large cerebral arteries in the subarachnoid space (anterior, middle and posterior cerebral arteries); 12, cerebral arteries after entering the brain substance.

Fig. 51. Diagrammatic representation of the vertebral artery subdivided according to structural differences of the wall: 1, vertebral artery proximal to entry into the costotransverse foramen of the 6th cervical vertebra; 2, vertebral artery between the 6th and 2nd cervical vertebrae; 3, vertebral artery between the axis and atlas; 4, vertebral artery between the arch of the atlas and the point of entry into the intracranial cavity; 5, vertebral artery within the skull; 6, basilar artery; 7, larger branches of the basilar artery, e.g. posterior cerebral artery and the superior cerebellar artery; 8, smaller cerebral and cerebellar arteries in the subarachnoid space; 9, intracerebral arteries.

cranial artery. These changes in the wall may be due to changes in surrounding structures. Extracranial arteries, unlike accompanying veins, are quite separate from adjacent tissues and are usually enveloped only in a layer of loose connective tissue. In contrast, the internal carotid artery enters the bony carotid canal accompanied by two veins on its convex and concave side (Teufel 1964). In the intraosseous segment these veins ramify with connections to the jugular vein, petrosal and cavernous sinuses, eventually completely enveloping the artery in a cushion of venous blood and at a distance, bone. Similarly, the vertebral artery is enveloped within the vertebral canal in a venous plexus which communicates with the internal vertebral plexus (Rickenbacher 1964, Zolnai 1964, Zanobio, Zanella 1968). It would appear that when the artery enters this fluid cushion, elastic, collagen and muscular elements of the wall are lost and the intravascular tension is supported in the intraosseous and intravenous parts by blood and beyond by cerebrospinal fluid. The very slow transformation of the vertebral artery into a typical intracranial vessel is apparently related to the prolongation of this cushioning segment. This hypothesis is supported by the studies of Goerttler (1953) who compared the cerebral with the extracerebral arteries of similar dimensions in human neonates and fetuses. He was unable to demonstrate the characteristic anatomical differences described in the walls of these two classes of vessels in the adult and therefore advanced the theory that the supporting layers of the cerebral arterial wall regressed after closure of the fontanelles. Hassler (1961) provided substantiation for this speculation when he demonstrated that the muscular layers of the cerebral arteries were more strikingly developed in rabbits submitted to craniotomy at birth than in control animals. Apart from this discrepancy in thickness of smooth muscle, there were no distinct morphological differences: the intima was thin, the elastic layer well developed and the adventitia not very thick. It is generally believed that the pattern assumed by most vessels depends upon mechanical factors. In his classic work, Thoma (1893)

stressed the paramount influence of the volume of blood, its rate of flow and its pressure in determining whether a capillary atrophies, remains a capillary or becomes a larger vessel, as well as in determining the thickness of its wall. Similarly, the Clarks (1940) observed that the differentiation of smooth muscle in the vessel wall is influenced by blood pressure. That the same must be true for elastic tissue is indicated by the following natural experiment, which indicates how markedly the morphology of the developing vessel wall is influenced by the blood stream. In an acardiac twin parasite, the aorta is subject to a pulse, blood pressure and speed of flow like those present in an ordinary peripheral artery; correlated with these peripheral conditions, such an aorta shows the structure of a typical muscular artery.

Important as these mechanical influences appear to be in the causal development of cerebral arteries, hereditary and chemical factors are undoubtedly also operative. To support both of these points of view, Scharrer (1939) observed that end arteries will develop in the dead brain tissue of the opossum. He interpreted this as evidence of the presence of a guiding factor inherent in the cerebral vessels themselves. In opposition to this view, Wislocki (1939) explained the result on the basis of chemical factors inherent in the brain tissue.

Recognition of these major variations in morphology of the arteries supplying the brain are of more than theoretical interest, for such differences must be considered if surgical reconstruction of diseased vessels is to be successful and the pathogenesis of such disease understood.

Studies of the special microscopic and ultra microscopic anatomy of the cerebral vessels remain largely incomplete, although useful information may be gained from the more systematic investigations of extracerebral vessels. Comparison of the basilar artery with the superior mesenteric artery, two muscular arteries of similar size, points out many of the pertinent differences. Clearly, the intracranial artery possesses a remarkably thin wall. The tunica adventitia of the basilar artery is usually 35—40 μ thick and consists of a delicate network of collagen fibers enveloping and containing an extensive ground plexus of autonomic nerve fibers, and a few myelinated presumably afferent fibers. Unlike the superior mesenteric artery there are no arterial or venous vasa vasorum, no lymphatics and no ganglionic cells in the adventitia of the basilar artery or indeed in most of the intracranial arteries (Fang 1961, Dahl et al. 1965). The tunica media of the basilar artery is 130—190 μ thick and contains 18—20 layers of spindle-shaped smooth muscle cells 20—50 μ in length and 5—10 μ in diameter arranged in a helical fashion but not forming the so-called 'ring muscle' of the external vessels. Tension muscles ('Spann-muskeln') are not found in the intracranial vessels and the muscular coat contains practically no elastic tissue (Pease, Molinari 1960). Throughout the body arterial smooth muscle shows qualities of spontaneous activity and independent conductivity and although the opposed double membranes of adjacent cells afford a high resistance, excitation is conducted slowly from cell to cell permitting the muscular wall to function as a syncitium. Smooth muscle cells although capable of regeneration are, after extensive damage (e. g. following surgical transection), usually replaced by collagen. Collagen fibers continuous with the subendothelial basement membrane are reflected over each smooth muscle cell and shared between adjacent cells to form a sarcolemmal envelope (Dahl et al. 1965). The collagen is fashioned by the ubiquitous fibroblast and made up of long protein chains linked with hydrogen and ionic bonds and surrounded by an amorphous ground substance of mucopolysaccharide. The collagen fiber, though less flexible, is 25 times as strong as elastic fiber and accounts for most of the structural integrity of the vessel wall. There is only 10% less collagen in the intracranial vessels as compared to the extracranial vessels. Furthermore, the collagen fibers are the only fibers replacing elastic and muscle fibers and are of prime importance in the healing and repair of damaged vessels. Elastic tissue is composed of the protein elastin and unlike collagen

contains no carbohydrate and is very insoluble. The elastic fibers are able to extend to twice their length but have little tensile strength and must be protected from excessive elongation and tearing by the collagen framework. The elastic fibers are condensed into fenestrated membranes lying concentrically over one another and serve as a foothold for the muscle layer as well as permitting elastic recoil of the wall. The external lamella of elastic tissue is entirely absent in intracranial vessels and the internal lamella, 5 μ thick and a striking feature in the circle of Willis, progressively decreases in the peripheral vessels, persisting only as a minor component of small arteries. Fewer differences are apparent in the tunica intima of intra- and extracranial vessels. Endothelial cells form the only cell population of the intima and this single layer of flat, polygonal cells rests on a reticulated, mucopolysaccharide basement membrane (Buck 1958). Vasa interna or intimal capillaries have not been described in intracranial vessels. In 1851 Virchow commented on the unusual morphology of the cerebral vessels and noted the similarity of these vessels to the umbilical artery. Both have thin walls without vasa vasorum and are surrounded by fluid.

A comparison of the structure of the intra- and extracranial vessels is provided in Table X and Figs. 52a—d.

Occasional divergencies from the basic structure have been described. Unusual

Table X. Differential Structure of the Walls of the Extra- and Intracranial Vessels

	Extra-cranial	Intra-cranial
Muscle layers	35 layers	20 layers
Collagen	33%	22%
Elastic fibers	4%	1—2%
Elastic external membrane	strong	absent
Tunica externa	strong	weak
Accompanying vein	present	absent
Lymphatic vessels	present	absent
Vasa vasorum	present	absent
Nerves	present	present
Vasomotor activity	strong	moderate

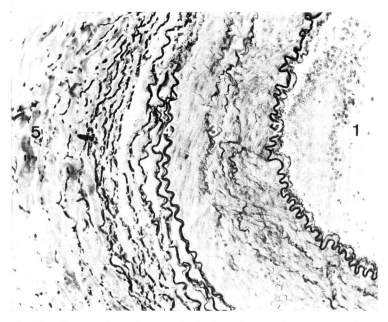

Fig. 52a. Cross-section of a mixed elastic and muscular extracranial artery. 1, lumen; 2, internal elastic lamina; 3, tunica media consisting of smooth muscle and elastic fibers; 4, external elastic lamina; 5, tunica adventitia. Photomicrograph; Elastic stain × 100.

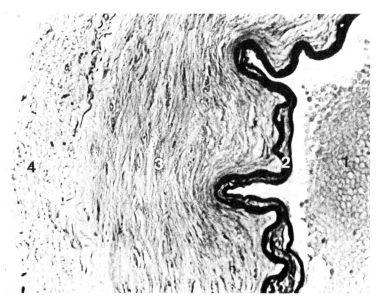

Fig. 52b. Cross-section of a middle cerebral artery from a 55-year-old male; 1, lumen; 2, internal elastic membrane; 3, tunica media; 4, adventitia. Duplication and layering of elastic lamella increases with advancing age. Photomicrograph; Elastic stain, × 200.

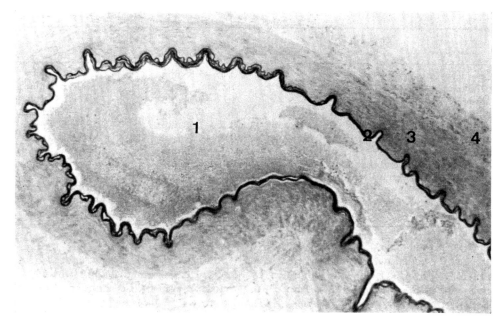

Fig. 52c. Cross-section of the basilar artery from a 55-year-old male; 1, lumen; 2, internal elastic membrane; 3, media; 4, adventitia. Photomicrograph; Elastic stain, × 100.

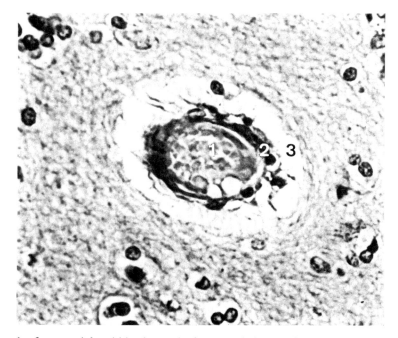

Fig. 52d. Photomicrograph of an arteriole within the cerebral cortex; 1, lumen; 2, vessel wall consisting of endothelium covered by a single layer of smooth muscle; 3, perivascular space artificially enlarged by fixation. H + E × 200.

Table XI

Vessel	Diameter	
	Right	*Left*
Internal carotid artery	3.70—4.55 mm.	3.72—4.51 mm.
Middle cerebral artery	1.87—3.10 mm.	1.94—3.16 mm.
Anterior cerebral artery	1.17—2.34 mm.	1.33—2.44 mm.
Anterior choroidal artery	0.17—0.60 mm.	0.13—0.62 mm.
Posterior choroidal artery	0.30—1.58 mm.	0.28—1.54 mm.
Vertebral artery	0.92—4.09 mm.	1.60—3.60 mm.
Basilar artery	2.70—4.28 mm.	
Posterior inferior cerebellar artery	0.70—1.76 mm.	0.65—1.78 mm.
Anterior inferior cerebellar artery	0.38—1.26 mm.	0.36—1.21 mm.
Superior cerebellar artery	0.73—1.50 mm.	0.72—1.49 mm.
Posterior cerebral artery	1.49—2.40 mm.	1.44—2.27 mm.
Cortical arteries	0.50—1.50 mm.	0.50—1.50 mm.

thinness or actual defects in the media were noted by Forbus (1930) and confirmed by many others (Voncken 1931, Glynn 1940, Richardson, Hyland 1941, Hassler 1961). Intravascular bridges (Figs. 53a—b) intimal cushions, breaches in continuity of elastic lamella and minute aneurysms are all seen frequently in relation to the origin of branches (Hassler 1961, Reuterwall 1923). The specific role of these variations in the pathogenesis of cerebrovascular hemorrhage and thrombosis remains controversial.

As noted, though thin-walled the cerebral arteries have a relatively large diameter. The detailed observations of Wollschlaeger et al. (1967) are of considerable importance to the microvascular surgeon (Table XI).

Nutrition

The components of the vascular organ system are in part cellular and therefore have a metabolic requirement of their own. Even non-cellular components such as collagen, elastin and basement membrane degenerate and regenerate and thus require mechanisms to ensure removal of metabolic products and a constant supply of the basic substances necessary for renewal. A number of problems involving the nutrition of the blood vessel wall remain unresolved. The intima and possibly the innermost layer of media may be supplied by diffusion of substances from within the vascular lumen, enhanced by the radical pressure gradient and probably active transport systems. Certainly, the latter mechanism would have to be operative to move substances from the wall to the lumen.

The arterial and venous vasa vasorum supply the tunica adventitia and outer one half of the tunica media of most extracranial vessels usually arising as rami of a first order branch and then doubling back to course in the adventitia of the parent artery and in turn giving off branches which penetrate the outer media. Occasionally, the arterial vasa originate as the first rami of a branch of the parent artery before the latter has penetrated beyond the adventitia of the parent artery.

In the vasa vasorum of arteries there is a paucity of anastomoses between the terminal branches although frequent collateral channels exist between the main branches of this supporting circulation in the adventitia. In contrast the walls of veins are nourished by two interconnecting networks of vasa vasorum; one lying in the adventitia and one in the outer layers of the media. These observations made by Smith (1966), are important as the commonly accepted practice of denuding the arterial wall of adventitia in arterial reconstructions is likely to deprive a segment of the wall of its circulation. This portion of the wall then functions as a free graft and indeed may undergo ischemic necrosis compromising the anastomosis.

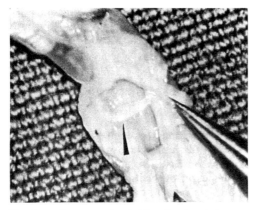

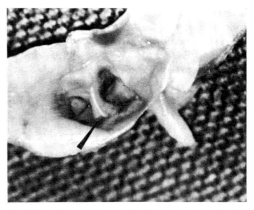

Fig. 53a. Intravascular bridge in the right vertebral artery at the level of the junction of both
vertebral arteries to form the basilar artery
(arrow).

Fig. 53b. Intravascular bridge in the Sylvian
bifurcation (arrow) of the middle cerebral artery.

Gimbert (1865) and more recently Clarke
(1965) have examined the vasa vasorum of
intra- and extracranial arteries. The intracranial segments of the internal carotid
artery, the vertebral arteries and occasionally
the proximal basilar artery all possess arterial
and venous vasa vasorum. Vasa vasorum are
absent on the remainder of the intracranial
arteries. In the course of micro-neurosurgical
operations the present authors have been able
to study the cerebral arterial vasa vasorum
and found them to be sparsely distributed

along the internal carotid to within 2—3 mm.
of the bifurcation where they come to an
abrupt end (Fig. 54). Vasa vasorum were not
observed on the middle or anterior cerebral
arteries or their branches nor on the posterior
communicating artery but on one occasion
were seen on the ophthalmic artery. On the
vertebrobasilar tree, vasa vasorum were found
regularly along the vertebral arteries to the
point of junction with the basilar artery
(Fig. 55). In one patient they were also observed on both posterior inferior cerebellar
arteries for a length of 2.0 cm. These vasa
vasorum on the vertebral artery have more
the appearance of the terminal branches of the
vertebral venous plexus than vessels carrying

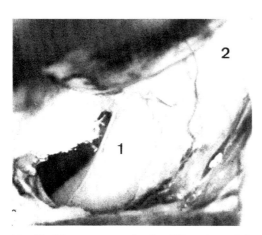

Fig. 54. Vasa vasorum in the C2 region of 1,
the left internal carotid artery; 2, optic nerve.

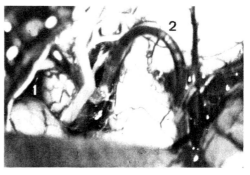

Fig. 55. Vasa vasorum along 1, the left vertebral
artery just distal to its entry into the skull;
2, posterior inferior cerebellar artery.

arterial blood to the wall. A definite pro-
liferation of vasa vasorum has been observed
on several occasions in the vicinity of athero-
sclerotic plaques in keeping with similar
observations on the aorta and coronary
vessels.

The question of how the major volume of the
cerebral arterial wall is nourished remains
unanswered. It is likely that diffusion through
endothelium supports the inner layers although the barrier of insoluble elastin in the
internal elastic membrane would probably
impede much of this flow to the media. One
may speculate that diffusion from the cerebrospinal fluid through the tunica adventitia to
the media is an important mechanism enhanced by the presence of the mucopolysaccharide in the ground substance of these
layers. The limits of this diffusion mechanism
would be determined by oxygen. Again, a
transport system may be operative. That such
an exchange with the cerebrospinal fluid is
significant for the functional activity of the
vessel is suggested by the known physiological
responses of vascular tone to variations in
cerebrospinal fluid ionic composition. Similarly, as yet unidentified substances in the
blood when released into the cerebrospinal
fluid appear to be important in the pathogenesis of vascular narrowing. This narrowing initially appears to be the result of severe
reactive contraction of the muscle layers in
response to vasoactive substances and mechanical deformation and may properly be
termed arterial spasm. This spasm is rapid in
onset, transient in duration and easily
counteracted by papaverine and probably
represents a functional part of the hemostatic mechanism. The more common and
clinically important vascular narrowing following subarachnoid hemorrhage may be
delayed 5—7 days after the ictus and may
persist for many days or even weeks. On
inspection these vessels appear opaque and
greyish-white and are frequently surrounded
by an inflammatory exudate. They dilate
poorly if at all to papaverine. Indeed, it may
well be that much of the significant persistent
vascular narrowing is not primarily vascular
hypertonus but edema and inflammation of the
vessel wall. This pathological alteration of the

wall may be due not only to the inflammatory
stimulus of the surrounding blood but also
from interference with the nutritive mechanisms of the wall.

The Relationship between Morphology and Flow*

The relationship between the structure of
vessels and the mechanisms regulating flow
remain controversial. Physiologic variations
in the caliber of the lumen of a vessel depend
upon the smooth muscle in the wall, and this
muscle possesses some degree of intrinsic
contractility and rhythmicity that is independent of its innervation and of specific
chemical or thermal factors. A basal vascular
tone in thus provided which varies greatly
in different parts of the peripheral circulation.
Obviously, vasoconstrictor mechanisms will
exert their greatest effect on vessels having
little intrinsic myogenic tone whereas
vasodilator substances or innervation will
be most effective in areas possessing a
high degree of tone. Although metabolic,
thermal, hormonal and nervous influences
all are capable of altering vascular tone, the
importance of any one or of combinations of
these factors differs depending on the site
of the vessel studied and its functional state
prior to stimulation. Thus, sympathetic
denervation of the head of a rabbit causes
marked vasodilatation of the skin of the ears
but apparently has little effect on the cerebral
vessels, the latter being regulated by the
interaction of their considerable intrinsic
tone, and the vasodilator products of metabolism especially carbon dioxide. Folkow's
(1955 and 1960) classification of vessels into
six functional types depending upon structure,
position in the circuit and reactivity is useful
and may be applied to considerations of the
cerebral circulation. These concepts, coupled
with the development of modern techniques
of determining blood flow, have made it
possible to express in fairly quantitative terms
changes in total resistance in the vascular

* This research work of Dr. S. J. Peerless has
been supported by Swiss National Funds (Credit
No. 4921).

system. However, no information is available as to the exact site or sites of the change in resistance, the possible related changes in capacitance vessels or of the range of influence of nervous, chemical and hormonal control.

Clearly vessel length and vessel radius are critical morphological dependent factors in the determination of resistance to blood flow through the vascular bed. In the central nervous system, changes in vessel length are important only in pathological situations (e. g. the elongation of perforating vessels of the brain stem with transtentorial herniation of the temporal lobe) and are otherwise considered to be relatively constant. Vessel radius is usually the most important factor in the regulation of flow as it is easily varied and subject to many controls and also bears a fourth power relationship to the flow rate. Vessel radius may be altered actively (i.e. an active change in the contractile state of the smooth muscle in the wall) or passively. Passive changes in radius result from alteration in the intra- and extraluminal pressure, organic change in the vessel wall or intraluminal occlusion. Variations in transluminal pressure are particularly important in the intracranial compartment (Langfitt et al. 1966). Regulation of flow by active contraction of the elements of the wall occurs principally at the arteriolar level but evidence is accumulating to indicate that macroscopic and microscopic muscular arteries are capable of influencing flow through active constriction and dilatation (Davis, Hamilton 1959, Haddy et al. 1957 and Haddy 1963).

The stimuli that produce an active change in radius may be physical, chemical or nervous. Thus, blood flow tends to remain constant through a vascular bed despite fluctuations of arterial pressure between 100 to 200 mm. Hg (auto regulation) and a large number of naturally occuring chemical substances ranging in structural complexity from ions to very large molecules are capable of locally altering radius and, therefore, flow. Similarly, vasoconstrictor and vasodilator nerves also actively effect vessel radius. Knowledge of how these stimuli are coupled to the contractile

mechanism and the relative importance of each in different organs remains obscure.

The rich perivascular nerve network of the cerebral arteries is largely limited to the superficial vessels, although the authors and others have observed adrenergic fibers associated with intracerebral arteries and deep cerebral veins (Carrato-Ibanez, Abadia-Fenoli 1966, Peerless, Yaşargil 1969). Of the great vessels at the base of the brain, the accompanying nerve plexus may be considered under four functional categories. The myelinated afferent and presumably sensory fibers which conduct centripetally with the cranial and upper cervical spinal nerves may be important in regulation of local axon reflexes (Bruce 1913, Celander, Folkow 1953). A second functional unit is the centrally controlled, vasoconstrictor, adrenergic nerves arising from the superior cervical ganglion. Another functional unit is the centrally regulated vasodilator fiber of both sympathetic and parasympathetic origin. The fourth group consists of the peripheral neural network in the vascular walls by which local mechanical, chemical as well as nervous stimuli may be integrated and propagated. Electronmicroscopic and histochemical studies have provided clear confirmation of previous light microscopic demonstrations of nerves in the adventitia of intracranial arteries (Dahl, Nelson 1964). Tentatively, afferent end organs in the form of diffuse arborizations of coarse fibers in baroreceptor and chemoreceptor areas, naked terminal branches and encapsulated structures similar to the end bulbs of Krause and Meissner's corpuscles have been identified (Penfield 1932, Hassin 1929). However, as in the skin, the functional significance of the latter structures is now open to serious question. The efferent fibers are unmyeliated and form a complex ground plexus on the outermost layer of the tunica media although in larger vessels they may accompany the vasa vasorum for a short distance into the muscle. Specialized neuromuscular endings of these autonomic fibers have not been found on arterial smooth muscle cells as have been described in the bladder and gut (Thaemert 1963). Rather, irregular varicosities bead the fibers and have been shown to consist of

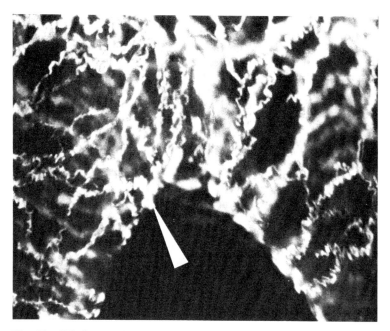

Fig. 56a. Whole stretch preparation of the anterior cerebral junction from a rabbit. White lines and varicosities are intensely fluorescent material (Noradrenalin) within nerve fibers and terminals. Note the size and density of catecholamine containing fibers in this region. Magnification 100 ×.

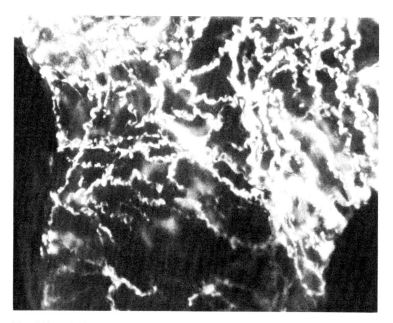

Fig. 56b. Whole stretch preparation of carotid bifurcation from the same rabbit illustrated in Fig. 56a and 56c. Fibers and varicosities containing the adrenergic transmitter are again seen but are not as numerous as in the anterior cerebral region. Magnification 100 ×.

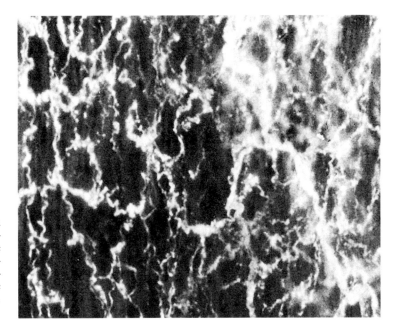

Fig. 56c. Whole stretch preparation of the basilar artery. Note the delicate fluorescent nerves and their arrangement into a typical wide meshed ground plexus. Magnification 100 ×.

vesicles with electron-dense cores. Autoradiographic and histochemical techniques strongly suggest these vesicles contain the transmitter noradrenalin (Falck 1962, Wolf et al. 1962). Fluorescent histochemical studies by Nielsen, Owman (1967) confirmed in our laboratories indicate that there are dense accumulations of large adrenergic fibers in the anterior parts of the circle of Willis and only a sparse ground plexus of fine fibers on the basilar artery and posterior segments of the circle (Figs. 56a–d). Curiously, these fibers are absent in the vessels of vascular malformations. Furthermore, these concentrated stores of adrenalin can be released by a variety of physiologic and pathologic stimuli including the presence of subarachnoid blood. It may well be that this adrenergic system plays an important role in the pathogenesis of cerebral arterial spasm possibly only after proximal fibers are disrupted by rupture of an aneurysm or atheroma formation making the terminal branches hypersensitive to circulating catecholamines.

The central control of the autonomic nervous system in relation to vasomotor tone is complex. It has long been known that afferent impulses are able to elicit reflex vasomotor

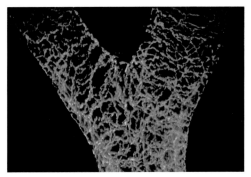

Fig. 56d. Color photomicrograph shows intense flourescense in same preparation as shown in 56b.

responses *via* the spinal cord. Integration is achieved by a network of reticular cells in the floor of the fourth ventricle known as the vasomotor or vasoconstrictor center. The more caudal part of this area seems to be primarily concerned with tonic discharge. Projections from this rather diffuse area in the medulla oblongata pass to the sympathetic spinal centers in the area between the dorsolateral and ventrolateral funiculi with a partial cumulative crossing of the fibers. Excitatory and inhibitory influences are known to project from the cerebellum, anterior and posterior hypothalamus and from diverse cortical areas of the forebrain. The importance of a central neural regulating mechanism for the cerebral circulation has been assumed to be negligible because of failure of autonomic denervation or stimulation to significantly affect cerebral blood flow. Nevertheless, the function of the rich plexus of nerves accompanying the cerebral vessels and their central connections is not understood. Recently, the work of Shalit et al. (1968) suggested that a central integrating mechanism may be functional in the control of cerebral circulation in response to changes in arterial CO_2 tension.

The further development and application of microtechniques to neurosurgery depend to a large extent on the precise manipulation of the cerebral and spinal vascular tree. To this end there is an urgent need for detailed studies of normal vascular metabolism and structure before the problems of regeneration and repair, inflammation and mechanisms of disease of this complex organ system can be elucidated.

References

Baker, A. B., A. Iannone: Cerebrovascular disease, I. The large arteries of the circle of Willis. II. The smaller intracerebral arteries. III. The intracerebral arterioles. Neurology (Minneap.) 9 (1959) 321 und 441

Bruce, A. N.: Vasodilator axon reflexes. Quart. J. exp. Physiol. 6 (1913) 339

Buck, R. C.: The fine structure of endothelium of arteries. J. Biophys. Biochem. Cytol. 4 (1958) 187

Carrato-Ibanez, A., F. Abadia-Fenoli: Morphology and origin of the perivascular fibres in the brain substance. Angiology 17 (1966) 771

Celander, O., B. Folkow: The nature and distribution of afferent fibres provided with an axon reflex arrangement. Acta physiol. scand. 29 (1953) 359

Clark, E. R., E. L. Clark: Microscopic observations on the extra-endothelial cells of living mamalian blood vessels. Amer. J. Anat. 66 (1940) 1

Clarke, J. A.: An X-ray microscopic study of the vasa vasorum of the intracranial arteries. Z. Anat. Entwickl.-Gesch. 124 (1965) 396

Clarke, J. A.: An X-ray microscopic study of the vasa vasorum of the human internal carotid and vertrebral arteries. J. neurol. Sci. 2 (1965) 301

Comèl, M., L. Laszt (Ed): Morphologie und Histochemie der Gefäßwand. Vol. I/II. Internat. Symposium, Fribourg, 21—22 June, 1965. Karger, Basel 1966

Dahl, E., E. Nelson: Electron microscopic observations on human intracranial arteries. II. Innervation. Arch. Neurol. (Chicago) 10 (1964) 158

Dahl, E., G. Flora, E. Nelson: Electron microscopic observations on normal intracranial arteries. Neurology (Minneap.) 15 (1965) 132

Davis, D. L., W. F. Hamilton: Small vessel response of the dog paw. Fed. Proc. 18 (1959) 34

Falck, B.: Observations on the possibilites of the cellular localization of monoamines by a fluorescent method. Acta physiol. scand. 56 Suppl. 1 (1962) 197

Fang, H. C. H.: Cerebral arterial innervation in man. Arch. Neurol. (Chicago) 4 (1961) 651

Flora, G., E. Dahl, E. Nelson: Electron microscopic observations on human intracranial arteries. Arch. Neurol. (Chicago) 17 (1967) 162

Folkow, B.: Nervous control of the blood vessels. Physiol. Rev. 35 (1955) 639

Folkow, B.: Role of the nervous system in the control of vascular tone. Circulation 21 (1960) 760

Forbus, W. D.: On the origin of miliary aneurysms of the superficial cerebral arteries. Bull. Johns Hopk. Hosp. 47 (1930) 239

Gimbert, J. L.: Structure et texture des artères. Thèse méd., Paris 1865

Glynn, L. E.: Medial defects in the circle of Willis and their relation to aneurysm formation. J. Path. Bact. 51 (1940) 213

Goerttler, K.: Die funktionelle Bedeutung des Baues der Gefäßwand. Dtsch. Z. Nervenheilk. 170 (1953) 433.

Haddy, F. J., M. Fleishman, D. A. Amanuel: Effect of epinephrine, norepinephrine and serotonin upon systemic small and large vessel resistance. Circulat. Res. 5 (1957) 247

Haddy, F. J.: Local Control of Vascular Flow in the Peripheral Blood Vessels. Ed. by J. L. Orbison, D. E. Smith. William and Wilkins, Baltimore 1963

Hassin, G. B.: The nerve supply of the cerebral blood vessels: A histologic study. Arch. neurol. Psychiat. 2 (1929) 375

Hassler, O.: Morphological studies on the large cerebral arteries. Acta psychiat. scand. Suppl. 154 (1961) 145

Hassler, O.: Physiological intima cushions in human meningeal arteries. Anat. Anz. 111 (1962) 370

Hassler, O.: Elastic tissue contents of the medial layer of the cerebral arteries. Arch. path. Anat. 335 (1962) 39

Hassler, O.: The perivascular nerve-plexus of human cerebral arteries in vascular disease. J. Neuropath. exp. Neurol. 22 (1963) 446

Langfitt, T. W., J. D. Weinstein, N. F. Kassell, J. L. Gagliardi, H. M. Shapiro: Compression of cerebral vessels by intracranial hypertension. Acta neurochir. 15 (1966) 212

Lansing, A. I. (Ed.): The arterial wall. William and Wilkins Baltimore 1959

Nielsen, K. A., C. Owman: Adrenergic innervation of pial arteries related to the circle of Willis in the cat. Brain Res. 6 (1967) 773

Pease, D. C., S. Molinari: Electron microscopy of muscular arteries; pial vessels of the cat and monkey. J. Ultrastruct. Res. 3 (1960) 447

Peerless, S. J., M. G. Yaşargil: 1969 (in press).

Penfield, W.: Intracerebral vascular nerves. Arch. Neurol. Psychiat. 27 (1932) 30

Platzer, W.: Die A. carotis interna im Bereich des Keilbeins bei Primaten. Morph. J. 97 (1956) 220

Platzer, W.: Die Variabilität der A. carotis interna im Sinus cavernosus in Beziehung zur Variabilität der Schädelbasis. Morph. J. 98 (1957) 227

Reuterwall, O. P.: Über bindegewebig geheilte Risse der Elastica interna der Arteria basilaris. Nordiska Bokhnaden, Stockholm 1923

Richardson, J. C., H. H. Hyland: Intracranial aneurysms. A clinical and pathological study of subarachnoid hemorrhage caused by berry aneurysms. Medicine (Baltimore) 20 (1941) 1

Rickenbacher, J.: Der suboccipitale und der intrakranielle Abschnitt der A. vertebralis. Z. Anat. Entwickl.-Gesch. 124 (1964) 171

Scharrer, E.: The regeneration of end arteries in the opposum brain. J. compl Neurol. 70 (1939) 69

Shalit, M. N., S. Shimojyo, O. M. Reinmuth, W. S. Lockhart, Jr., P. Scheinebrg: The mechanism of action and carbon dioxide in the regulation of cerebral blood flow. In: Cerebral Circulation. Elsevier, Amsterdam 1968

Smith, J. W.; Microsurgery: Review of the literature and discussion of microtechniques. Plast. reconstr. Surg. 37 (1966) 227

Teufel, J.: Einbau der Arteria carotis interna in den canalis caroticus unter Berücksichtigung des transbasalen Venenabflusses. Gegenbauers Morphologisches Jahrbuch 106 (1964) 188

Thaemert, J. C.: The ultrastructure and nerve deposition of vesiculated processes in smooth muscle. J. Cell. Biol. 16 (1963) 361

Thoma, R.: Untersuchungen über die Histogenese und Histomechanik des Gefäßsystems. Enke, Stuttgart 1893, p. 91

Virchow, R.: Über die Erweiterung kleinerer Gefäße. Arch. Anat. Physiol. 3 (1851) 439

Voncken, J.: Über histologische Eigenarten der basalen Hirnarterien. Frankf. Z. Path. 42 (1931) 481

Voncken, J.: Über Atherosklerose der Gehirnarterien. Beitr. Path. Anat. 91 (1933) 515

Wislocki, G. B.: The unusual mode of development of the blood vessels of the opossum's brain. Anat. Rec. 74 (1939) 409

Wolf, D. E., L. I. Petter, K. C. Richardson, J. Axelrod: Localizing tritiated norepinephrine in sympathetic axons by electron microscopic autoradiography. Science 138 (1962) 440

Wollschlaeger G., P. B. Wollschlaeger, F. U. Lucas, V. F. Lopez: Experience and results with postmortem cerebral angiography performed as routine procedure of autopsy. Amer. J. Roentgenol. 101 (1967) 68

Zanobio. B., L. Zanella: Morfologia e morfogenesi delle formazioni venose del canale transversario nell'uomo. I. T. E. C., Milano 1968, p. 35

Zolnai, B.: Die zwischen der A. vertebralis und den vertebralen Venen bestehende Verbindung am atlantookzipitalen Abschnitt beim Menschen. Anat. Anz. 114 (1964) 400

B. Diagnosis and Indications for Operations in Cerebrovascular Occlusive Disease

Since 1953 lesions of the extracranial segments of the cerebral arteries have come to be operated upon routinely in many surgical centres (De Bakey et al. 1961, Rob 1961, Edwards, Gordon 1962, Murphey, Maccubbin 1965, Clauss et al. 1965, Clark, Perry 1966, Callow 1966, Blaisdell et. al. 1966, Davie, Richardson 1967). With microvascular operative techniques it is possible to operate upon the intracranial segments of the cerebral vessels as well. A prerequisite is experience in microsurgical methods, i.e. exposure of the cerebral arteries under the operating microscope, correct use of the micro-instruments and the suture material, and mastery of the suturing techniques.

Although satisfactory technical progress has been made, the indications for operation in occlusive cerebrovascular diseases remain somewhat ill-defined. The pathomorphology of these diseases has been exhaustively analysed by means of angiographic and morbidanatomical studies. Sufficient statistics are available concerning the sites of predilection, as well as the incidence and extent of the morphological changes, but knowledge of the pathogenesis and resultant pathophysiology of occlusive cerebrovascular disease remains very deficient. Clinical experience shows that

neither the extent nor the number of the occlusions is entirely responsible for the symptoms or the course of the disease: the performance of the heart, blood pressure, the cerebral collateral circulation and not least the integrity of the cerebral parenchyma are all contributory factors. A partial and apparently insignificant stenosis of a cerebral artery may in one patient lead to a complete paralysis, while in another a complete occlusion of the same artery may provoke only mild symptoms — or none at all. Unfortunately there are no measuring techniques available which allow a prognosis to be ventured on whether spontaneous recovery will follow vascular occlusion or whether further progression of the disease with concomitant neuronal damage can be expected.

Carotid angiography is unfortunately recommended earlier in patients with a complete insult than in those with mild, transient and intermittent insults. The increasing frequency and intensity of the attacks finally forces the decision to perform cerebral angiography; indeed, this usually occurs only when irreversible parenchymal damage is already present. Routine four-vessel angiography is theoretically highly justifiable but in practice it is seldom achieved: the more trivial the symptoms, the less often are the indications for angiography fulfilled. This unsatisfactory situation cannot be solved by angiography: a safe, painless and bloodless examination technique is required. It should indicate that morphological changes are present, and that cerebral angiography is specifically indicated. Definite investigation of arterial occlusions would make operation in such patients a prophylactic measure, before the circulatory disturbances cause irreversible parenchymal damage. Statistics show that it is precisely in these patients that the better results are to be expected.

After the onset of a complete paralysis as a result of stenosis or occlusion of a cerebral artery, 3—5 minutes are available before irreversible hypoxic damage occurs. This interval is too short: even under ideal circumstances (prompt referral, angiography, preparation and performance of the operation) 2—3 hours are necessary. The author believes that in cases of complete neurological deficit emergency operation fails to benefit the patient; on the contrary it frequently aggravates the situation. Secondary hemorrhages and aggravation of the edema of the ischemic area of the brain are well recognized complications (Bruetman et al. 1963, Wylie et al. 1964, Gonzales, Lewis 1966). After 2—3 weeks of recovery the indications for operation should be tested individually in each case. Focal and perifocal edema in the infarcted area regresses within three weeks, so that recanalization of the diseased vascular channel carries less risk of provoking secondary hemorrhage than operation during the acute stage. Apart from recanalization of occluded arterial segments, it is now also possible to provide new arterial channels, e.g. anastomoses between the superficial temporal artery and cortical branches of the middle cerebral artery.

Familiarity with microvascular techniques and their application in the central nervous system is of considerable value to the neurosurgeon dealing with traumatic vascular lesions resulting from a variety of head injuries as well as inadvertently occurring during surgical manipulation of the brain. One need not necessarily despair when an aneurysm is accidently torn off the parent vessel for simple or patch angioplasty is feasible and has been carried out in three cases in this clinic.

Reconstructive Operations on the Cerebral Arteries

Endarterectomy

Occlusion of the Internal Carotid Artery in its Extracranial Part

A skin incision 6—7 cm. in length is made along the anterior margin of the sternomastoid muscle at the level of the thyroid cartilage, and the common carotid artery and its bifurcation exposed. The internal carotid artery is dissected for 2—3 cm. in a cranial direction. The common carotid and both internal and external carotid arteries are occluded with bulldog clamps applied 1—1.5 cm. below and above the bifurcation respectively. The anterior wall of the artery is incised lengthwise at the level of the carotid bulb and one limb of a T-tube inserted downwards for a distance of 3—4 cm. into the common carotid and secured by a sling ligature around the artery. The two other limbs of the T-tube are occluded with artery clamps. Now the internal carotid is incised above the level of the stenosis and the distal limb of the T-tube inserted for a length of 2—3 cm. cranially, and secured with a sling ligature as before. The bulldog clamps are removed and the interrupted blood flow restored. The whole procedure — occlusion of the arteries, incision of the wall and insertion of the T-tube, its fixation and removal of the clamps — should take no longer than 3 minutes. The incision is extended over the site of the stenosis and the mural thrombus, and the sclerotic plaques in the vicinity of the carotid bulb and in the internal carotid artery are removed by subintimal dissection. Smoothing out and repair of the damaged intima and media of the internal carotid is then undertaken, so that when blood flow is restored turbulence and thrombosis are not produced. In order to eliminate all irregular-

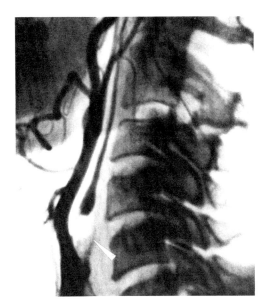

Fig. 57a

Fig. 57a—b; a, Subtotal occlusion of the internal carotid artery (arrow); b, angiography four weeks later after carotid endarterectomy. The dilated segment was patched (arrow).

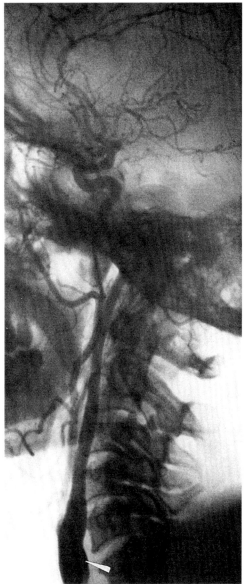

Fig. 57b

ity and to suture the intima precisely, it is advisable to use the operating microscope with 6–10-fold magnification. The site of the incision may be closed with a patch (a graft taken from the anterior tibial vein over the medial malleolus) or directly with Dacron. The patch is secured at its upper and lower ends with single sutures, then sutured continuously along one side to the level of the exit of the T-tube. Before the last few sutures are tightened, the bulldog clamps are reapplied to the common, internal and external carotid arteries, the sling threads removed and the T-tube pulled out of the artery. For a brief moment the clamps are momentarily released, one after the other — first the one on the external carotid, then that on the internal carotid and finally the one on the common carotid — and then immediately reapplied, so that any free plaque, air or thrombus can be washed from the lumen. The last opening of the arteriotomy is then closed by pulling and knotting

the ends of the suture. The clamp on the external carotid artery is then opened in order to disperse all gas bubbles from the operating area in the relatively low pressure blood reaching it from this retrograde source. When this has been done, the common

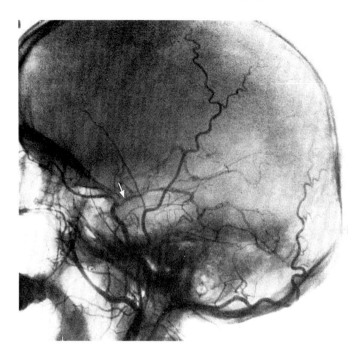

Fig. 58a. *Left carotid angiogram* in a 19-year-old male patient with a progressive right hemiparesis and aphasia since November 1968 (i.e. for six months), shows stenosis of the upper siphon of the internal carotid artery (arrow) and poor visualization of the middle cerebral artery.

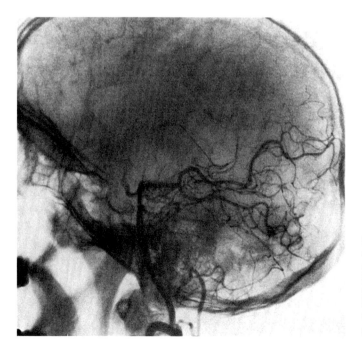

Fig. 58b. *Vertebral angiogram* demonstrates a collateral circulation to the anterior cerebral artery through dilated posterior communicating artery but with no connection to the left middle cerebral atery.

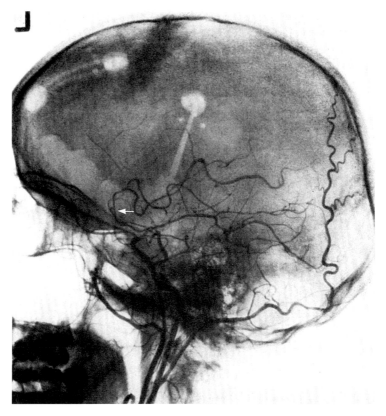

Fig. 58c. *Left carotid angiogram* in same patient who 9 days previously (i.e. March 17th, 1969) had an end-to-side anastomosis of the left superficial temporal artery to a cortical artery on the left temporal pole performed. The angiogram shows patency of the anastomosis (see arrow).

carotid clamp is removed and the blood diverted for several seconds through the external carotid artery only, in order to isolate the smaller remaining clots and gas bubbles in the external carotid tree. Finally the internal carotid clamp is removed and the patch site is superficially compressed with the index and middle finger without compromising the blood flow. If after 3 minutes any site is found to be insecure, additional single sutures are now applied. An atraumatic round needle is used with 6.0 or 7.0 silk or 8.0 nylon. Anticoagulants are not used pre- and postoperatively. During the operation, 1 ml. of heparin (5000 U) is injected intravenously following the insertion of the T-tube (Figs. 57a—b).

Occlusions of the Internal Carotid Artery in its Intracranial Part

Up to now in the author's material, no case has occurred in which indications for operation on the intracranial portion have been present: either a severe neurological deficit was already present or an adequate collateral circulation through the anterior or posterior communicating arteries was demonstrated by angiography. In case of incomplete occlusion (stenosis) of the internal carotid in its intracranial portion with clearly demonstrable inadequate collateral channels and transient symptomatology, the internal carotid artery may be approached by the subfrontal route (frontotemporal craniotomy) with sparing of

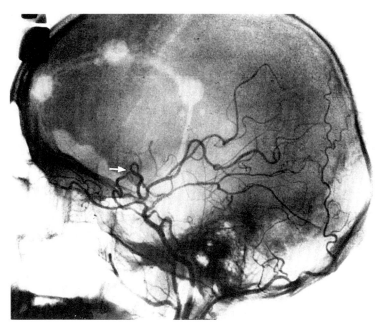

Fig. 58d. *Left carotid angiogram* 8 weeks postoperatively shows dilatation of the superficial temporal artery (see arrow) together with better filling of the branches of the middle cerebral artery.

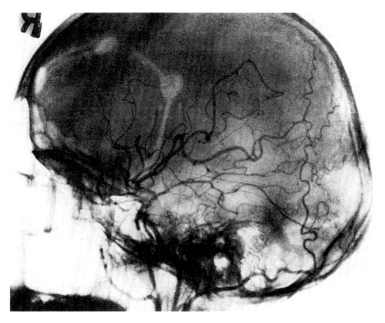

Fig. 58e. Late phase of left carotid angiogram as shown in Fig. 58d demonstrates a filling of the distal branches of the middle cerebral artery.

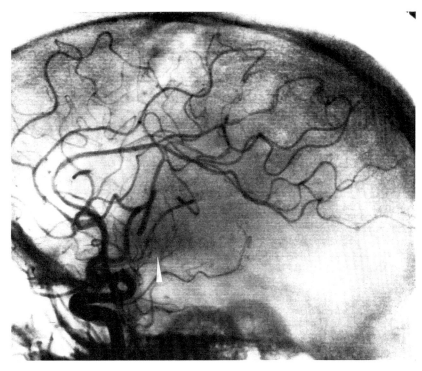

Fig. 59a. Occlusion (arrow) of the posterior branches of the left middle cerebral artery in a 32-year-old male who presented with acute hemiparesis and aphasia.

the origins of the anterior choroidal artery. Clamps are applied proximal and distal to the stenotic segment, the artery is incised, the thrombus is removed and the incision closed with microsutures.

In one instance of intracranial carotid stenosis in a 19-year-old man an attempt was made to carry out an endarterectomy. This was abandoned, however, because of insufficient room to safely occlude the vessel because the stenosis extended from the origin of the ophthalmic artery to the middle cerebral artery. Temporary occlusion of the carotid would, therefore, endanger the flow to the anterior choroidal artery. Accordingly a superficial temporal — temporal cortical artery anastomosis was carried out (see fig. 58a—e).

Occlusions of the Middle Cerebral Artery

Embolectomy or thrombectomy of the middle cerebral artery have been carried out in single

cases without the use of the microscope (Welch 1956, Shillito 1961, Scheibert 1962, Driesen 1962, Chou 1963) and with microtechniques (Jacobson et al. 1962, Lougheed et al. 1965, Lougheed 1967). In our clinic, the following procedure has been used for removal of middle cerebral artery emboli or thrombi in 11 cases.

A frontotemporal craniotomy is performed placing the Sylvian fissure in the center of the operative field. The superficial arachnoid is opened in the immediate vicinity of the Sylvian vein with the aid of the operating microscope, and the numerous arachnoid fibers between the convolutions of the frontal and temporal lobes are successively severed. With careful dissection between the invaginated layers of pia it is possible to expose the middle cerebral artery from the bifurcation of the internal carotid artery, along the Sylvian fissure and even further

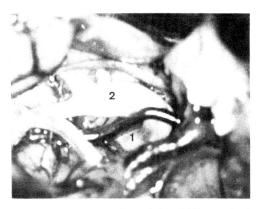

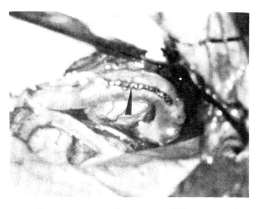

Fig. 59b. Exposure of the left middle cerebral artery in the Sylvian fissure: 1, middle cerebral artery; 2, thrombotic segment of a main branch of the middle cerebral artery.

Fig. 59c. The operated segment of the artery after thrombectomy and the insertion of twenty-two separate sutures (8.0 Davis and Geck) (arrow).

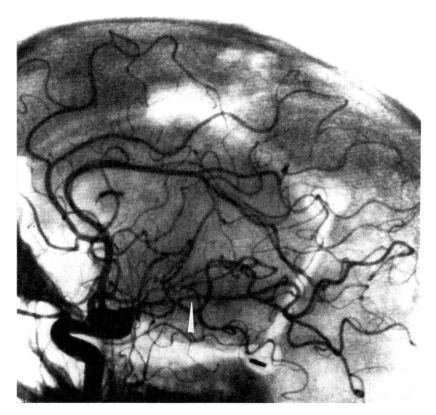

Fig. 59d. Left carotid angiogram two months after the operation showing the operated segment patent, and the posterior Sylvian branches opacified.

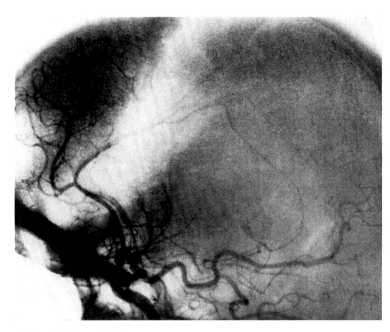

Fig. 60a. Total occlusion of left middle cerebral artery distal to lenticulostriate branches in a 43-year-old woman.

distally, without damaging the cerebral cortex. Microclamps are applied proximal and distal to the site of the thrombus in the middle cerebral artery, taking care to spare lenticulostriate arteries if possible. A rubber dam is laid under the exposed and mobilized artery. Depending on the extent of the thrombus — which sometimes presents as a yellowish-white shiny column of plasma — the artery is incised for 5—15 mm. of its length. The thrombus is then carefully freed from the inner surface of the artery with a blunt probe and removed. After ensuring that the thrombus has been extirpated from the lumen and all irregularities smoothed out, first the distal and then the proximal forceps are momentarily removed, so that all residual thrombotic remnants can be flushed out. The thin, almost transparent walls of the cerebral arteries collapse easily and adhere to each other. In order to apply the suture accurately, a 5—10 mm. length of Silastic tubing (diameter, 1.5—2 mm.) is inserted into the opened artery and the edges of the incision closed with single sutures. The tube is withdrawn

before the last two sutures are tied. If the artery possesses a diameter of less than 2 mm., closure with a patch is advised, the patch being taken from an artery in the skin flap and suitably prepared. Nylon monofilament 8.0—9.0 or 10.0 is used as suture material. The sutures are applied under 10—25-fold magnification of the microscope precisely 0.4—0.5 mm. apart. In cases of complete occlusion of more than 2—3 weeks the T-tube is not used because restoration of the cerebral blood flow 1—2 hours earlier is no longer important. In such cases embolectomy can be undertaken without urgency and the blood flow re-established as soon as the sutures have been completed. The T-tube should be used in cases of subtotal occlusion of the middle cerebral artery. The technique used in human cerebral arteries is essentially the same as that used in experimental animals.

The following details should be noted: the distal clamp is released first, in order to disperse air pockets from the artery by means of the retrograde blood flow; at the same

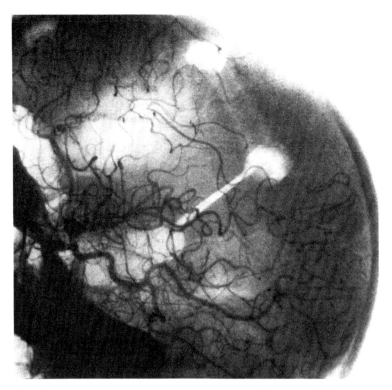

Fig. 60b. Postoperative angiogram three weeks following middle cerebral endarterectomy showing complete filling of middle cerebral artery.

time the wound is inspected for leaking sutures and additional sutures applied if necessary. Bleeding seldom occurs from the suture site. It is then covered with a rubber dam (1.5–2 cm. × 0.5 mm.) and a cotton-wool pledget on which light compression is applied with the cannula of the sucker for 2–3 minutes. Inversion of the adventitia into the wound, or of the patch into the lumen of the artery, is particularly to be avoided.

Of our experience with 11 cases of occlusion of the middle cerebral artery, nine cases were operated upon one week or more following onset of symptoms. Five of these cases have subsequently been studied with angiography and all operated vessels were patent (see Table XII, page 106—107).

Neurologically, two cases had improved considerably prior to surgical intervention and six cases improved during the weeks

following the procedure. One case died of pulmonary embolus three days postoperatively.

One case was operated upon within two hours of occlusion of the middle cerebral artery after an attempt to embolize a carotid cavernous fistula and although vessel patency was restored he remains hemiparetic (see p. 149). Another case, operated upon twelve hours after occlusion suddenly became much worse six hours postoperatively and reoperation demonstrated a large area of hemorrhagic infarction in the territory of the lenticulostriate branches of the restored middle cerebral artery. This patient died three months after operation of meningitis but at autopsy the middle cerebral artery was found to be patent.

Our experience with these few cases is of course of no statistical significance. Certainly we make no claims that restoration of blood flow and subsequent neurological improvement or recovery are in any way causally related. Nevertheless, this group of cases has shown it is technically possible to restore flow in an occluded vessel and restoration of patency, theoretically at least, would seem to be of value in the total cerebral irrigation particularly in the young individual. We are the first to realize that rational indications for this operation are totally lacking and depend on a clear understanding and measurement of the oxygen requirement of the neurone in the insulted area. With this data one would be able to assess the possible value of improving flow to hypoxic but not infarcted areas rather than depend entirely on restoration of vascular morphology.

Constructive Operations on the Cerebral Blood Vessels

Anastomosis between the Superficial Temporal artery and a Branch of the Middle Cerebral Artery

(see Fig. 58 a—e, 61 a—h, 62 a—h)

In cases of stenosis or occlusion of the internal carotid or middle cerebral artery that show an inadequate collateral circulation, the creation of a new collateral vascular channel is now technically feasible. Henschen (1950) in 1944 transplanted a pedicle of temporalis muscle over the surface of the brain, in a type of 'encephalo-myo-synangiosis', in order to improve the cerebral blood flow in a 44-year-old male with bilateral (extracranial) stenosis of the internal carotid artery. This procedure, similar in concept to Vineberg's and Jewett's operation for revascularization of the myocardium (1947), was unfortunately never documented angiographically although the patient was said to have been improved. Direct anastomosis of an extracranial to an intracranial vessel has the distinct advantage of not depending on the development of new collateral vessels.

The superficial temporal artery crosses the zygomatic arch about 3—4 mm. anterior to the tragus of the ear on the surface of the temporal region, lying over the temporalis fascia immediately beneath the subcutaneous layer. The artery, which is spread during preparation of the skin flap, is everted downwards with the latter. After removal of the bone flap and opening of the dura, the superficial temporal artery is freed from its subcutaneous situation: it is freed distally from the underlying layers from about the level of the upper rim of the zygomatic arch for a length of about 5—7 cm. together with the periarterial connective tissue; the smaller branches are coagulated, the larger ligated. At this stage the artery has not yet been divided. In the next stage of the operation, a superficial cortical artery on the temporal lobe, in the immediate vicinity of the Sylvian fissure, is chosen. After opening the arachnoid close to the artery, the latter is held up, together with its arachnoid covering, by means of a pair of microforceps, so that the arachnoid and adventitial fibers under it can be divided. In this way the artery is mobilized for a length of 10—20 mm. A rubber dam of appropriate size is laid under the artery in order to avoid touching or damaging the cerebral cortex with the instruments during further manipulations. Now 3—4 cm. length of the distal end of the superficial temporal artery is carefully stripped free of the connective tissue and adventitia. About 1—1.5 cm. proximal to this a microclamp is applied to the artery, which is divided obliquely at the level of the prepared segment. The free end of the artery is then pushed through a defect in the temporalis muscle so that it lies in the vicinity of the mobilized cortical artery. The latter artery is then clamped at two levels and its wall incised longitudinally between the clamps. The wound is widened somewhat so that the opening is not too narrow and the walls do not collapse. The obliquely incised end of the superficial temporal artery is then anastomosed end-to-side to the cortical artery with single sutures. Since the superficial temporal artery has a breadth of 1.8—2 mm. and the oblique incision allows an addition 0.2—0.3 mm. to be gained, the incision into the cortical artery must be 2.0—2.2 mm. in length. In all, 10—12 solitary sutures of 10.0 monofilament

Table XII. Direct Middle Cerebral Artery Reconstruction

Name Age Sex	Date of Vascular Accident and Clinical Description	Angiography	Date Operation Length of Clot
M. E. 48 Male	August, 7, 1966 Hemiparesis, aphasia, homonymous hemianopsia	Occlusion Left middle cerebral artery	January 7, 1967 Thrombectomy 4 cm.
A. A. 31 Male	August 12, 1967 Hemiparesis, aphasia and homonymous hemianopsia	Occlusion Left middle cerebral artery	August 14, 1967 Thrombectomy 1 cm.
R. H. 44 Male	August 11, 1967 Myocardial infarct in 1960 Hemiparesis and aphasia	Occlusion Left middle cerebral artery	August 27, 1967 Embolectomy 3 cm.
G. A. 29 Male	January 19, 1967 Hemiplegia, left	Occlusion Right middle cerebral artery	January 27, 1967 Thrombectomy 2 cm.
W. E. 43 Male	February 9, 1967 Hemiplegia and aphasia	Stenosis left internal carotid artery in neck Occlusion left middle cerebral artery	March 10, 1967 Carotid Endarterectomy April 4, 1967 Embolectomy 3 cm.
M. A. 42 Male	August 28, 1967 Hemiplegia	Occlusion Right middle cerebral artery	September 9, 1967 Thrombectomy 1 cm.
H. T. 44 Male	Starr-Edwards Valve in 1965 December 21 and 26, 1968 Hemiplegia worsening suddenly five days later	Occlusion Right middle cerebral artery	December 26, 1968 Embolectomy Two 0.5 cm. emboli
K. R. 43 Male	July 20, 1968 and December 5, 1968 Hemiplegia and aphasia, homonymous hemianopsia	Occlusion Left middle cerebral atrery	December 12, 1968 Thrombectomy 1 cm.
M. R. 46 Male	March 28, 1969 Hemiparesis and aphasia	Occlusion Left middle cerebral artery	April 4, 1969 Embolectomy 1 cm.
K. H. 44 Male	February 13, 1969 Hemiparesis, right and aphasia	Occlusion Left middle cerebral artery	February 21, 1969 Thrombectomy 1 cm.
P. L. 62 Male	April 21, 1969 Carotid — cavernous sinus fistula treated surgically by muscle embolization resulted in middle cerebral occlusion	Occlusion Left middle cerebral artery	April 21, 1969 40 minutes after onset muscle embolus removed 0.5 cm.

Time Elapsed from Vascular Accident	Early-Follow up Clinical Status	Angiography	Late Follow-up Status
5 Months	Marked improvement for 4 months	Not done	Died 6 months later of glioblastoma multiforme, left parietal
12 Days	Rapid improvement	Patent	No paresis Slight speech impairment
11 Days	Rapid improvement	Patent	No paresis No aphasia
2 Days	No improvement	Not done	Hemiplegia unchanged
1 Month	Moderate improvement	Patent	Moderate improvement Speech good
2 Months		Patent but stenosed	Hemiparesis remains
2 Months	No change for 3 days, then fatal pulmonary embolus	Not done	Died No post-mortem
18 Hours	Improvement 10 hours, then coma due to intracranial hemorrhage — Reoperation — infection	Not done	Died 3 months postoperatively of cerebral infection. Post-mortem showed patent artery
7 Days	Moderate improvement	Patent	Moderate improvement — walks alone but speech difficult
7 Days	Moderate improvement	Patent	Moderate improvement — walks alone, arm paresis persists, speech better but impaired
9 Days	Moderate improvement	Not done	Paresis improved — speech impairment
40 Minutes	Moderate improvement	Not done	Paresis better Speech impairment

Table XIII. Superficial Temporal-to-Temporal Cortical Artery Shunt

Name Age Sex	Date Onset Vascular-Accident and Clinical Description	Angiography	Operation and Date
N. K. 20 Male	August 7, 1967 Hemiplegia, right Aphasia	Occlusion of left middle cerebral artery; no collaterals	October 30, 1967 Shunt
St. E. 61 Male	October 22, 1967 Syncope on turning head Hemiparesis and homonymous hemianopsia	Occlusion right and left internal carotid arteries and right vertebral artery	November 7, 1967 Shunt
F. G. 51 Male	December 5, 1967 Left hemiplegia and homonymous hemianopsia	Occlusion of right internal carotid artery in siphon — no collaterals	January 4, 1968 Shunt
R. L. 66 Female	January 29, 1968 Subarachnoid hemorrhage	Aneurysm of posterior communicating artery, right	February 2, 1968 Shunt — clipping of aneurysm with narrowing of internal carotid artery
K. W. 39 Male	May 17, 1968 Severe hemiparesis Left homonymous hemianopsia	Occlusion of right internal carotid artery in siphon. No collaterals	June 17, 1968 Shunt
H. J. 19 Female	Progressive weakness of left side — most marked in forearm and hand since 1964	Aneurysm of internal carotid bifurcation, occlusion of right middle cerebral artery — poor collaterals	December 18, 1968 Shunt
P. A. 56 Male	Vertigo and dysphagia for 2 years	Occlusion of left internal carotid in siphon	March 3, 1969 Shunt
W. R. 19 Male	Progressive right hemiparesis and aphasia starting November 8, 1968	Progressive stenosis of left internal carotid artery; no collaterals	March 17, 1969 Shunt
S. M. 42 Male	May 19, 1969 Left hemiplegia with homonymous hemianopsia	Occlusion of left middle cerebral artery — segment too long (6 cm.) for embolectomy — poor collaterals	June 10, 1969 Shunt

Time Elapsed from Vascular Accident	Follow-up Clinical Status	Follow-up Angiography	Pulsation of Superficial Temporal Artery
3 Months	Moderate improvement	Refused	Good
2 Months	Marked improvement in hemiparesis; can turn head freely	Bypass Patent	Good
1 Month	Slight improvement	Poorly visualized ? stenotic	Poor
3 Days	Left hemiparesis Moderately improved	Refused	Good
1 Month	Hemiparesis completely disappeared	Bypass Patent	Good
4 Years	Hemiparesis completely disappeared	Bypass Patent	Good
2 Years	Worse initially, slightly improved at present	Closed Bypass — Basilar artery stenosis not appreciated preoperatively	Absent
4 Months	Marked improvement	Bypass Patent	Good
1 Month	Slight improvement	To be done	Good

nylon are inserted, spaced at regular intervals from each other under 25-fold magnification of the microscope, which takes 10—15 minutes. When the wound is closed, the microclamps on the superficial temporal artery are briefly released in order to wash air bubbles from the lumen. Thereafter the distal and proximal clamps in the cortical artery are released, and finally those on the superficial temporal artery. (Figs. 61 a—g).

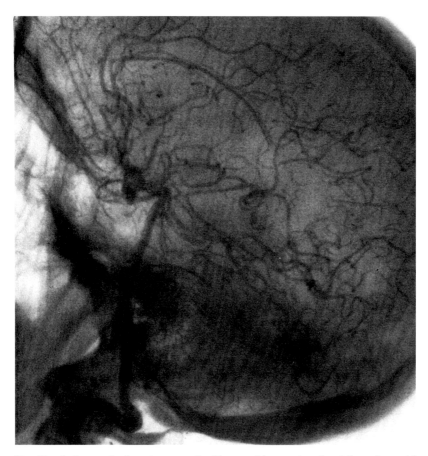

Fig. 61 a. Left vertebral angiogram of a 65-year-old man showing bilateral opacification of the infra- and supratentorial arteries. Occlusion of both internal carotid arteries and the right vertebral artery.

Fig. 61 c. Right temporal craniotomy: 1, exposure of a 1 mm.-diameter cortical artery (branch of the anterior temporal artery); 2, previously prepared superficial temporal artery.

Fig. 61 d. End-to-side anastomosis between 1, a cortical artery and 2, the superficial temporal artery.

Fig. 61 e. Complete end-to-side anastomosis between 1, the superficial temporal artery, and 2, cortical artery.

Fig. 61 f. Right carotid angiogram twelve weeks after the operation, revealing patency of the site of the anastomosis and opacification of cortical vessels; 1, posterior temporal artery; 2, angular artery; 3, posterior parietal artery; (see Fig. 61 g).

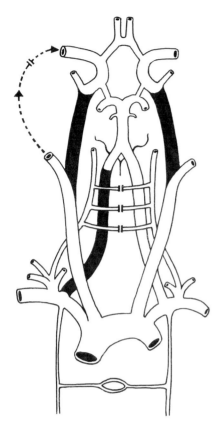

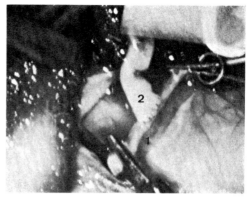

Fig. 61 d

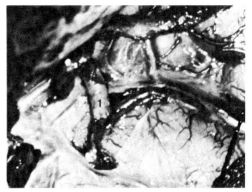

Fig. 61 e

Fig. 61 b. Diagram of the arterial occlusion in the case described. Blackened vessels indicate occluded segments. Dotted line indicates extra-cranial-intracranial anastomosis surgically constructed.

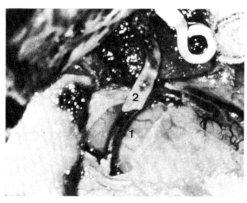

Fig. 61c

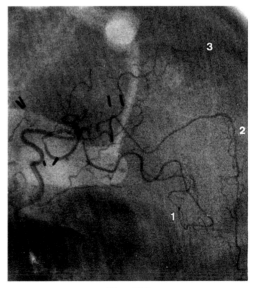

Fig. 61 f

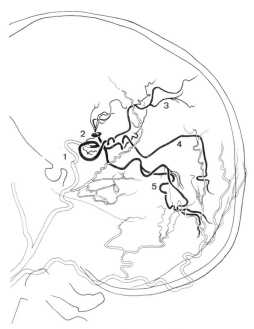

Fig. 61g. See Fig. 61f: 1, superficial temporal artery; 2, site of anastomosis; 3, posterior parietal artery; 4, angular artery; 5, posterior temporal artery.

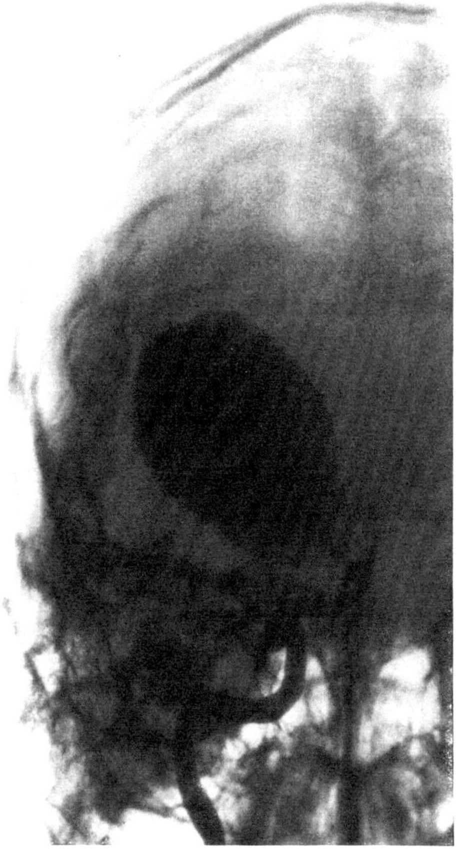

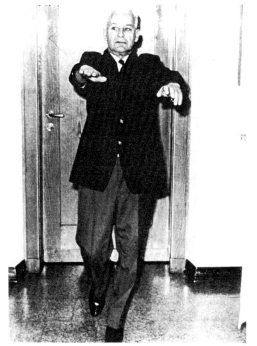

Fig. 62a. Giant saccular aneurysm arising from bifurcation of right carotid artery as demonstrated by an anteroposterior angiogram in a 20-year-old woman. Patient presented with focal epilepsy and slight distal paresis of the left arm.

Fig. 61h. Patient postoperatively, balancing on one leg: mild paresis of distal part of left arm and left upper quadrantic field defect, but no other neurological signs. The patient, who was incapacitated by restricted head movements due to attacks of vertigo and visual disturbances before the operation, could now move his head freely.

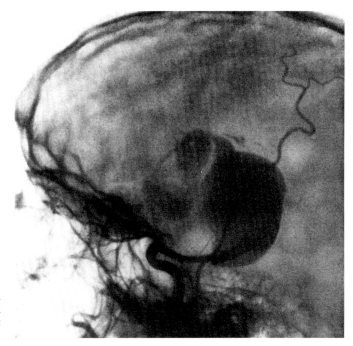

Fig. 62b. Lateral angiogram of same case showing partial thrombosis of anterior part of aneurysm.

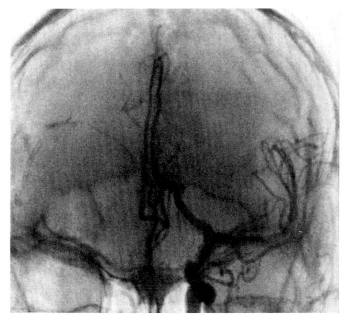

Fig. 62c. Antero-posterior angiogram following left carotid injection shows bilateral opacification of the anterior cerebral arteries. The aneurysm is not filled.

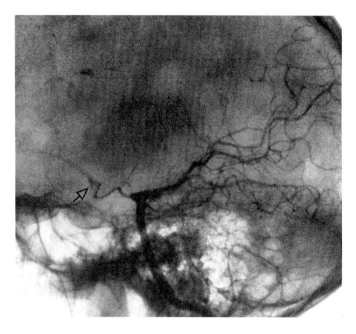

Fig. 62d. Vertebral angiogram demonstrates a small posterior communicating artery on the right side showing minimal filling of the middle cerebral artery (arrow) without opacifying the aneurysm.

In the author's experience to date with nine patients, hemorrhage has not been encountered at the site of the anastomosis. If oozing occurs, the site is covered with a rubber dam and then a cotton-wool pledget, for light compression and also to absorb the blood. During closure of the dura, a gap is left in the inferior temporal region for entry of the superficial temporal artery.

Of the nine cases operated upon with this technique, six were subsequently studied angiographically. Four of these anastomoses are patent and furthermore, appear to be supplying the major amount of the cortex, in the middle cerebral artery territory. These patients, all of whom showed progressive or repeated intermittent neurologic dysfunction, are now entirely free of symptoms. This is in contrast to the 2 cases in which the shunt was occluded as shown by angiography. Three cases have not as yet completed their postoperative study (see table XIII).

The fact that a small cortical artery is used for the anastomosis, and not a Sylvian artery or even the middle cerebral trunk, was occasioned by the desire to minimize the risks of a new operating technique. In particular, the danger of exposing the entire middle cere-

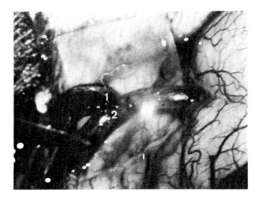

Fig. 62e. End-to-side anastomosis between 1, the superficial temporal artery and 2, cortical artery.

bral artery territory to a blood flow disturbance, if only for a brief period, was to be avoided. Personal experience to date suggests that more proximal anastomoses are indeed a possibility. The time cannot now be far distant when an autograft between the common carotid artery and the middle cerebral artery or intracranial carotid artery will be clinically feasible (Woringer, Kunlin 1963, Loew 1968). This depends only on the development of methods of evaluating the cerebral blood flow and metabolism, which will permit objective indications for operation to be defined.

Anastomosis between the Anterior Cerebral Arteries

Aneurysms of the internal carotid in the cavernous sinus cannot be approached di-

rectly: the operation of choice is ligation of the internal carotid in the neck and also intracranially, i. e. distal to the aneurysm. Such ligation presupposes an intact circle of Willis. Patients with cerebral aneurysms not infrequently show congenital anomalies of the circle of Willis (Baptista 1964, Fisher 1965), including complete absence of the anterior communicating artery (Kirgis et al. 1966). In such a case, an anterior communicating artery should first be constructed before the internal carotid is ligated. The author has personal experience of one case of this type: a walnut-sized aneurysm of the left internal carotid was present in the cavernous sinus, producing a left exophthalmos with involvement of the oculomotor, trochlear and abducent nerves, and leading to blindness (Fig. 63a). Right carotid and left vertebral angiography failed to visualize the vessels

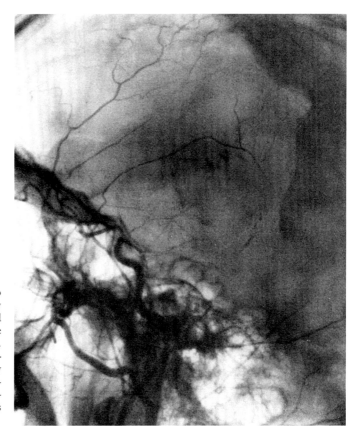

Fig. 62f. Angiogram two weeks following craniotomy and creation of a superficial temporal — cortical (middle temporal) artery anastomosis. At this operation the aneurysm was found to be totally thrombosed. Note the internal carotid artery is occluded and the anastomosis is not opacified.

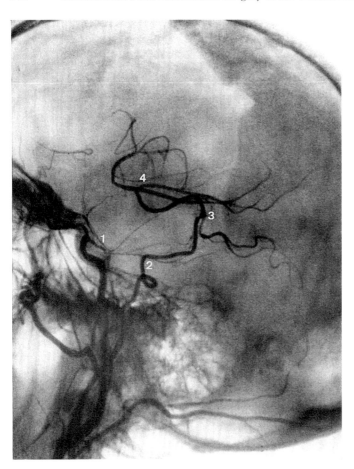

Fig. 62g. Angiogram three months following operation demonstrating the superficial temporal-cortical anastomosis functioning with opacification of the distal branch of the middle cerebral artery; 1, occluded internal carotid artery; 2, superficial temporal artery; 3, site of anastomosis; 4, branches of middle cerebral artery.

of the left cerebral hemisphere. The patient did not tolerate left carotid compression, exhibiting a transient hemiparesis and aphasia after a few seconds. It was therefore decided to reconstruct a communication between the two anterior cerebral arteries. Through a left frontal craniotomy, the anterior cerebral arteries were exposed at the level of the origin of the frontopolar artery, on the anterior aspect of the inter-hemispheric fissure. No communication was in fact found between the anterior cerebral arteries. In order to safeguard the circulation of the frontal lobe, an end-to-end anastomosis between two branches of the frontopolar arteries (outer diameter 0.8 mm.), instead of a side-to-side anastomosis between the two anterior cerebral arteries themselves, was

performed. On both sides, 1 cm. lengths of the arteries were prepared and mobilized. A Scoville clamp was applied to the origin of each frontopolar artery and the artery obliquely sectioned 1 cm. distal to the clamp. Both oblique ends were then carefully dilated by inserting a microforceps into the mouth of each. A 5 mm.-long tube (outer diameter 0.6 mm.) was inserted as a bridge between the two arteries. The end-to-end anastomosis was carried out with 10.0 monofilament nylon, and twelve single sutures were tied after removing the tube. No hemorrhage from the suture line occurred when both Scoville clamps were released. The newly-fashioned anterior communicating artery immediately filled with blood and was seen to pulsate vigorously during the half-hour before the dura was closed (Fig. 63b). Initially, the postoperative course was unremarkable: the patient awoke without any difficulty from the anesthetic, with intact sensory modalities and no neurological deficit. Digital compression of the left common carotid artery was tolerated without neurological incident on the first three days. On the fourth day a phlebitis developed from the caval catheter which rapidly progressed to a cellulitis of the left arm and shoulder and left side of the neck, and then to an osteomyelitis of the frontal bone flap and signs of meningitis. The bone flap had to be removed. During the pyrexial phase the patient remained markedly somnolent. Two weeks later he again showed a transient right hemiparesis on carotid compression. Follow-up carotid angiography subsequently revealed that the anastomosis was no longer functioning (Fig. 63c).

The postoperative infection in this patient was a most unfortunate complication. In retrospect, it is impossible to know whether the anastomosis was patent before the infection occurred. From a purely technical point of view, this type of anastomosis is quite feasible. In this case it would have been better to have performed a wide side-to-side anastomosis between the anterior cerebral arteries themselves.

In the future it is likely that constructive and reconstructive vascular surgery will come to have a useful application in aneurysms and vascular malformations in the immediate vicinity of the circle of Willis.

Repair of the Intracranial Venous Sinuses

So far two patients in the author's series have been submitted to microsurgical operations on the venous sinuses. In the first case during the removal of an acoustic neurinoma the sigmoid sinus was damaged: after the application of two bulldog clamps the 4 mm. long tear in the wall was repaired with

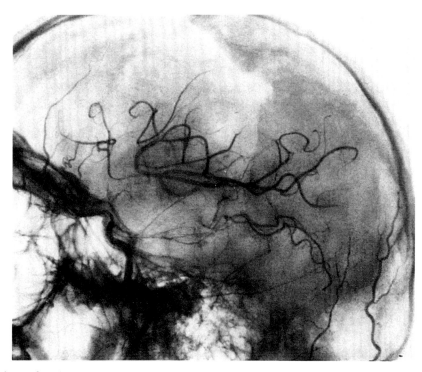

Fig. 62h. Later phase of angiogram showing more complete filling of middle cerebral artery branches.

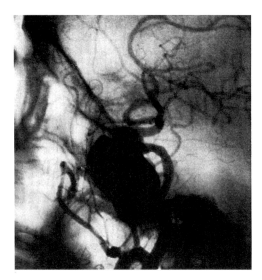

Fig. 63a. Large saccular aneurysm of the internal carotid artery in the cavernous sinus. The patient could not tolerate compression of the left common carotid artery, immediately developing a transient right hemiparesis and aphasia.

five single sutures (8.0 Davis & Geck). The suture line remained intact after removal of the clamps.

In the second patient, a 5-year-old girl, the sigmoid sinus was damaged during mastoidectomy, but the bleeding could be controlled

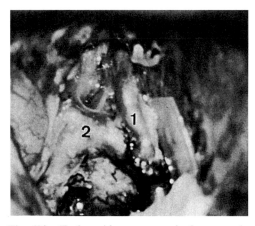

Fig. 63b. End-to-side anastomosis between 1, the right frontopolar artery, and 2, the left frontopolar artery.

by packing the wound with muscle and fatty tissues. In the succeeding months recurrent subgaleal hematomas appeared in the operation site, and eventually with the aid of the microtechnique the damaged sinus was patched with fascia. No further hemorrhage occurred.

References

Bakey, M. E. De, E. S. Crawford, G. C. Morris, Jr., D. A. Cooley: Surgical considerations of occlusive disease of the innominate, carotid, subclavian and vertebral arteries. Ann. Surg. 154 (1961) 698

Baptista, A. G.: Studies on the arteries of the brain. III. Circle of Willis: morphologic features. Acta psychiat. scand. 40 (1964) 398

Blaisdell, W. F., A. D. Hall, A. Thomas: Surgical treatment of chronic internal carotid artery occlusion by saline endarterectomy. Ann. Surg. 163 (1966) 103

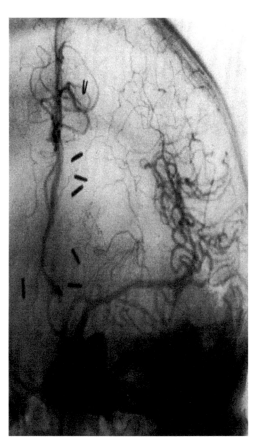

Fig. 63c. Repeated carotid angiography showing non-function of the anastomosis.

Bruetman, M. E., W. S. Fields, E. S. Crawford, M. E. De Bakey: Cerebral hemorrhage in carotid artery surgery. Arch. Neurol. Psychiat. (Chic.) 9 (1963) 458

Callow, A. D.: Surgical management of varying patterns of cerebral artery and subclavian artery insufficiency. New. Engl. J. Med. 270 (1966) 546

Chou, S. N.: Embolectomy of middle cerebral artery. Report of a case. J. Neurosurg. 20 (1963) 161

Clark, K., M. D. Perry: Carotid vertebral anastomosis. An alternate technic for repair of the subclavian steal syndrome. Ann. Surg. 163 (1966) 414

Clauss, R. H., W. K. Hass, J. Ransohoff: Simplified method for monitoring adequacy of brain oxygenation during carotid-artery surgery. New Engl. J. Med. 273 (1965) 1127

Davie, J. C., R. Richardson: Distal internal carotid thrombembolectomy using a Fogarty catheter in total occlusion. J. Neurosurg. 27 (1967) 171

Driesen, E.: Erfolgreiche Naht der linken A. cerebri media nach Verletzung bei Tumorresektion. Acta Neurochir. 10 (1962) 462

Edwards, C. H., N. S. Gordon: Surgical treatment of narrowing of the internal carotid artery. Brit. Med. J. 1 (1962) 1289

Fisher, C. M.: The circle of Willis: Anatomical variations, Vasc. Dis. 2 (1965) 99

Gonzales, L. L., C. M. Lewis: Cerebral hemorrhage risk stressed after endarterectomy. Surg. Gynec. Obstet. 122 (1966) 773

Henschen, C.: Operative Revascularisation des zirkulatorisch geschädigten Gehirns durch Anlegen gestielter Muskellappen. (Encephalo-Myo-Synangiose). Langenbecks Arch. klin. Chir. 264 (1950) 392

Jacobson, II, J. H., L. J. Wallman, G. A. Schumacher, M. Flanagan, F. L. Suarez, R. M. P. Donaghy: Microsurgery as an aid to middle cerebral artery endarterectomy. J. Neurosurg. 19 (1962) 108

Kirgis, H. D., W. L. Fisher, R. C. Llewellyn, F. M. C. Peebles: Aneurysms of the anterior communicating artery and gross anomalies of the circle of Willis. J. Neurosurg. 25 (1966) 73

Krayenbühl, H., M. G. Yaşargil: Die Anwendung des Operationsmikroskops in der Behandlung der vaskulären zerebrospinalen Erkrankungen. Münch. med. Wschr. 110 (1968) 1931

Kulenkampff, W., W. Dorndorf (Ed.): Die chirurgische Behandlung der Carotis- und Vertebralisinsuffizienz. Thieme, Stuttgart 1966, p. 86

Loew, F.: Personal communication 1968

Lougheed, W. M.: The surgery of intracranial vascular occlusion. In: Micro-Vascular Surgery. Ed. by R. M. P. Donaghy, M. G. Yaşargil. Thieme, Stuttgart 1967, pp. 142—147

Lougheed, W. M., R. W. Gunton, H. J. M. Barnett: Embolectomy of internal carotid, middle and anterior cerebral arteries. J. Neurosurg. 22 (1965) 607

Murphey, F., D. A. Maccubbin: Carotid endarterectomy. A long-term follow-up study. J. Neurosurg. 23 (1965) 156

Rob, C.: The surgical treatment of stenosis and thrombosis of the extracranial parties of the carotid arteries. J. cardiovasc. Surg. (Torino) 2 (1961) 336

Scheibert, C. D.: Middle cerebral artery surgery for obstructive lesions. Presented at the Meeting of Harvey Cushing Society, New Orleans, La, 2 May, 1962

Shillito, Jr., J.: Indications for surgery in cerebrovascular accidents. Postgrad. med. J. 30 (1961) 537

Shillito, Jr., J.: Intracranial arteriotomy in three children and three adults. In: Micro-Vascular Surgery. Ed. by R. M. P. Donaghy, M. G. Yaşargil. Thieme, Stuttgart 1967, pp. 138—142

Stevenson, G. C.: Transclival exposure of basilar artery. A case presentation of basilar artery embolectomy in man. In: Micro-Vascular Surgery. Ed. by R. M. P. Donaghy, M. G. Yaşargil. Thieme, Stuttgart 1967, pp. 148—149

Vineberg, A., B. L. Jewett: Anastomoses between coronary vessels and internal mammary artery. Canad. med. Ass. J. 56 (1947) 609

Vineberg, A.: Clinical and experimental studies in the treatment of coronary artery insufficiency by internal mammary artery implant. J. Int. Coll. Surg. 22 (1954) 503

Welch, K.: Excision of occulusive lesions of the middle cerebral artery. J. Neurosurg. 13 (1956) 73

Woringer, E., J. Kunlin: Anastomose entre la carotide primitive et la carotide intracranienne de la sylvienne par greffon selon la technique de la suture suspendue. Neurochir., Paris 9 (1963) 181

Wylie, E. J., M. F. Hein, J. E. Adams: Intracranial hemorrhage following surgical revascularization for treatment of acute strokes. J. Neurosurg. 21 (1964) 212

C. Aneurysms, Arteriovenous Malformations and Fistulae

1. Operations on Saccular Aneurysms

Aneurysms of the Internal Carotid Artery

A small frontotemporal craniotomy is undertaken with the patient's head turned slightly to the side opposite to the aneurysm. The bony opening should be centered over the pterion so that the outermost part of the wing of the sphenoid may be conveniently removed extradurally. The sphenoid ridge is *the key landmark* in the approach to the circle of Willis. A preliminary lumbar puncture is performed, and during opening of the dura, cerebrospinal fluid is drained off so that the brain diminishes considerably in volume within 5—10 minutes. After attaching the dura to the bony rim of the wound, the operating microscope is assembled and positioned. The frontal pole is covered with a strip of gutta-percha and lightly retracted with a metal spatula (1.5 cm. in breadth) so that the optic nerve is brought into view. Using 10-fold magnification, the arachnoid layer between the base of the frontal lobe and the optic nerve is now opened, and a sucker applied to remove the cerebrospinal fluid that gushes out, until the basal cisterns are virtually empty. Normally numerous arterioles and small-caliber veins run within the arachnoid network, and these are individually grasped with the microforceps and coagulated then sectioned with the microscissors. Any disturbing hemorrhagic oozing from the retracted frontal lobe may be avoided in this way. The arachnoid layer is thin but very elastic and tough, so that it is best sectioned with a microscissors, rather than the use of a blunt hook. Next the arachnoid should be opened medially to the level of the tuberculum sellae, and laterally towards the Sylvian fissure, including its anterior third. Exposure of the Sylvian fissure opens up the ideal lateral approach to the internal carotid artery for lateral or posterolateral aneurysms. The temporal pole, after opening of the Sylvian fissure, can be retracted laterally and backwards, so that a conical cavity of 2—2.5 cm. in extent is produced between the frontal and temporal poles, and the internal carotid artery can be well visualized. The arachnoid fibers surrounding the internal carotid are sectioned with the microscissors, using 10—16-fold

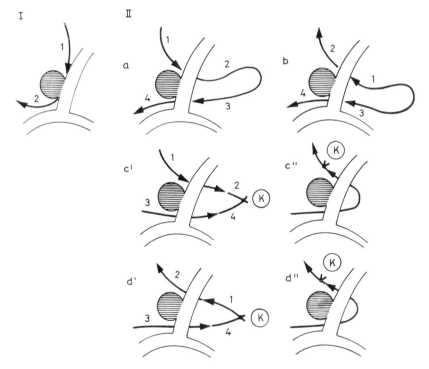

Fig. 64. Technique of ligation of aneurysms with silk thread: I. Direct ligation of the neck of the aneurysm, the thread passing around the neck in the direction of the arrows. This technique is not without danger, since it may cause tearing and rupture of the aneurysmal sac. II. Indirect ligation of the neck of the aneurysm: a, the thread is passed in the direction 1—2—3—4 indicated by the arrows; b, the thread may be inserted in the direction 1—2 and then in direction 3—4; c1, when the thread can be inserted only from one side, two separate threads are passed through and knotted (k); c2, the knotted thread is then withdrawn in the direction entailing the least risk, and the neck of the aneurysm is ligated; d, another variation, in which the two threads are inserted in different directions, then knotted and drawn back, and finally pulled tight around the neck of the aneurysm.

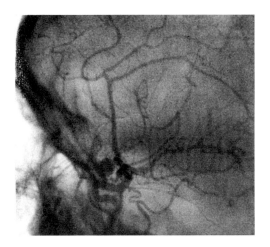

Fig. 65a. Carotid aneurysm just distal to origin of ophthalmic artery.

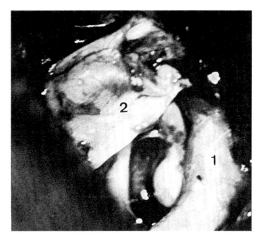

Fig. 65b. Operative exposure of same case showing 1, carotid artery; 2, clipped aneurysm overlying optic nerve.

magnification. On three occasions the author has observed the presence of very fine arterioles (0.05–0.1 mm.) arising from the carotid artery and running towards the dura of the anterior clinoid process (see Fig. 69b); these are coagulated and sectioned. The internal carotid artery is stripped from the root of the anterior clinoid process to its bifurcation (Sections C2–C1). The arachnoid fibers around the pedicle of the aneurysm are then sectioned, until a blunt hook can be passed around its base. The apex of the aneurysm sac is left undisturbed, if possible, for fear of dislodging the blood clot at the site of rupture. During this dissection in the immediate vicinity of the aneurysm, the systolic blood pressure is reduced to 70 or 80 mm. Hg by means of Arfonad. The silk ligature is not applied directly around the neck of the aneurysm, because this manipulation moves the apex of the aneurysm and may dislodge the blood clot plugging its wall. Instead it is passed, together with the holder, under the internal carotid artery and around the aneurysm, and then tied firmly around the neck of the aneurysm. When technical difficulties (lack of space, etc.) prevent passage of the ligature in the appropriate site, both ends are threaded along the most accessible path and knotted together on the desired side,

then applied to the neck of the aneurysm (Figs. 64, 65a–c, 66a–d).

During the introduction of the thread it is necessary to avoid the anterior choroidal artery. In order to ensure that the thread is correctly placed, the shorter end (1–1.5 cm.)

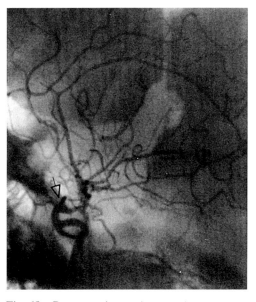

Fig. 65c. Postoperative angiogram. Arrow points to clip across obliterated aneurysm.

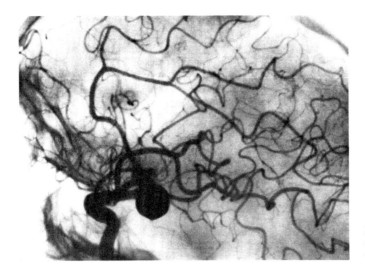

Fig. 66a. Large saccular aneurysm at the bifurcation of the internal carotid artery.

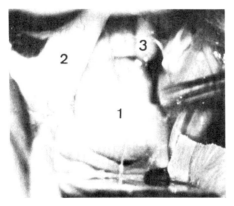

Fig. 66b. Operative exposure showing aneurysm at the termination of 1, the internal carotid artery; 2, optic nerve; 3, oculomotor nerve.

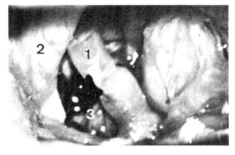

Fig. 66d. After tying the ligature, puncture of the aneurysmal sac and application of 3, a Samuel clip; 1, internal carotid artery; 2, optic nerve.

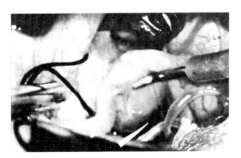

Fig. 66c. Application of silk ligature around the aneurysm with sparing of the lenticulostriate arteries (arrow).

is twisted around the longer end and slowly knotted around the neck of the aneurysm. In the presence of large aneurysms and severe arteriosclerotic changes in the internal carotid artery, the knot is not completely tied — only 4/5ths secured, then the aneurysm neck coagulated with bipolar forceps, and finally the knot tightened around the collapsed neck. This technique prevents narrowing of the lumen in sclerotic internal carotid arteries. Exclusion of the aneurysm is assured by the application of 1 or 2 hemostatic clips (Samuel clips) immediately after the ligature. (Figs. 67a—b).

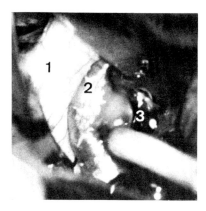

Fig. 67a. Saccular aneurysm of right internal carotid artery proximal to the origin of the posterior communicating artery; 1, optic nerve; 2, internal carotid artery; 3, aneurysm.

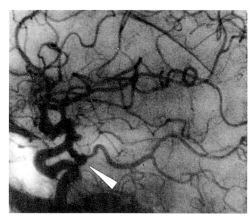

Fig. 68a. Lateral carotid angiogram showing the position of an aneurysm on the posterior communicating artery (arrow).

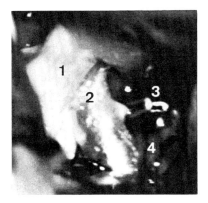

Fig. 67b. Obliteration of the aneurysm with two Samuel clips; 1, optic nerve; 2, internal carotid artery; 3, ligated aneurysm; 4, posterior communicating artery.

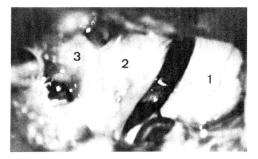

Fig. 68b. Operative dissection of the aneurysm: 1, optic nerve; 2, internal carotid artery; 3, aneurysm.

Aneurysms of the Posterior Communicating Artery

Exposure is effected by the same technique and methods described above, viz. opening of the arachnoid layer with sparing of the Sylvian veins and sectioning of the arachnoid fibers between the frontal and temporal lobes in the region of the Sylvian fissure. This enables a direct approach to be made to the internal carotid artery in the lateral plane, especially when the patient's head is rotated slightly to the opposite side and the temporal pole is retracted laterally. This maneuver involves merely the risk of transient compression of the Sylvian vein which, in the author's experience, is well tolerated. Resection of the temporal pole is avoided by the use of this technique. A hemostatic clip or a thread ligature or the coagulation technique is applied to the neck of the aneurysm, according to the findings in situ. The posterior communicating artery should be sought in the direction of the basilar artery and ligated if it is connected with the mouth of the aneurysm (Figs. 68a–d).

Aneurysms of the Carotid Bifurcation

These aneurysms are approached in the same fashion as the aneurysms arising at the origin of the posterior communicating artery. It is necessary, however, to open the Sylvian fissure for a longer distance so as to fully visualize the lenticulostriate arteries and avoid excessive traction on the frontal lobe and thereby on the fundus of the aneurysm. Furthermore, the ligature should be passed indirectly (i.e. around the anterior cerebral, internal carotid and middle cerebral arteries) so as to avoid including the lenticulostriate and anterior choroidal arteries with the neck (Figs. 69a—d).

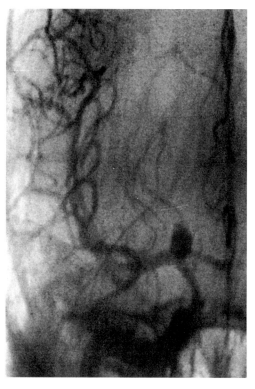

Fig. 69a. Saccular aneurysm at the bifurcation of the right internal carotid artery.

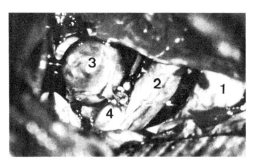

Fig. 68c. Obliteration of the aneurysm with Samuel clips: 1, optic nerve; 2, internal carotid artery; 3, aneurysm; 4, clips.

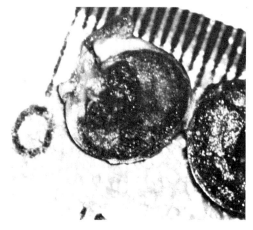

Fig. 68d. Cross-section of the dissected aneurysm.

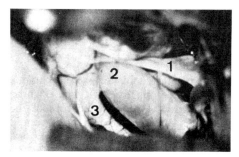

Fig. 69b. A fine branch of the right internal carotid artery 1, passing into the dura at the level of the anterior clinoid process; 2, internal carotid artery; 3, optic nerve.

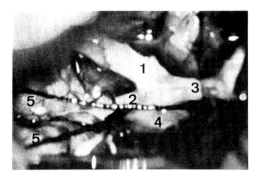

Fig. 69c. Dissection of the neck of the aneurysm, with a silk ligature applied around it; 1, internal carotid artery; 2, anterior cerebral artery; 3, middle cerebral artery; 4, aneurysm; 5, silk thread.

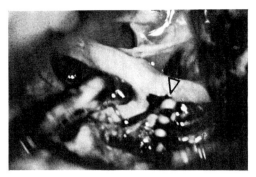

Fig. 69d. View of the obliterated aneurysm following ligation, evacuation of the contents and application of three Samuel clips (arrow).

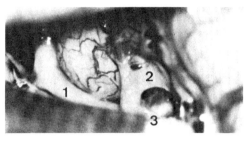

Fig. 70b. Dissection of the aneurysm in the Sylvian fissure; 1, trunk of middle cerebral artery; 2, a branch of the middle cerebral artery; 3, part of the aneurysm.

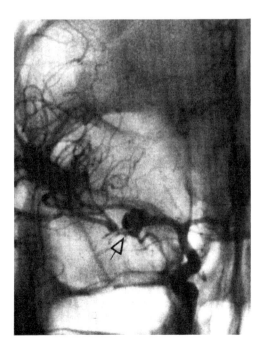

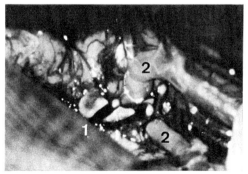

Fig. 70a. Bilobular aneurysm (arrow) at the right Sylvian trifurcation.

Fig. 70c. After ligation of the aneurysm: 1, clipped aneurysm; 2, middle cerebral artery branches.

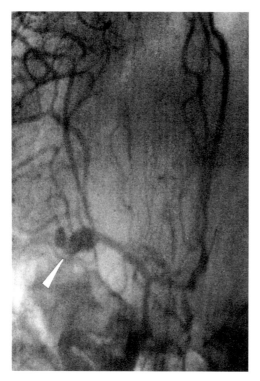

Fig. 71a. Aneurysm at right Silvian trifurcation (arrow). Note medial shift of lenticulostriate arteries due to intracerebral hematoma.

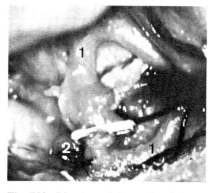

Fig. 71b. Ligation of the neck of the aneurysm and resection of sac: 1, middle cerebral artery and branches; 2, clip on the remnant of the neck of the aneurysm.

Aneurysms of the Middle Cerebral Artery

The same operating approach as has been described is used, irrespective of whether the aneurysm is situated in the sphenoidal part or in the bi- or trifurcation region of the middle cerebral artery. Next the arachnoid over the optic nerve is opened and the internal carotid identified and freed of arachnoid fibers as far as the bifurcation. From here the middle cerebral artery is followed distally by careful dissection of the arachnoid fibers, to within a few millimeters of the presumed site of the aneurysm. The site itself is left alone, and the Sylvian fissure is opened further distally and the Sylvian arteries exposed as far as the immediate vicinity of the aneurysm. The aneurysm is then freed from basal adhesions, so that its neck is clearly exposed and coagulated for clipping or ligation, and it is then ligated (Figs. 70a—c, 71a—b, 72a—d, 73a—c).

Aneurysms of the Anterior Cerebral and Anterior Communicating Arteries

Unilateral, fronto-temporal craniotomy is fashioned similar to that described for aneurysms of the internal carotid artery. Again, the lateral part of the sphenoid wing is removed so as to permit exposure of the suprachiasmal region without undue elevation of the frontal lobe. This fronto-basal-lateral approach to the anterior communicating artery allows one to preserve the olfactory tract and the integrity of the frontal sinus. Furthermore, compared to the medial-subfrontal approach the depth of the exposure will be decreased by 2—3 cm. Next the arachnoid coverings of the optic nerve and internal carotid artery are opened and reflected laterally towards the Sylvian fissure, as well as medially over the chiasm towards the opposite side. The internal carotid artery is exposed as far as its bifurcation, and the anterior cerebral artery then followed up to the level of the anterior communicating artery. Before the sac of the aneurysm is dissected free from its concealed position between the frontal lobe convolutions, it is

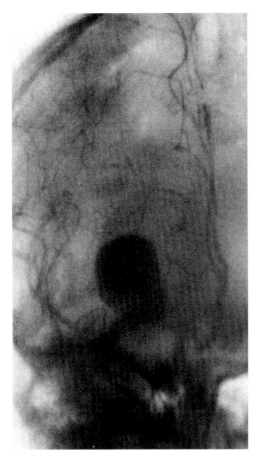

Fig. 72a. Large saccular aneurysm of middle cerebral artery; antero-posterior projection.

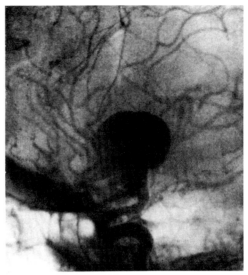

Fig. 72b. Large saccular aneurysm of the middle cerebral artery; lateral projection.

advisable to open the arachnoid layer between the undersurface of the frontal lobe and the optic nerve on the opposite side to the level of the anterior communicating artery. The origin of Heubner's artery can be defined precisely with the operating microscope, so that when temporary clamps are applied to one or both anterior cerebral arteries, it is possible to avoid damaging either the lenticulostriate arteries or Heubner's artery.

An attempt is now made indirectly to encircle the neck of the aneurysm. If this fails, the neck is cleared of arachnoid fibers, then coagulated and occluded with hemostatic clips (Figs. 74a—c, 75a—b).

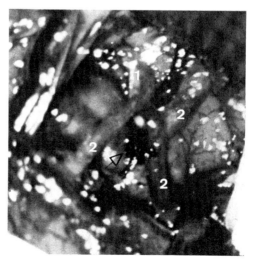

Fig. 72c. Operative exposure showing ligation of neck of aneurysm (arrow); 1, middle cerebral artery; 2, branches of middle cerebral artery.

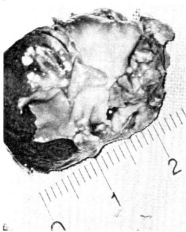

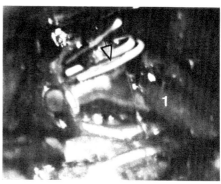

Fig. 73b. Operative exposure showing sac obliterated with 3 clips (arrow); 1, main trunk of
middle cerebral artery.

Fig. 72d. The resected aneurysm.

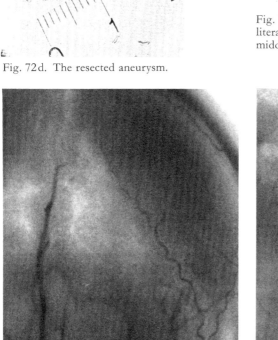

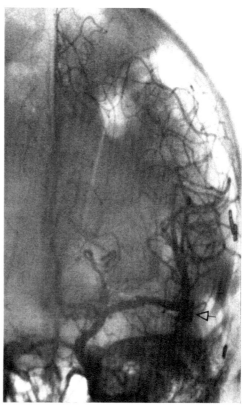

Fig. 73a. Aneurysm (arrow) at bifurcation of
middle cerebral artery. Note narrowing of distal
branches.

Fig. 73c. Postoperative angiogram showing excellent filling of middle cerebral vessels and
absence of aneurysm six months after operation;
Samuel clips (arrow).

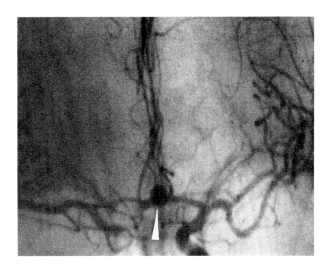

Fig. 74a. Saccular aneurysm of the anterior communicating artery (arrow).

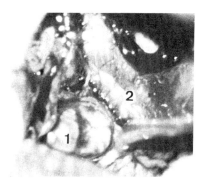

Fig. 74b. Saccular aneurysm of the anterior communicating artery, seen through the dissecting microscope: 1, aneurysm; 2, optic chiasm.

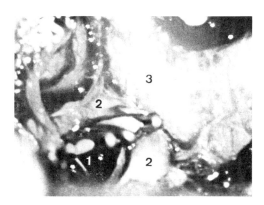

Fig. 74c. Clipping of the aneurysm with three Samuel clips 1, with sparing of 2, the anterior cerebral arteries; 3, optic chiasm.

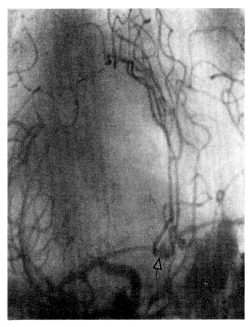

Fig. 75a. Saccular aneurysm of anterior communicating artery (arrow).

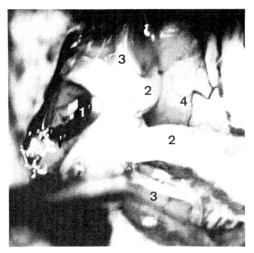

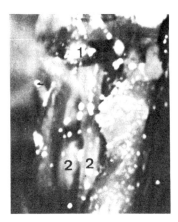

Fig. 75b. Clipped and resected aneurysm 1, of anterior communicating artery; 2, anterior cerebral arteries; 3, Heubner's arteries; 4, chiasm.

Fig. 76b. Operative exposure (interhemispheric) with obliteration of pericallosal aneurysm; 1, clipped aneurysm; 2, pericallosal arteries.

Hemoclip (Samuel)

We prefer hemoclip for aneurysm surgery. The hemoclip applicator has been modified, which now provides a "double action" and has bayonet grips (Aesculap, Tuttlingen, Germany).

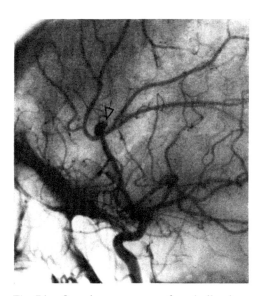

Fig. 76a. Saccular aneurysm of pericallosal artery (arrow).

Aneurysms of the Pericallosal Artery

Aneurysms situated at the origin of the callosomarginal and the pericallosal arteries are exposed through a frontomedial craniotomy and opening of the interhemispheric fissure. Any artery emerging from the latter is followed backwards to the trunk of the artery, and from there forwards until the aneurysm is found (Figs. 76a–b).

Aneurysms of the Basilar Artery

Subtemporal Approach:

Aneurysms situated at the distal bifurcation of the basilar artery are approached through a lateral frontotemporal craniotomy along the subtemporal route (under the temporal pole). Resection of the temporal lobe is unnecessary. The basal cisterns are opened and the posterior communicating artery followed backwards: in most cases the aneurysm will be very obvious in the field of dissection. Aneurysms directed forwards and laterally have necks that are accessible for ligation (Jamieson 1964 and 1968, Drake 1965, Rand, Jannetta 1967, Housepian et. al. 1967).

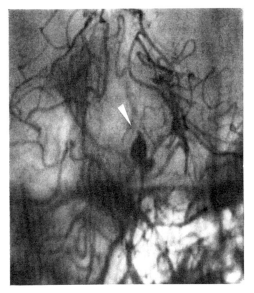

Fig. 77a. Bilocular aneurysm (arrow) at the bifurcation of the basilar artery.

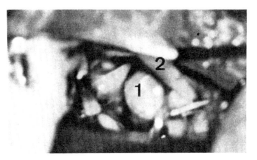

Fig. 77b. Subtemporal exposure of 1, the aneurysm beneath 2, the oculomotor nerve. Clipping of the neck of the aneurysm impossible due to adherence of its posterior wall to the perforating arteries. The aneurysmal sac was wrapped with adhesive (Biobond). No recurrence of hemorrhage.

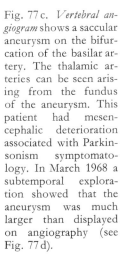

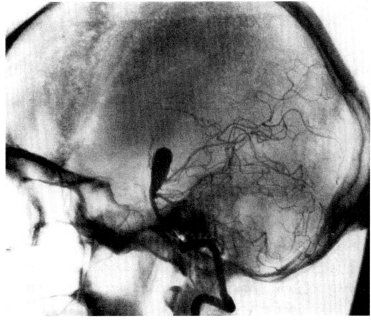

Fig. 77c. *Vertebral angiogram* shows a saccular aneurysm on the bifurcation of the basilar artery. The thalamic arteries can be seen arising from the fundus of the aneurysm. This patient had mesencephalic deterioration associated with Parkinsonism symptomatology. In March 1968 a subtemporal exploration showed that the aneurysm was much larger than displayed on angiography (see Fig. 77d).

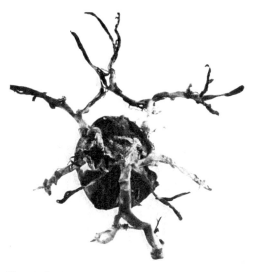

Fig. 77d. Autopsy specimen shows that the aneurysm at the bifurcation of the basilar artery is massive and involves both posterior cerebellar arteries as well as thalamic vessels. The patient died 6 months after the initial hemorrhage.

Aneurysms directed backwards into the interpeduncular fossa and those associated with the very fine mesodiencephalic perforating arteries and covered by blood clot are probably best managed by coating externally with adhesives. Three of the author's patients were treated in this way (Figs. 77a—d). Even with the most meticulous care in the exposure of aneurysms at this site spasm of the perforating vessels can be induced with resulting ischemia in the vital midbrain centers (Fig. 78).

Aneurysms of the distal two-thirds of the basilar artery are approached subtemporally (Drake 1965, Jamieson 1968).

Transoral (Transmesopharyngeal) Clivectomy:

Aneurysms in the junction area of the vertebral arteries and in the proximal one-third of the basilar artery are explored by the transcervical-transclival route, which was pioneered by Fox (1967) and Wissinger et al. (1967) (Fig. 79).

This route has been used twice by the author for ligation of the saccular aneurysm on the basilar artery at the junction of the vertebral arteries (Figs. 80a—b). Following intubation anesthesia, a prophylactic tracheotomy is performed to manage any postoperative

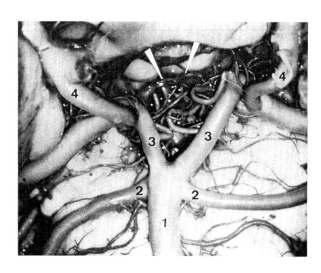

Fig. 78. Anatomical preparation to show the perforating arteries in the interpeduncular fossa (arrows); 1, basilar artery; 2, superior cerebellar arteries; 3, posterior cerebral arteries; 4, posterior communicating artery.

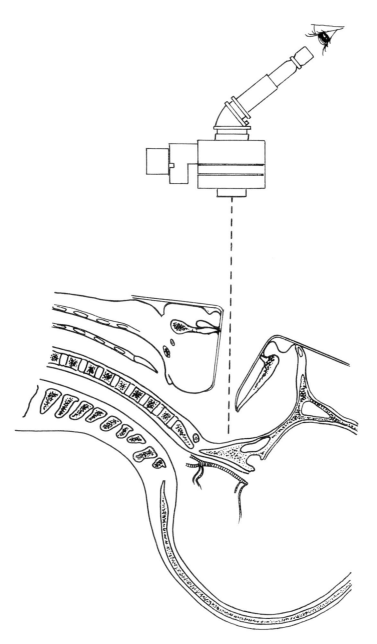

Fig. 79. Method of utilizing the operating microscope during transoral clival exposure of the basilar artery.

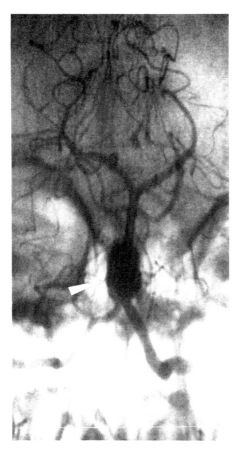

Fig. 80a. Aneurysm at the junction of the two vertebral arteries with the basilar artery (arrow); antero-posterior projection.

laryngeal edema, that may occur. The patient is then placed supine on the operating table, the head somewhat extended and the back of the neck supported on narrow pillows (Figs. 80c—d). The Negus retractor is used to draw the patient's tongue downwards and laterally, so that opening of the mouth gives generous access to the mesopharynx. Under microscope the soft palate is incised on the right side and the incision extended diagonally to the midline to the vomer process. The soft parts are separeted laterally to the left side from the hard palate, partly by the use of a periosteal elevator, partly by an electrocautery, and then fixed with holding

sutures. The soft parts of the mesopharynx are isolated in the same way and reflected caudally in the direction of the oesophageal opening, the hypopharyngeal entrance to the oesophagus and trachea being occluded with the soft tissues. The hard palate is hollowed out to the level of the choanae with a diamond drill. The choanae are packed cranially with Oxycel and cotton wool. The soft tissues of the mesopharynx have a thickness of 4—5 mm.; immediately beneath them there is a similar sheet of muscle and connective tissue 5—8 mm. thick which is stripped from the anterior surface of the clivus with an electrocautery only. The tubercle of the anterior arch of the atlas serves as a landmark for judging the level of the exposure. The clivus is now excavated with the diamond drill from the level of the vomer process to the level of the anterior rim of the foramen magnum in a length of 2—2.5 cm. and a breadth of 8—12 mm. The outer and inner tables of the clivus are about 2—3 mm. thick. These two layers of compact bone are separated by cancellous bone 3—4 mm. thick. In the author'a cases, bleeding from the bone was minimal and could be controlled by the application of bone wax. During incision of the dura (about 2 mm. thick) numerous fine arterioles and venules are coagulated. There is no venous plexus on the inner aspect of the dura. On the right side the dura is sutured to the muscle layer. On the left side in one of the author's cases adhesions were present between the inner surface of the dura and the anterior surface of the aneurysm. The aneurysm lay behind the basilar artery in the junction region of the vertebral arteries, with a bulge to the right alongside the basilar artery and another large one to the left below and behind it. Under these circumstances, direct clipping was out of the question. Instead, a silk thread was carefully applied stepwise, the one end being passed first under the right, then under the left vertebral artery, and the other end between the basilar artery and the sac of the aneurysm; both the anterior and the posterior inferior cerebellar arteries were spared bilaterally by this maneuver. After separating the adhesions between the aneurysm and the

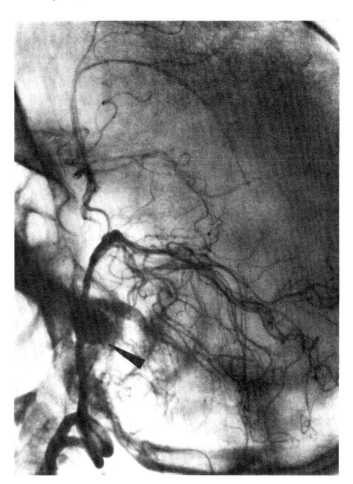

Fig. 80 b. Aneurysm at the junction of the two vertebral arteries with the basilar artery (arrow); lateral projection.

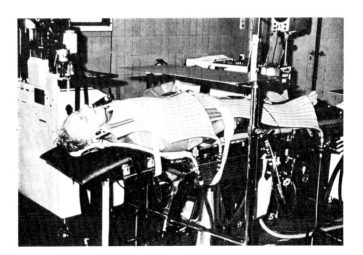

Fig. 80 c. Position of patient on operating table.

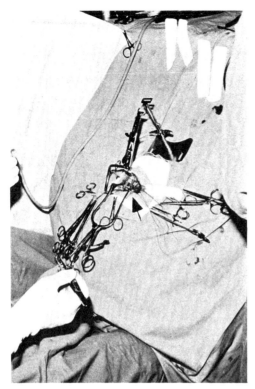

Fig. 80 d. Position of the oral (Negus) retractor (arrow).

basilar artery in the direction of the base of the aneurysm, the suture ends were tied instrumentally (Figs. 80 e, f). Neither the vertebral artery nor the basilar artery or any of its branches were occluded. Just before applying the ligature, the patient was given Arfonad and the blood pressure maintained at 50—60 mm. Hg for fifteen minutes. For two and a half minutes during the actual ligation, the larger left vertebral artery was occluded with a Scoville clamp. No attempt was made to re-suture the dura which was somewhat shrivelled by the electrocoagulation. It would have been an easy matter to apply a fascial layer to the opening but it was decided to dispense with this fascioplasty in order not to prolong the six and a half hour operation. Instead, Oxycel spread with Biobond adhesive was applied in layers over the opening. The preclival muscles, connective tissue layer, and finally the pharyngeal mucosa, were carefully closed in layers.

The patient tolerated the operation well, and regained full consciousness after the anesthetic. No cranial-nerve disturbances were present but the patient's right limbs showed a pure motor spasticity which, after two days, developed into a flaccid paralysis. The reflexes

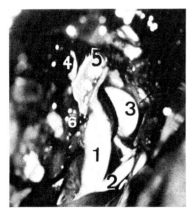

Fig. 80 e. Transoral-transclival exposure of the aneurysm. Application of a silk ligature to the neck of the aneurysm; 1, basilar artery; 2, anterior inferior cerebellar artery; 3, aneurysm on the right side; 4, left vertebral artery; 5, right vertebral artery; 6, aneurysm on the left side of basilar artery.

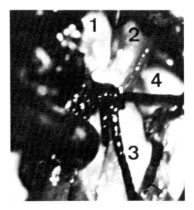

Fig. 80 f. After ligating the neck of the aneurysm; 1, and 2, vertebral arteries; 3, basilar artery; 4, aneurysm.

were not increased, and neither plantar reflex was extensor. The paralysis began to clear rapidly from the right leg on the third day, the arm recovering more slowly. During the first two and a half weeks the patient made excellent progress, asked to get up, and walked about in his room. The wound in the pharynx and palate healed by primary intention. No leakage of cerebrospinal fluid occurred. The patient resumed eating normally, although his speech remained somewhat nasal in quality.

On the seventeenth postoperative day, an acute gastrointestinal hemorrhage occurred. This did not respond to treatment and the patient died the following day.

Autopsy examination revealed duodenal ulceration with frank hemorrhage into the gastrointestinal tract. The brain and the circle of Willis appeared macroscopically normal. Histological examination revealed that the aneurysm had thrombosed completely and that the basilar and both vertebral arteries were patent (Figs. 80g, h).

The second case, a 23-year-old woman, presented with a subarachnoid hemorrhage and partial loss of sensation over the left side of the face. Angiography demonstrated a huge saccular aneurysm arising from the

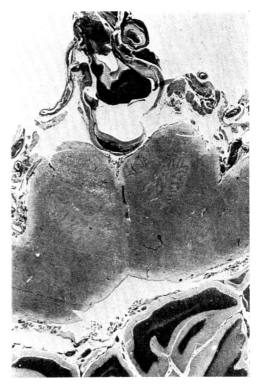

Fig. 80g. Postmortem findings: cross-section of the brain stem; thrombosed aneurysm. Vertebral and basilar arteries are patent. No infarction on the brain tissue.

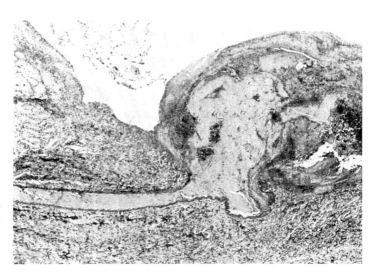

Fig. 80h. Duodenal ulcer showing aneurysm of duodenal artery which led to the exsanguinating hemorrhage.

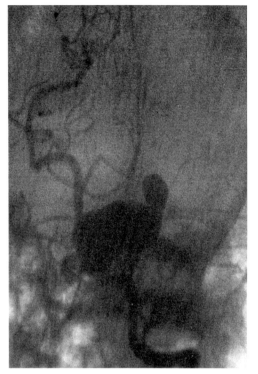
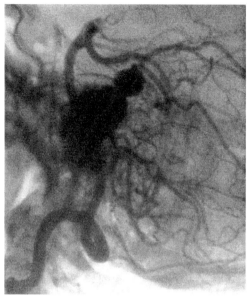

Fig. 81 a—b. Giant saccular aneurysm of basilar artery:

Fig. 81 a) antero-posterior projection;   Fig. 81 b) lateral projection.

proximal basilar artery on its dorsal surface so that the fundus projected into the pons. (Figs. 81 a—b). Through a subtemporal, transtentorial approach it was not possible to visualize the aneurysm nor the lower basilar artery because the brain stem had been markedly expanded by the aneurysmal mass. Accordingly, this craniotomy was closed and although her neurological status remained unchanged her postoperative course was complicated by a staphylococcal septic-aemia. Three weeks after the first procedure she was re-explored through a transoral, transclival approach. With this exposure (8 mm. in width and 2.0 cm. in length) the aneurysm could be clearly visualized and the neck was dissected free and clipped. The neck was however, unusually large and with closing of the 1.0 cm. long hemostatic clip the basilar artery kinked constricting the flow.

In an attempt to overcome this intolerable situation the basilar artery was temporarily occluded between two Scoville clips and then the clip on the neck of the aneurysm re-moved. In its place a silk ligature was passed and tied after opening of the aneurysmal wall and emptying the mass. The wound was closed in the same manner as in the previous case. Immediately, postoperatively she was well, with no increase in her neurological deficit despite the fact that the basilar artery had been occluded for twenty minutes. Nevertheless, twelve hours postoperatively she slowly developed a complete tetraplegia and although she remained conscious her course over the next month until her death was complicated by a recurrence of the infection and communicating hydrocephalus for which a ventriculo-atrial shunt was performed.

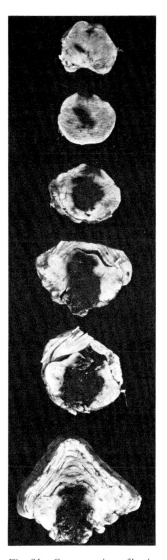

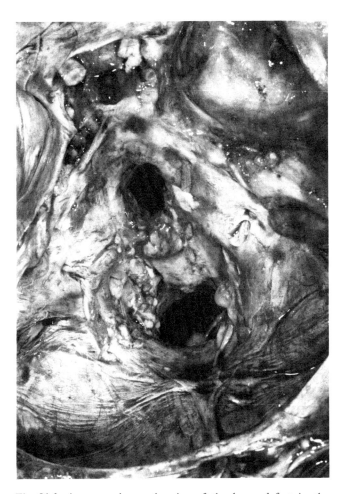

Fig. 81 c. Cross-section of brain stem showing extensive central hemorrhagic infarction.

Fig. 81 d. Autopsy shows the size of the bony defect in the clivus made for exposure of a basilar aneurysm during a transclival approach.

Postmortem examination revealed extensive hemorrhagic infarction of the brain stem extending from the midbrain to the medulla. One can only assume that the period of occlusion was sufficient to cause local edema with subsequent failure of the microcirculation, ischemia and infarction (Fig. 81 c).

Aneurysms of the Branches of the Basilar Artery

Posterior and posterolateral aneurysms of the vertebral artery, including those on the posterior inferior cerebellar artery, are approached by the suboccipital route (Rizzoli,

Hayes 1953, Logue 1958, De Saussure et al. 1958, Poppen 1959, Paulson et al. 1959, Norlén et al. 1960, Abbott et al. 1961, Höök et al. 1963, Sedzimir 1963), while those on the superior cerebellar and posterior cerebral arteries are approached subtemporally. The author to date has had no opportunity of utilizing the microsurgical technique for aneurysms in these sites.

Value and Limitation of Microsurgery in the Treatment of Saccular Aneurysms

The exploration of arteries, and particularly aneurysms on both the anterior and posterior parts of the circle of Willis by means of the operating microscope undoubtedly represents a great advance and offers many advantages (Adams, Witt 1964, Pool 1965, Pool, Colton 1966, Rand, Janetta 1967, Sundt, Nofzinger 1967):

With the microtechnique procedures are possible in a deep and narrow field, so that retraction of the frontal and temporal lobes is reduced to a minimum and resection of either pole avoided. The operating field is well illuminated and all structural details are seen stereoscopically improving the visualization in the depths of the wound. The Sylvian fissure may be opened without damage to the adjacent structures and easy access gained to both the middle cerebral artery and the lateral aspect of the internal carotid artery. Exposure of an artery with sparing of its smaller, as well as its larger branches is ensured with 10—16-fold magnification of the operating microscope. The arachnoid and adventitial fibers may be sectioned individually with the microscissors and microscalpel and traction on adjacent vital structures thus avoided. In the immediate vicinity of the aneurysm, normal and abnormal relationships can be clearly defined. The thin walls of the aneurysm, sites of rupture, and the fine arterioles occasionally emerging directly from the aneurysm sac are clearly visible, so that further manipulation of these sites can be avoided. Exceptional operative precision can be exercised in the vicinity of cranial nerves (optic nerve, and especially oculomotor nerve).

We feel strongly that the combined use of the microscope and the bipolar microcoagulator represents the most significant advantage of microtechnique in aneurysm surgery. After careful exploration of the neck of the aneurysm it is possible with gentle bipolar coagulation to shrink the neck of the aneurysm permitting easier ligation of clipping. Preliminary coagulation toughens the adjacent wall and by shrinking the neck size provides room to apply the clip or ligature without deforming the wall of the parent vessel or destroying adjacent perforators.

Table XIV. Results of the Surgical Treatment of Patients with Intracranial Saccular Aneurysms

Localization	No. of Cases	Good	Poor	Death	
Int. car. art.	16	15	1	—	
Post. com. art.	28	23	3 (1)	2 (2)*	(7.1%)
Ant. com. art.	43	35	6 (4)	2 (1)**	(4.65%)
Middl. cer. art.	17	14	2 (2)	1*	(5.8%)
Basilar. art.	5	2	—	3***	(60.0%)
	109	89 (82.0%)	12 (11.0%)	8	(7.36%)

( ) Preoperative hemiparesis
  * Preoperative rebleeding
 ** Infection
*** Hemorrhagic infarction of metencephalon in one case (see Figs. 81a—c), bleeding from a duodenal ulcus in another case after ligation of the aneurysm (see Figs. 80a—b) and preoperative mesodiencephalic deterioration in the third case (see Figs. 77c—e).

The coagulation of an aneurysm neck requires complete familiarity with the bipolar microcoagulator achieved in the animal laboratory. The following points should be carefully observed. The tip of the forceps must be absolutely clean and smooth and moistened with saline. The vessel or aneurysmal neck should be gently touched with the forceps and not squeezed. Finally it is hazardous to attempt to coagulate the lesion with a single passage of current. Rather, one must repeatedly apply short, low voltage bursts of current across the aneurysmal neck over 3—4 minutes. Using this graduated intermittent coagulation system it is possible to progressively diminish the diameter of the neck with safety.

Our results in the microsurgical approach to intracranial aneurysms are shown in Table XIV. Although the surgical manipulation of an aneurysm appears to be significantly improved with microtechnique there remain many problems in the total management of the individual with a ruptured cerebral aneurysm which remain unresolved. Recurrent hemorrhage preoperatively or at operation, narrowing of vascular channels (spasm or edema of arterial wall) and disturbances of the cerebrospinal fluid circulation (low, normal or high pressure hydrocephalus) continue to adversely affect the outcome.

In three cases we observed unilateral hydrocephalus after successful clipping of an aneurysm and an immediate smooth postoperative course which then deteriorated with progressive drowsiness and a strikingly contralateral hemiparesis. Each of the 3 cases made a gratifying recovery following cerebrospinal fluid diversion though a ventriculo-atrial shunt. In another 6 cases, also after successful surgical management of the aneurysm we observed deterioration on the second or third day with a progressive somnolence, small unreactive pupils and in three instances contralateral hemiparesis. In all six cases the cerebrospinal fluid pressure as measured with lumbar puncture manometrics was zero or apparently below the zero mark. These cases made a dramatic

improvement of their level of consciousness and focal neurologic dysfunction following injection of 50—100 cc of saline into the lumbar subarachnoid space. This injection of saline was repeated 3—4 times daily for 3—4 days in combination with parenteral administration of hypotonic saline. In no instance was there a visible loss of cerebrospinal fluid into or from the wound and we have no rational explanation for this clinical syndrome.

Rupture of the aneurysm at operation is frequently a disastrous complication making it necessary to temporarily occlude the parent artery. The effects of short term occlusion of a cerebral artery remain entirely uncertain. However, the perfection of an external or internal bypass would permit prolonged occlusion of the parent vessel providing the time necessary to resect and repair with precision the site of origin of an aneurysm. Even a fusiform aneurysm at the bifurcation of the middle cerebral artery would then be surgically accessible. It is vitally necessary to perfect these cerebral bypass techniques. The ideal solution to this problem would present a turning point in neurosurgery.

Bypass-Techniques

a) External Bypass

During the fashioning of a frontotemporal skin flap, care is taken to ensure that the temporal limb of the incision is placed immediately above the tragus so that the superficial temporal artery is not damaged. After eversion of the skin flap the artery is exposed under the microscope for a length of 2—3 cm. and prepared for a drainage tube. If, later in the operation temporary occlusion of an essential artery is considered necessary (e.g. internal carotid if angiography reveals inadequate collateral filling from the other side, or the middle cerebral artery), one limb of a T-tube is inserted retrograde for 2—3 cm. into the exposed superficial temporal artery and secured with a circular ligature. The second limb of the T-tube, provided with a special needle, is closed with a Scoville clamp. The third limb remains attached to a syringe with a 3-way system. The T-tube is filled with a heparin and saline solution. At the moment in which the artery (internal carotid, middle cerebral or anterior cerebral) is temporarily interrupted, the needle attached to the second limb of the T-tube is inserted into a cortical temporal artery and fixed there, and the Scoville clamp is released, so that blood from the superficial temporal artery can flow into the cerebral artery. The third limb of the T-tube serves as a circulation monitor and it may be used as pathway for the injection of papaverine (Figs. 37 a–b).

Although this preparation has been carried out in 31 cases the shunt has never been completed because either the obliteration of the aneurysm was uncomplicated and a bypass not required or the situation was so desperate that time and hands were not available to insert the tube into the cortical artery.

Future developments with regard to hypothermic anesthesia, transient induced cardiac arrest, and continuous measurement of oxygen uptake and other metabolic parameters, should permit technical perfection of the bypass technique, in order to make full use of reconstructive and constructive microvascular surgery in the treatment of cerebral aneurysms.

b) Internal Bypass

Dolce (1964) inserted a fine-caliber catheter *via* the common carotid artery, the carotid bulb and the internal carotid in a cephaled direction, and demonstrated that the carotid siphon, and anterior and middle cerebral arteries can be selectively catheterized. He used this technique for selective cerebral angiography. Luessenhop and Velasquez (1964) developed a catheter technique utilizing a somewhat thicker catheter which was advanced from the common carotid artery into the internal carotid through which he injected muscle, glass or plastic emboli into the vicinity of large arteriovenous malformations.

One of the disadvantages of the internal bypass technique lies in the difficulty of advancing the catheter smoothly and quickly to the level of the siphon: beyond this point to the carotid bifurcation, the manipulation is even more uncertain. Yodh et al. (1968) developed an electro-magnetic control system for this intravascular manipulation. They have demonstrated that a Silastic catheter of 1–3 mm. diameter tipped with a platinum-cobalt bullet of corresponding size may be navigated along the artery to the desired position and also be withdrawn without any difficulty. Further development of this technique promises to be a significant step forward in the application of microvascular surgery to neurosurgery.

More recently, Hilal (1969) describe a similar although more sophisticated magnetic navigation technique for intravascular catheterization. A small diameter Silastic tube, perforated at the end and tipped with a magnet is inserted into the cerebral circulation through a proximal vessel. The tip of the tubing is controlled by means of an external electromagnet which when powered by alternating current causes the tip to oscillate. This oscillation tends to keep the tip away from the vessel wall and prevents intimal damage. When the external magnet is powered by direct current, intravascular manipulation and navigation of the advancing tip is possible. Hilal has successfully used this technique for the injection of radio-opaque compounds and chemotherapeutic agents into selected portions of the cerebrovascular tree but a similar device may well be useful in establishing an internal bypass.

New approaches to aneurysms

We recognize that any exposure or retraction of the brain, no matter how gentle, causes a degree of focal cerebral edema and that in a brain insulted by an injection of subarachnoid blood, vascular spasm and impaired cerebrospinal fluid flow conventional surgical manipulation may precipitate disaster. We would suggest that there is a great need for the development of new surgical approaches to the aneurysm.

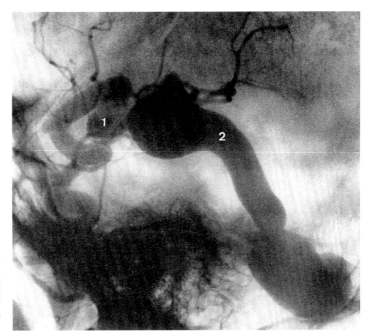

Fig. 82a. Arteriovenous malformation with a fistulous connection between 1, the right middle cerebral artery (which is markedly enlarged) and 2, the vein of Labbé.

One such approach would be the exposure of the anterior communicating region through a transnasal-transsphenoidal or ethmoidal method. These techniques, already proven by otorhinolaryngologists, should permit direct exposure of an aneurysm of the anterior communicating region and the pre- and post-communicating anterior cerebral arteries without displacement or retraction of the brain. Using established microtechniques the aneurysm may then be safely excluded from the circulation, the dura sutured and the wound closed with cartilage or fat grafts. We have not, as yet, had the opportunity to test this concept.

2. Operations on Intracranial Arteriovenous Malformations

The value of the microtechnique is especially emphasized in the resection of cerebral arteriovenous malformations; the feeding vessels are exposed at a distance from the malformation, then traced towards it and ligated a short distance before they penetrate into its substance, so that as many cortical

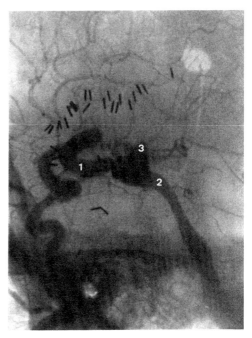

Fig. 82b. Following ligation, 1, the middle cerebral artery and 2, the vein of Labbé are of normal caliber. However, a further fistulous connection 3, has developed.

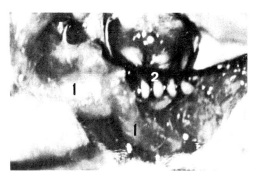

Fig. 82c. Ligation of the fistulous connection and clipping of the varices; 1, middle cerebral artery; 2, site of interrupted fistulous connection.

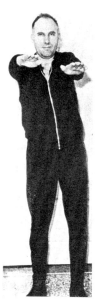

Fig. 83b. The patient following total removal of the malformation using microtechniques.

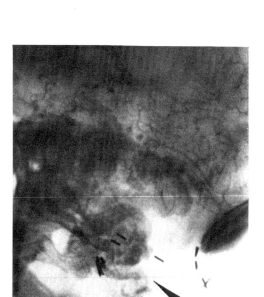

Fig. 83a. Angiogram showing large arteriovenous malformation of right cerebellar hemisphere (arrow) following an initial unsuccessful operation using standard operative technique.

arteries as possible are spared. Numerous small feeding and draining vessels can be clearly seen with the operating microscope in the immediate vicinity of the malformation, and these can be isolated and eliminated by ligation, clipping or coagulation.

To date the author has resected fourteen cerebral and cerebellar arteriovenous malformations with the aid of the operating microscope. Disregarding one frontalpole malformation twelve of the cerebral malformations and the single cerebellar lesion were unique in terms of site, size or morphology and therefore inoperable with standard lobectomy techniques (Figs. 82a—c, 83a—b, 84a—d, 85a—c). Of these thirteen cases eleven malformations were successfully removed without significant neurological deficit, two have disabling paralysis and one died during the operation (Tbl. XV). The operative death occurred as a result of massive intraventricular hemorrhage extending into the right ventricle during mobilization of a huge malformation originating on the medialbasal part of the left temporal lobe and extending into the temporal horn of the ventricle and mesencephalon. In retrospect this tragedy may have been averted by a more generous exposure of the lesion prior to mobilization rather than the small cortical incision used (Fig. 86a—b).

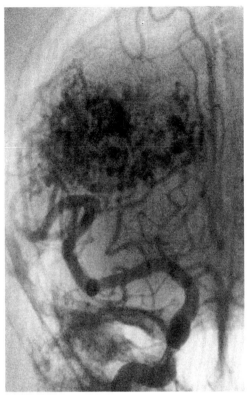

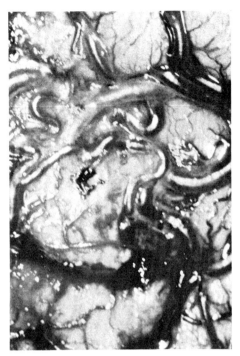

Fig. 84a. Large arteriovenous malformation of the right frontoparietal region.

Fig. 84b. Operative exposure.

Table XV. Results of the Surgical Treatment of Patients with Intracranial Arteriovenous Malformations

Localization	No. of Cases	Good	Poor	Death
Cerebellare	1	1	—	—
Frontalpole (left)	1	1	—	—
Sylvian (right)	3	3	—	—
Sylvian (left)	2	2	—	—
Frontoparietal (right)	2	1	1 (1)	—
Frontoparietal (left)	2	1	1	—
Splenium (left)	2	2	—	—
Hippocampal (left)	1	—	—	1
	14	11	2	1

( ) preoperative hemiparesis

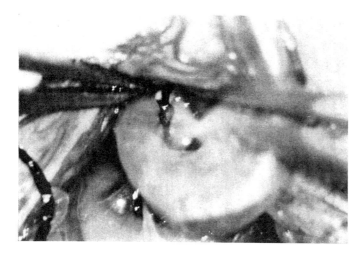

Fig. 84c. Ligature of feeding vessels under the microscope.

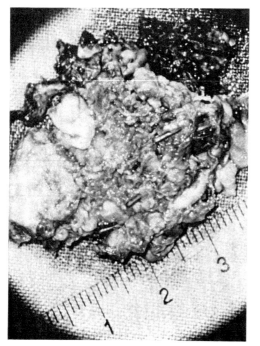

Fig. 84d. Operative specimen.

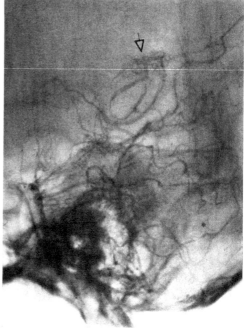

Fig. 85a. Lateral angiogram showing small arteriovenous malformation lying on the left side of the splenium (arrow).

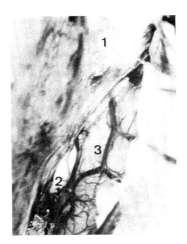

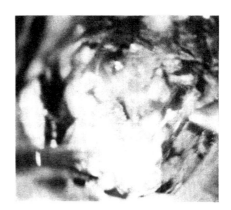

Fig. 85 b. Operative exposure (interhemispheric); 1, tentorium; 2, splenium; 3, cortex with angioma.

Fig. 85 c. After removal of angioma.

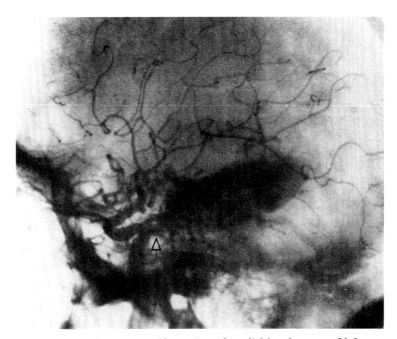

Fig. 86. Lateral angiogram showing arteriovenous malformation of medial basal aspect of left temporal lobe: Note intracavernous branches supplying the lesion (arrow). The attempt of removal failed.

References

Abbott, K. H., D. V. Hubbell, P. J. Vogel: The surgical treatment of vertebral aneurysms. Report of case. Bull. Los Angeles neurol. Soc. 26 (1961) 79

Adams, J. E., J. Witt: The use of otologic microscope in the surgery of aneurysms. Presented at the Meeting of the Neurological Society of America 25 January, 1964

Dinsdale, H., V. Logue: Ruptured posterior fossa aneurysms and their surgical treatment. J. Neurol. Neurosurg. Psychiat. 22 (1959) 202

Dolce, G.: Über eine neue Methode. Der Arterien-Katheterismus des Gehirns. Psychopharmacol. (Brl.) 5 (1964) 313

Drake, C. G.: On the surgical treatment of ruptured intracranial aneurysms. Clin. Neurosurg. 13 (1965) 122

Drake, C. G.: Surgical treatment of ruptured aneurysms of the basilar artery. Experience with 14 cases. J. Neurosurg. 23 (1965) 457

Fox, J. L.: Obliteration of midline vertebral artery aneurysm via basilar craniotomy. J. Neurosurg. 26 (1967) 406

Hamby, W. B.: Intracranial Aneurysms. Thomas, Springfield, Ill. 1952, p. 303

Hilal, S. K.: Catheter with a magnetic tip for cerebral angiography. Med. Tribune 2 (1969) 1

Höök, O., G. Norlén, J. Guzman: Saccular aneurysms of the vertebral-basilar arterial system. A report of 28 cases. Acta psychiat. scand. 39 (1963) 271

Housepian E. M., F. O. Bowman, A. J. Gissen: Elective circulatory arrest in intracranial surgery. Successful treatment of an aneurysm of the basilar artery with a method of open-chest circulatory arrest. J. Neurosurg. 26 (1967) 594

Jamieson, K. G.: Aneurysms of the vertebrobasilar system — surgical intervention in 19 cases. J. Neurosurg. 21 (1964) 781

Jamieson, K. G.: Aneurysms of the vertebrobasilar system. Further experience with nine cases. J. Neurosurg. 28 (1968) 544

Krayenbühl, H., M. G. Yaşargil: Die Anwendung des Mikroskops bei Operationen des Zentralnervensystems. Praxis 57 (1968) 214

Logue, V.: The surgical treatment of aneurysms in the posterior fossa. J. Neurol. Neurosurg, Psychiat. 21 (1958) 66

Luessenhop, A. J., M. Gibbs, A. C. Velasquez: Cerebrovascular response to emboli. Arch. Neurol. (Chic.) 7 (1962) 264

Luessenhop, A. J., A. C. Velasquez: Observations on the tolerance of the intracranial arteries to catheterization. J. Neurosurg. 21 (1964) 85

Norlén, G., S. N. Paly: Aneurysms of the vertebral artery. Report of two operative cases. J. Neurosurg. 17 (1960) 830

Paulson, G., B. S. Nashold Jr., G. Margolis: Aneurysms of the vertebral artery. Report of 5 cases. Neurology (Minneap.) 9 (1959) 590

Pool, J. L.: Personal communication (1965)

Pool, J. L.: Excision of cerebral arteriovenous malformations. J. Neurosurg. 29 (1968) 312

Pool, J. L., R. P. Colton: The dissecting microscope for intracranial vascular surgery. J. Neurosurg. 25 (1966) 315

Pool, J. L., D. G. Potts: Aneurysms and Arteriovenous Malformations of the Brain. Hoeber, New York 1965

Poppen, J. L.: Vascular surgery of the posterior fossa. Clin. Neurosurg. 6 (1959) 198

Rand, R. W., P. J. Jannetta: Micro-neurosurgery for aneurysms of the vertebral-basilar artery system. J. Neurosurg. 27 (1967) 330

Rizzoli, H. V., G. J. Hayes: Congenital berry aneurysm of the posterior fossa. Case report with successful operative excision. J. Neurosurg. 10 (1953) 550

Samuels, P. B.: The use of metal clips in the surgery of blood vessels. Bull. Soc. int. Chir. 21 (1962) 21

Samuels, P. B., H. Roedling, R. Katz, J. J. Concotti: A new hemostatic clip. Ann. Surg. 163 (1966) 427

Saussure, R. L., De, S. E. Hunter, J. T. Robertson: Saccular aneurysms of the posterior fossa. J. Neurosurg. 15 (1958) 385

Sedzimir, C. B.: Surgical teatment of aneurysms of the vertebral artery. J. Neurosurg. 20 (1963) 597

Sundt, Jr., T. M., J. D. Nofzinger: Clip-grafts for aneurysm and small vessel surgery. 1: Repair of segmental defects with clip-grafts: Laboratory studies and clinical correlations. 2: Clinical application of clip-grafts to aneurysms: technical considerations. J. Neurosurg. 27 (1967) 477

Wissinger, J., D. Danoff, E. S. Wisiol, L. A. French: Repair of aneurysm of the basilar artery by a transclival approach. J. Neurosurg. 26 (1967) 417

Yodh, S., N. T. Pierce, R. J. Weggel, D. B. Montgomery: A new system for "intravascular navigation". Med. biol. Eng. 6 (1968) 143

3. Operations on Caroticocavernous Fistulae

Parkinson (1964, 1965, 1966 and 1967) showed, on the basis of personal studies of the anatomical relationship in the cavernous sinus, that fistulae may develop not only between the internal carotid artery itself and the cavernous sinus, but also between branches of the internal carotid artery and the cavernous sinus (Fig. 87). Since these intracavernous branches anastomose (Schnürer, Stattin 1963) through numerous dural branches with the ipsilateral external carotid and vertebral arteries on the one hand, and with intracavernous branches of the opposite internal carotid on the other, it is understandable why extra- and intracranial ligation of the internal carotid artery or even muscle embolization may fail to eliminate the fistula. Parkinson consequently explored the cavernous sinus under conditions of cardiac arrest (35 minutes at 12° C) and successfully ligated the internal carotid artery and its intracavernous branches in the cavernous sinus. No opportunity has yet presented itself to the

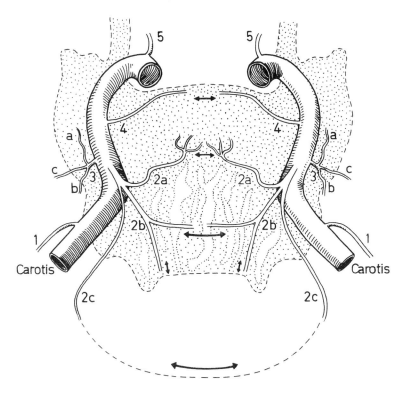

Fig. 87. The intracavernous branches of the internal carotid artery (modified from Parkinson, 1967); 1, caroticotympanic arteries; 2, meningohypophyseal trunk: a) inferior hypophyseal artery; b) posterior meningeal artery; c) tentorial artery; 3, inferior cavernous sinus artery: a) branches for the 3rd, 4th and 5th nerves; b) branches for the Gasserian ganglion, direct anastomosis with the middle meningeal arteries; 4, capsular artery (McConnell's artery); 5, ophthalmic arteries.

author to open the cavernous sinus under the operating microscope. Nonetheless, it is apparent that the microscope will prove to be of value in carrying out the necessary minute dissection successfully. Future developments may permit repair of the fistulous opening without occlusion of the internal carotid artery.

Instead of extracranial ligation of the internal carotid artery at the neck or simultaneous intracranial ligation (trapping) a muscle embolus may be directed at the fistulous connection. Brooks (1930), and Lang, Bucy (1965) recommend that, following insertion of the muscle embolus into the internal carotid artery, the artery to be left unligated and merely the incision in its wall closed with sutures. The author has used a modification of this method in patients by introducing the muscle emboli through the external carotid to the internal carotid artery.

In one, the third embolus lodged in the petrosal part of the carotid artery completely occluding this vessel, but fortunately closing the fistula and with no ischemic complications. In the second case, the second of two emboli stopped at the fistula but the first embolus of muscle was dislodged into the right proximal middle cerebral artery. A craniotomy was rapidly performed and the embolus removed and the middle cerebral artery repaired. Although the embolectomy took only 14 minutes, 35 minutes were required to set up for and turn a bone flap and the patient woke from anesthesia with a hemiparesis. The fistula was ultimately closed by ligation of the intra- and extracranial carotid artery and the ophthalmic artery.

In the third case a frontolateral craniotomy was previously carried out and the upper siphon of internal carotid artery temporarily clipped. The muscle embolus marked with a one millimeter clip closed successfully only the fistula, leaving the blood flow in the internal carotid artery free.

References

Brooks, B.: The treatment of traumatic arteriovenous fistula. Sth. med. J. (Bgham, Ala.) 23 (1930) 100

Hamby, W. B.: Carotid-Cavernous Fistula. Thomas, Springfield, Ill. 1966, pp. 139

Krayenbühl, H.: Treatment of carotid-cavernous fistula consisting of a one stage operation by muscle embolization of the fistulous carotid segment. In: Micro-Vascular Surgery. Ed. by R. M. P. Donaghy, M. G. Yaşargil. Thieme, Stuttgart 1967, pp. 151—167

Lang, E. R., P. C. Bucy: Treatment of carotid-cavernous fistula by muscle embolization alone. J. Neurosurg. 22 (1965) 387

Parkinson, D.: Collateral circulation of cavernous carotid artery: Anatomy. Canad. J. Surg. 7 (1964) 251

Parkinson, D.: A surgical approach to the cavernous portion of the carotid artery. Anatomical studies and case report. J. Neurosurg. 23 (1965) 474

Parkinson, D.: Persistent carotid cavernous fistula. Transcavernous repair. Presentation to Harvey Cushing Society, 18 April, 1966

Parkinson, D.: Transcavernous repair of carotid cavernous fistula. J. Neurosurg. 26 (1967) 420

Schnürer, L. B., S. Stattin: Vascular supply of intracranial dura from internal carotid artery with special reference to its arteriographic significance. Acta radiol. (Stockh.) 1 (1963) 441

CHAPTER 5

A. Intracranial Tumors

The tumors most amenable to resection under the operating microscope are those situated within the ventricles and on the surface of the brain and brainstem; meningiomas, neurinomas, chordomas, astrocytomas, oligodendrogliomas and ependymomas in the vicinity of vessels and cranial nerves which are vital to conserve.

It is apparent that the improved magnification and illumination afforded by the operating microscope makes access to deep structures possible. The successful application of this instrument in the transsphenoidal, translabyrinthine and transclival approaches to basal structures is well known. Moreover, improved vision and micro-operative technique frequently permits dissection between normal and neoplastic tissue (Fig. 88).

Sellar and Parasellar Tumors

By means of the microtechnique, intrasellar tumors as well as parasellar ones can be radically resected and adjacent structures better protected.

The transsphenoidal Approach

The sublabial transsphenoidal approach to the sella was first used successfully by Cushing in 1907. However, it claimed few adherents among neurosurgeons — presumably because of the narrow and long passage of entry. Later, the otorhinolaryngologists exploited the transethmoidal and intranasal transsphenoidal routes (Schloffer 1907, Kanavel 1909, Halstead 1910, Hirsch 1910, Mixter, Quackenbass 1910, Chiary 1912). Hardy and Wigser (1965), Hardy (1967) reintroduced the sublabial-transsphenoidal approach, utilizing the operating microscope and monitoring the operation by means of an image amplifier (see Chapter VII).

The Subfrontal Approach

The author has not yet performed a hypophysectomy by the transsphenoidal route by means of the operating microscope. In a case in which the diagnosis was not certain, the subfrontal route was used with the aid of the microscope because a meningioma of the tuberculum sellae was suspected. Instead, a chromophobe adenoma was found at operation showing extrasellar extension. The tumor was shelled out, and then the adhesions between the tumor capsule and both anterior cerebral arteries separated. In this manner a radical resection was carried out.

Craniopharyngioma

The large suprasellar craniopharyngioma that abuts on the third ventricle and spreads retro- and suprasellarly towards the pons and middle cranial fossae presents ideal material for visualization, localization and extirpation under the operating microscope. The optic nerve, optic chiasm, oculomotor nerve, internal carotid artery, posterior communicating artery, posterior cerebral artery and basilar artery, which may be surrounded by overgrowth of tumor, can be carefully dissected free. Exposure of the chiasmal region is carried out through a lateral subfrontal craniotomy. Using the operating microscope, precise visualization of the individual adhesions between the surface of the tumor and the nerves, floor of the third ventricle, cerebral peduncle, pons and blood vessels allows

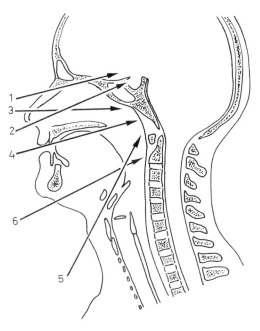

Fig. 88. The various surgical routes to the base of the skull; 1, transnasal — transethmoidal; 2, transnasal — transsphenoidal; 3, transnasal — transclival; 4, transoral — transclival; 5, transcervical — transclival; 6, transcervical approach for the atlas and axis.

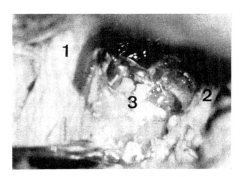

Fig. 89a. Extensive supra- and retrosellar craniopharyngioma; 1, left optic nerve; 2, right optic nerve; 3, tumor tissue with calcified foci.

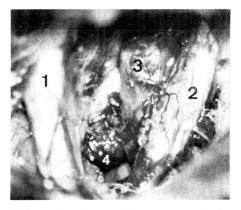

Fig. 89b. Following partial resection of the tumor between both optic nerves (1 and 2): under the right optic nerve the internal carotid artery can be seen displaced to the left. 3. Deeper in the tumor tissues, a large artery 4, was identified, which proved to be a displaced posterior cerebral artery (see Fig. 89d).

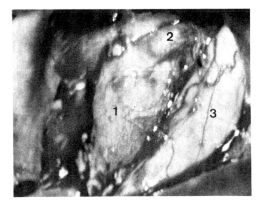

Fig. 89 c. After stripping the remaining tumor tissue from 1, the right internal carotid artery, 2, the ophthalmic artery and 3, right optic nerve were exposed.

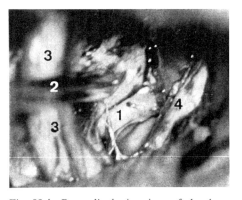

Fig. 89 d. Retroclival situation of 1, the posterior cerebral artery, 2, sucker; 3, left optic nerve; 4, right optic nerve.

one to carefully divide them with micro-instruments (Figs. 89 a—e).

When the intrasellar craniopharyngioma extends basally against the sphenoidal and ethmoidal sinuses rather than upwards and retrosellarly, the following operative technique is advisable (Rand): After subfrontal exposure of the chiasmal region, the dura over the tuberculum sellae is incised length-wise and reflected laterally; the tuberculum sellae and the anterior wall of the sella turcica are then opened with the microdrill. As soon as the mucus membrane of the sphenoidal sinuses comes into view, it is separated from the bone with a micro-spatula and the cavity filled with bonewax; this does not interfere with the drilling and at the same time it protectively forces the mucus membrane further forwards and downwards. It is best not to use pledgets of cotton wool during the actual drilling, because the strands are liable to be caught in the drill and clog it.

After drilling away the anterior part of the floor of the sella and then enlarging the opening laterally towards the cavernous sinuses, an excellent view is obtained of the ventrobasal and ventrolateral aspects of the tumor, so that it can be freed from adhesions along the cavernous sinus and extirpated under direct vision. This operation was performed successfully in three patients with recurrent craniopharyngiomas.

Sphenoid-wing-Meningiomas

A highly vascular meningioma situated either medially or laterally on the sphenoidal wing, with basal or retrosphenoidal extension under the frontal or temporal lobes and apparently adherent to the internal carotid and middle cerebral arteries, is suitable for removal under the operating microscope. The dorsal layers of the tumor are first exposed through a fronto-temporal craniotomy, the surface co-agulated, and the center cored out. After this space-gaining maneuver, the operating micro-scope is used to free the tumor, millimeter by millimeter, from the base of the brain and skull, the tumor vessels being individually dealt with and eliminated. Finally, the tumor tissue adherent to the optic and oculomotor nerves, and the internal carotid and middle cerebral arteries is detached and removed. In one of the author's cases operated upon in this way (Fig. 90) a thumb sized mass of tumor tissue extended backwards under the anterior rim of the tentorium towards the peduncle, where adhesions between the tumor and the posterior communicating and superior cerebellar arteries and the oculo-motor nerve had to be separated.

By utilizing the bypass system to carry blood from the superficial temporal or the main trunk of external carotid arteries to the distal branches of the middle cerebral artery, reconstructive surgery can be carried out successfully and the hazard of possible damage of the middle cerebral artery made less critical.

Clivus Tumors

Tumors such as chordomas, chondromas, epidermoids, dermoids and meningiomas that lie in a retrosellar and parasellar situation and spread backwards to parapontine or paracerebellar, as well as sideways into parapetrosal and subtemporal situations, can be removed with the aid of the operating microscope — through the subfrontal, subtemporal (Bonnal et al. 1964) or transclival (Klingler 1960, Mullan et al. 1966) routes. The actual route depends on the extent of the tumor, and on its direction of growth. The topography of the tumor can be determined by the neurological presentation and the results of radiological examination (tomograms, carotid and vertebral angiography, pneumoencephalography, pneumo- and positive contrast cisternography). The author has utilized the subtemporal route for the removal of two basal dermoids which extended from the olfactory bulb to the cerebellar

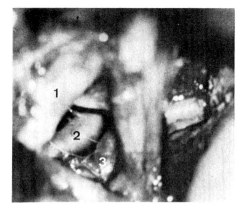

Fig. 89e. After removal of the tumor mass behind the clivus; 1, the left optic nerve and 2, the basilar artery appeared behind it. Note markedly displaced 3, posterior cerebral artery.

tonsil on the right side, also of two clivus meningiomas that had spread supra- und infratentorially as well as into the retropetrosal space.

Two retro- and parasellar chordomas were removed through the subfrontal route, through the 1.5 cm. gap between the right optic nerve and the internal carotid artery. It was possible to free the basilar and superior cerebellar arteries from the tumor surface and to remove the tumor completely (Figs. 91a—b, 92).

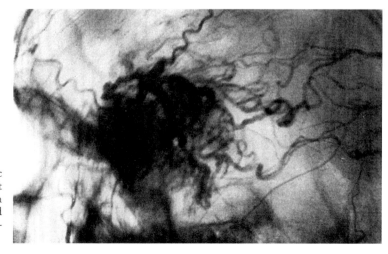

Fig. 90. Angioblastic meningioma of the left sphenoidal wing, which was radically resected without damage to arteries or nerves.

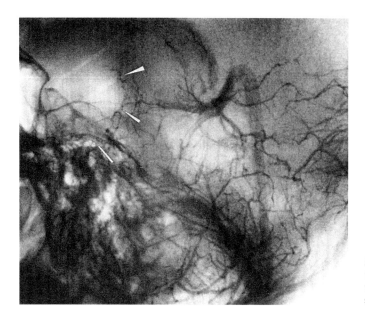

Fig. 91 a. Retrosellar avascular tumor, clearly visible in the venous phase of the vertebral angiogram (arrows).

The transcervical approach to the clivus utilizing the operating microscope and drill should be used for the pure parapontine clivus tumor (Stevenson et al. 1966). The author has no experience with this operation.

Acoustic Neurinomas

Operations on the cerebellopontine angle commenced in the early part of this century.

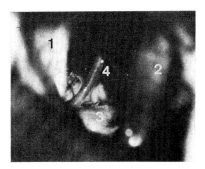

Fig. 91 b. Exposure and resection of the tumor through a right frontal craniotomy, subfrontally between 1, the right optic nerve and the 2, right internal carotid artery. Between two structures the 3, basilar artery and 4, superior cerebellar artery can be seen in the depth of the wound.

In 1904 Panse recommended the translabyrinthine approach, and he received support from Quix (1912), Kümmel (1912) and Hegner, Zange (1916). In 1915 Schmiegelow utilized this approach in two patients to remove small extradural tumors.

Fraenkel et al. (1904), Borchardt (1905) and von Eiselsberg (1907) chose the suboccipital transpetrosal route with the patient's head in a lateral position. Frazier (1905) recommended the bilateral occipital suboccipital approach with ligation of the transverse sinus. Ballance (1908) first totally removed an acoustic neurinoma successfully, the mortality at that time being about 80%. Cushing (1917) achieved significantly better results by restricting himself to intercapsular removal of the tumor, but the course of his patients was nonetheless disappointing.

The next advance was the bilateral — and later unilateral — suboccipital technique with total extirpation developed by Dandy (1922, 1925) which was adopted by most neurosurgeons in the 1930's. Using a modification of Dandy's total extirpation technique, McKenzie, Alexander (1955) reported 142 cases with a mortality of 12.5%.

Many advocates have been found for both the prone position, or the sitting position introduced by de Martel (1931) for this operation. Cairns (1931) first reported preserving the facial nerve during removal of an acoustic neurinoma. Olivecrona (1940) reported sparing of the facial nerve in 14 out of 23 patients, (in whom only a transient facial paresis occurred).

House (1961) and Kurze, Doyle (1962) introduced a microtechnique, and by utilizing the transpetrosal route from the middle cranial fossa were able to remove small intracanalicular acoustic neurinomas without damaging the facial nerve. House and House (1964), Hitselberger, House (1966 and 1968) developed the translabyrinthine approach which previously had been used successfully without the microscope by Quix (1912), Kümmel (1912) and Schmiegelow (1915) as well as Hegner, Zange (1916) Zange (1934) and Mayer (1934) (Figs. 93a—b). The work of House and his colleagues has vigorously stimulated neurosurgeons in this field. Kurze (1963) and Rand, Kurze (1965 and 1968) developed the suboccipital-transmeatal technique for use with the operating microscope with the patient in the sitting position, while Drake (1967) performed the same operation with magnifying spectacles.

Further developments in otological and radiological methods of investigation (Scanlan 1964, Ziedses des Plantes 1968) offer the possibility of diagnosing smaller tumors with certainty. A study of the literature reveals that the early protagonists of the translabyrinthine approach (Quix, Kümmel, Zange), 50 years and again 30 years before modern vestibular testing and radiological techniques of examining petrous bone, were extremely optimistic in regard to the early diagnosis of acoustic neurinomas. The intervening 50 years has not seen the fulfilment of these expectations, in that most cases only present when the tumor is already quite large. Perhaps in the future the use of cisternal myelography and subtraction techniques will enable smaller tumors to be diagnosed with certainty.

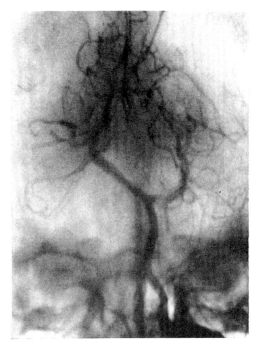

Fig. 92. Large meningioma arising from the right side of the tentorium and growing into both the supra- and infratentorial compartments. Note simultaneous displacement of posterior cerebral and basilar arteries. Tumor was totally removed through a suboccipital craniotomy in sitting position with complete recovery of patient.

At the present time the following methods of operating on the cerebellopontine angle with the microscope are available to surgeons: (Fig. 94a—c).

(1) Subtemporal-transpetrosal Approach (see Chapter VIII)

(2) Transtentorial Approach

Fay, in 1931, described resection of an acoustic neurinoma by the transtentorial route. Using the subtemporo-occipital approach, the laterobasal aspect of the temporal and occipital lobes are elevated, the tentorium is incised parallel to the petrous bone and the tumor removed through this opening. The disadvantages of retracting the cerebral hemi-

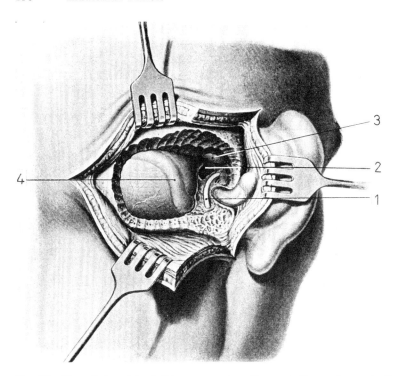

Fig. 93a. Zange's translabyrinthine approach to the cerebellopontine angle (In: Kirchner's *Operations-lehre* Vol. III/1, Springer, Berlin, 1934). Resection of the mastoid. Radical operation on the middle ear. Dissection of the horizontal and vertical parts of 1, the facial nerve, opening into 2, the laby-rinthine system above it, as well as into 3, the cochlea immediately below it, exposure of the dura of the middle cranial fossa, and extensive reflection downwards of the cerebellar dura including 4, the transverse and sigmoid sinus, after removal of the bone flaps.

sphere and the inadequate view of the caudal pole of the tumor are obvious. For these reasons, this method has not found general acceptance. It remains to be seen whether the use of the operating microscope combined with simultaneous ligation of the superior petrosal sinus and excavation of the petrous bone will provide a better view of the cere-bellopontine angle.

Nevertheless we have used this approach in two cases of posterior fossa epidermoid tumors localized lateral to the brain stem and running through the tentorial hiatus from the olfactory nerves to the vagus nerve and filling all of the basal cisterns. Micro-surgical techniques permitted total removal of these tumors, including capsule, with complete preservation of cranial nerves.

(3) Translabyrinthine Removal of the Relatively Small Tumor (1—1.5 cm. diameter)

The translabyrinthine approach developed by House (1964) allows the surgeon to expose the dura in the retromeatal trigone (Traut-mann's triangle) between the sigmoid sinus jugular bulb and superior petrosal sinus. This permits removal of neurinomas up to 1.0—2.5 cm. in diameter. The translaby-rinthine route requires cooperation between otologists and neurosurgeons, in that the otologists opens the entrance to the trigone under the operating microscope through a retroauricular skin incision, and opens a narrow transmastoid translabyrinthine path-way to the internal auditory canal with the diamond drill. Then, after exposure of the facial nerve and freeing of the adhesions between the tumor and the nerve up to the porus acousticus, the neurosurgeon takes over the operation. The dura in the retro-meatal trigone is 1.5–1.8 cm. long and 1.0–1.5 cm. broad. After surface coagulation of the dural vessels, the dura is opened in a cross incision, reflected laterally and fixed. Before the tumor is freed medially from the acoustic-facial nerve group, the tumor is dissected free from the cerebellar hemisphere,

so that the arachnoid fibers between the tumor and the inferolateral aspect of the cerebellar hemisphere can be sectioned, especially those running from the upper pole into the superior petrosal sinus. The petrosal vein is exposed and isolated against the tumor with a cotton-wool pledget. It is very important to visualize the caudal pole of the tumor clearly, at the point where the anterior inferior cerebellar artery enters the tumor frequently describing an arc, from which originate one or more branches. Before the

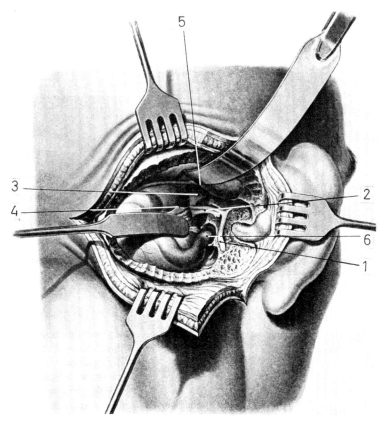

Fig. 93 b. Zange's translabyrinthine approach to the cerebellopontine angle (1934). Complete sacrifice of the inner ear with the removal of the larger part of the petrous pyramid and exposure of the cerebellopontine angle: 1, vertical part of the facial nerve which divides higher in the region of the geniculate ganglion, and the trunk of which then passes into the internal auditory canal, in which 2, the stump of the acoustic nerve can be seen directly beneath it. Above 3, the trigeminal nerve can be seen over the apex of the pyramid; 4, the dura of the cerebellum, split in the region of the internal auditory canal; 5, superior petrosal sinus; 6, exposed jugular bulb. In practice even more pyramidal apex is sacrificed than is shown here, where it is preserved to demonstrate the topography.

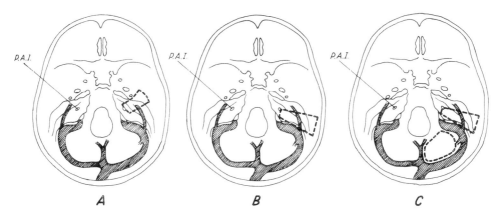

Fig. 94a—c. The various surgical approaches to the cerebellopontine angle: a) subtemporal-trans-petrosal; b) translabyrinthine; c) translabyrinthine-suboccipital. PAI = porus acousticus.

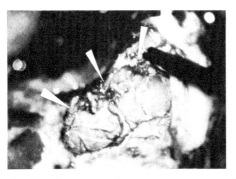

Fig. 95a. Exposure of a tumor about the size of a walnut by the translabyrinthine approach. The tumor is seen in its full size through the dural opening in the retromeatal triangle (arrows).

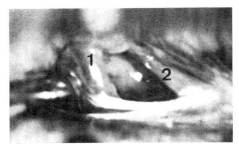

Fig. 95c. Magnified view of 1, the anterior inferior cerebellar artery and 2, facioacoustic nerve trunks.

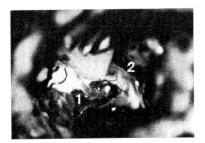

Fig. 95b. After removal of the tumor: 1, the anterior inferior cerebellar artery and 2, the facioacoustic nerve trunks can be seen in the depth of the wound.

use of the operating microscope, this artery was viewed as a tumor vessel and either ligated or coagulated often with disatrous pontine infarction. After careful separation of the adhesions between the caudal pole of the tumor and the artery on the one hand, and the glossopharyngeal-vagus nerve group on the other, the dorsal aspect of the tumor capsule is coagulated and the tumor tissue removed piecemeal through a small incision. The resulting reduction in size allows the tumor to be reflected medially and to be better freed from the nerve groups (Figs. 95a—c, 96a—d).

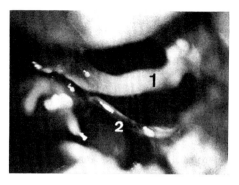

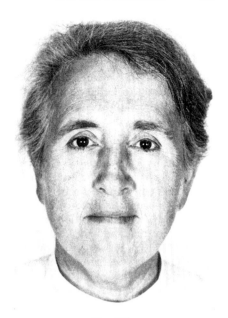

Fig. 96a. Facial nerve after removal of a pea-sized acoustic neurinoma by the translabyrinthine route; 1, facial nerve; 2, anterior inferior cerebellar artery.

Fig. 96b—d. Facial nerve function preserved after removal of a left acoustic neurinoma.

Fig. 96b

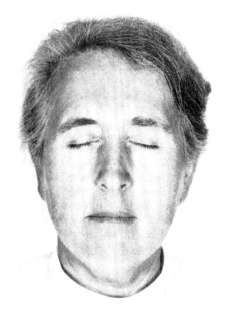

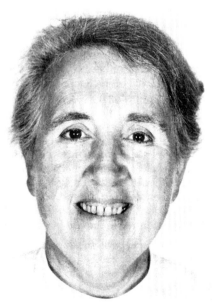

Fig. 96c

Fig. 96d

(4) Combined Translabyrinthine and Suboccipital Approach for larger Tumors (4—9 cm. diameter)

If during a translabyrinthine operation the tumor is found to be larger than anticipated from the preoperative neurological and radiological investigation, it is advisable to do no more than prepare the meatal aspect of the facial nerve to perform a two-stage procedure. A 1 cm. length of silk thread is tied loosely around the facial nerve which is then covered with a strip of Teflon so that it can be recognized later. The wound is then closed after the insertion of fatty tissue taken from the abdomen. At the second session 4—7 days later, the retroauricular skin incision is enlarged towards the occipital midline. The skin and muscle flap is lifted from the one half of the occipital squama, reflected downwards and fixed with fish-hooks. The posterior arch of the atlas is removed to a width of 1.5 cm. and the occipital squame opened as far as the foramen magnum. It is important to remove the bone over the sigmoid sinus as far as the jugular bulb. The dura is then opened over the cisterna magna releasing the cerebrospinal fluid, and then extended dorsolaterally, parallel to the course of the sigmoid and transverse sinuses, so that the posterior surface of the cerebellar hemisphere remains covered by dura. The cerebellopontine angle is then examined under the operating microscope along the dorsolateral border of the cerebellar hemisphere. It is not necessary to ligate or section either the transverse sinus or the sigmoid sinus: at the first session the dura was opened retromeatally, and now it is deflected medial to the sinus, which remains in the middle as a bridge and can be displaced either laterally or medially. If the relationships demand it, the sigmoid sinus may be sectioned between two bulldog clamps and then resutured at the end of the operation.

The dorsal aspects of the tumor are defined in relation to the cerebellar hemisphere and especially the petrosal vein, and the surface coagulated. After the tumor has been shelled out, the capsule can be dissected free from the anterobasal aspect of the pons and deflected

towards the center of the tumor. After reduction in its size, the glossopharyngeal-vagus-accessory nerve group comes into view on the ventral surface of the caudal pole of the tumor. The arachnoid fibers between the tumor tissue and the nerve group are sectioned and the nerve group isolated and covered with cotton wool. The anterior inferior cerebellar artery is constantly encountered at the level of the flocculus, running in an anterobasal direction at the caudal pole of the tumor and often forming a loop, from which large branches run to supply it. After elimination of these branches with sparing of the anterior inferior cerebellar artery itself, the vertebral artery is better visualized: it also may give fine branches to the tumor, and these are obliterated with the Malis coagulator. The tumor capsule must now be separated from the pons and from the facial and auditory nerves. The preliminary dissection carried out on the lateral aspect of the tumor during the first operative session is fully utilized at this stage, in that the dural opening in the retromeatal trigone provides the surgeon with access to the internal auditory canal and enables him to identifiy the facial nerve within it. This is done quickly by finding the black silk thread and Teflon strip left behind at the first session, and the tumor is then dissected free from the nerves. After extirpation of the tumor the extradural space of the mastoid process is packed with fatty tissue and the operative wound closed in layers.

(5) Suboccipital Transmeatal Approach

The suboccipital technique is performed with the patient in the sitting position which reduces venous and cerebrospinal fluid stasis. (The risk of air embolism is nonetheless to be remembered: if this accident occurs, the patient should immediately be placed in the left lateral decubitus position and the gas sucked out of the right auricle with a catheter).

The occipital squama is opened up to the midline, down to the foramen magnum and as far laterally as possible. The posterior arch of the atlas is removed if raised intra-

cranial pressure is present. After opening
and tethering the dura, the ipsilateral cerebellar hemisphere is retracted upwards and
somewhat to the opposite side. Then the
tumor is carefully freed dorsomedially from
the cerebellum, dorsocranially from the
petrosal vein and dorsocaudally from
the glossopharyngeal-vagus-accessory nerve
group. The capsular blood vessels are coagulated and the center of the tumor cored
out. Bleeding points are packed with Oxycel.
Space is made by the coring out process so
that the porus acousticus is more easily
located and the posterior wall of the internal
auditory canal is excavated with a diamond
drill to expose the facioacoustic nerve group.
The facial nerve lies along the anterior wall.
The bulk of the tumor is freed from the facial
and cochlear nerves by microdissection as
far as the internal auditory meatus. In the
next phase, the tumor capsule is dissected
free of the brainstem, starting at the lower
pole where the vagus and glossopharyngeal
nerves have already been mobilized. Anterior
to the lower pole is the loop of the anterior
inferior cerebellar artery which lies in the
space between the foramen of Luschka and
the porus acousticus, usually between the
facioacoustic nerve group and the flocculus.
Adhesions between the artery and tumor
capsule are best freed under the operating
microscope. The branches of the artery
supplying the tumor are microcoagulated and
sectioned. After exposure of the artery, the
tumor capsule is freed from its connections
with the brainstem and then deflected upwards by compression with a pledget of
cotton wool. At the level of the flocculus the
facial nerve appears as a narrow white filament
which runs 1–10 mm. caudally and then
winds laterally under the tumor. As the next
step, the upper pole of the tumor is freed
under the petrosal vein, the adhesions separated and the trigeminal nerve freed.
Tumor deposits attached to the facial nerve
are removed (Figs. 97 a–b).
In large tumors producing raised intracranial pressure it is advisable to perform a
shunt one week before attacking the tumor.
By this means, the pressure is relieved preoperatively and free drainage of the cerebro-

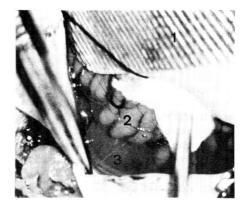

Fig. 97a. Large left acoustic neurinoma. Operation with the patient in the sitting position; 1,
spatula; 2, cerebellar hemisphere; 3, edge of
the tumor.

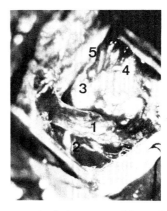

Fig. 97b. After removal of the tumor. View of
the left cerebellopontine angle with 1, the facioacoustic nerve trunks; 2, abducent nerve; 3,
trigeminal nerve; 4, the pons and 5, the superior
cerebellar artery.

spinal fluid reestablished improving the
patient's general condition and enhancing
the operative removal of the tumor.

To date twenty-nine cases of acoustic neurinomas have been operated upon, by four
different routes:

(1) Transtemporal approach (two cases),
(2) Translabyrinthine approach (ten cases),
(3) Translabyrinthine and suboccipital ap-
    proach (six cases),
(4) Suboccipital transmeatal approach
    (eleven cases).

In the cases in group (2) and (3) the tumors were resected in cooperation with Dr. Fisch of the Department of the Otorhinolaryngology. In group (2), it was possible to resect completely four small (1—2 cm. diameter) and six large (2—3 cm. diameter) neurinomas through the small opening in the retromeatal trigone, and to preserve the facial nerve anatomically. Postoperatively six patients (three with small tumors) showed no evidence of facial palsy, and four showed a severe paralysis. Improvement of the paralysis occurred in three cases within 2—6 months.

In each of the group (3) cases, the mass of the tumor was first freed from the facial nerve in the internal auditory meatus. Then 7—14 days later, a suboccipital operation was performed (four with the patient prone, two with the patient on his side), and large tumors (5—8 cm. in length, 3—4 cm. in breadth) were radically removed in four and partially removed in two. It was possible to preserve anatomically the facial nerve in all six patients. Of the four patients in whom the tumor was radically resected, three cases showed slight facial palsy postoperatively and one a severe facial palsy. Of the two patients undergoing partial resection, two showed a total facial paralysis.

The prone position of the patient (four cases) was found to be very tiring and permitted an inadequate microsurgical examination of the cerebellopontine angle, despite prior mastoidectomy and ligation of the sigmoid sinus (two cases). The lateral position with slight elevation of the head (two cases) prevents venous congestion. This position is recommended for smaller tumors. In none of sixteen cases was cerebrospinal fluid leakage produced. The mastoidectomy cavity is filled with fatty tissue taken from the subcutaneous layers of the abdomen and covered with muscle and fascia from the pedicle flap of the temporal region.

Three huge neurinomas (bulging of the tentorial opening, extending to the foramen magnum and hollowing out of the pons medially), and seven moderate sized and one small tumors were removed by the suboccipital route with the prone position (two cases) and in the sitting position (nine cases). A ventriculoatrial shunt had been inserted in one case with a large tumor ten days previously to relieve the obstructive hydrocephalus (severe papilledema). The sitting position with the head tilted forwards and slightly to the opposite side provides ideal visualization while the uncongested cerebellar hemisphere can be raised and retracted upwards and to the opposite side. The postoperative course was without complications in all those eleven cases. Slight or moderate facial paralysis improved within some weeks. Permanent facial paralysis resulted in three cases; one the individual with the largest tumor in the series, the other a small tumor measuring only 4—5 mm. in diameter and a third in which the facial nerve was mixed with a tumor of moderate size.

On the basis of personal experience to date, the author is of the opinion that only small neurinomas in the internal auditory meatus

Table XVI. Result of Different Surgical Approaches to Acoustic Neurinomas

Approaches	No. of Cases	Good	Poor	Death	Facial Paralysis Permanent	Facial Paralysis Transient	None
Transtemporal	2	2	—	—	—	—	2
Translabyrinthine	10	9	—	1**	1	3	6
Translabyrinthine and suboccipital	6	4	—	2*	2 (1)	3	1
Suboccipital	11	11	—	—	3	8	—
( ) preoperative paresis	29	26	—	3	6	14	9

  * one case of v. Recklinghausen's disease with bilateral acoustic, trigeminal neurinomas and a frontal meningioma with severe neurological defects preoperatively.
** second case died three months later postoperatively from myocardial failure (68-year-old female).

(up to 1—1.5 cm. in diameter) should be removed by the translabyrinthine approach while larger tumors should be dealt with by the suboccipital routes. Of cardinal importance is the fact that the anterior inferior cerebellar artery must not be damaged or coagulated during removal of the tumor. In all the author's cases, this artery could be identified and preserved, so that no case of postoperative paresis was observed.

Other Tumors of the Posterior Fossa

The microtechnique were also found to be of considerable value in removing three meningiomas, one medulloblastoma, one glioma of the pons and one ependymoma from the cerebellopontine angle and one astrocytoma and two hemangioendotheliomatas from the cerebellar hemisphere. In each case the patient was in the sitting position. The author feels that these techniques permit a more complete and precise removal of the neoplasm while protecting nearby vital structures. This would be particularly true of tumors of the fourth ventricle. (Figs. 98, 99).

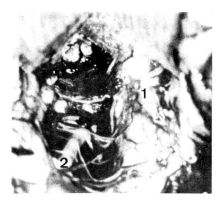

Fig. 98. Medulloblastoma of left cerebellar tonsil with expansion into the left cerebellopontine angle. Following removal of tumor lower cranial nerves are preserved; 1, pons and medulla; 2, vertebral artery.

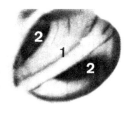

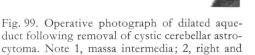

Fig. 99. Operative photograph of dilated aqueduct following removal of cystic cerebellar astrocytoma. Note 1, massa intermedia; 2, right and left foramina of Monro.

References

Ballance, C. A.: A case of division of the auditory nerve for painful tinnitus. Lancet 2 (1908) 1070

Bonnal, J., R. Louis, A. Combalbert: L'abord temporal transtentoriel de l'angle ponto-cérébelleux et du clivus. Neuro-chir., Paris 10 (1964) 3

Borchardt, R.: Zur Operation der Tumoren des Kleinhirnbrückenwinkels. Berl. klin. Wschr. 42 (1905) 1033

Cairns, H.: Acoustic neurinoma of right cerebellopontine angle. Complete removal. Spontaneous recovery from postoperative facial palsy. Proc. ray. Soc. Med. 25 (1931) 35

Chiary, O.: Über eine Modifikation der Schloffer'schen Operation von Tumoren der Hypophyse. Wien. klin. Wschr. 25 (1912) 5

Cushing, H.: Partial hypophysectomy for acromegaly. With remarks on the function of the hypophysis. Ann. Surg. 50 (1909) 1002

Cushing, H.: The Pituitary Body and its Disorders. Clinical States produced by Disorders of the Hypophysis Cerebri. Lippincott, Philadelphia 1912, p. 314

Cushing, H.: Surgical experience with pituitary disorders. J. amer. med. Ass. 63 (1914) 1515

Cushing, H.: Tumors of the Nervus Acousticus and the Syndrome of the Cerebellopontine Angle. Saunders, Philadelphia 1917, p. 296

Dandy, W. E.: An operation for the total extirpation of tumors in the cerebellopontine angle. Bull. Johns Hopk. Hosp. 33 (1922) 344

Dandy, W. E.: An operation for total removal of cerebellopontine (acoustic) tumors. Surg. Gynec. Obstet. 41 (1925) 129

Drake, C. G.: Total removal of large acoustic neurinomas. A modification of the McKenzie operation with special emphasis on saving the facial nerve. J. Neurosurg. 26 (1967) 554

Drake, C. G.: Surgical treatment of acoustic neurinoma with preservation or reconstruction of the facial nerve. J. Neurosurg. 26 (1967) 459

Eiselsberg, A. F., von: Über die chirurgische Behandlung der Hirntumoren. Trans. Internat. Cong. Med. London. 7 (1913) 203

Fay, T.: The management of tumors of the posterior fossa by the transtentorial approach. Surg. Clin. N. Amer. 10 (1931) 1427

Fraenkel, J., S. R. Hunt, G. Woolsey, C. A. Elsberg: Contribution to the surgery of neurofibroma of the acoustic nerve, with remarks on the surgical procedure. Ann. Surg. 40 (1904) 293

Frazier, C. H.: Remarks upon the surgical aspect of tumors of the cerebellum. N. Y. St. J. Med. 18 (1905) 272 and 332

Halstead, A. E.: Remarks on the operative treatment of tumors of the hypophysis. With the report of two cases operated on by an oro-nasal method. Trans. amer. Surg. Ass. 28 (1910) 73

Hardy, J., S. M. Wigser: Transsphenoidal surgery of pituitary fossa tumors with televised radiofluoroscopic control. J. Neurosurg. 23 (1965) 612

Hardy, J.: La chirurgie de l'hypophyse par voie transsphénoidale. Étude comparative de deux modalités techniques. Un Méd. Canad. 96 (1967) 702

Hegner, C. A., J. Zange: Über translabyrinthäre Operationen von Tumoren im Kleinhirnbrückenwinkel, zugleich ein Beitrag zur operativen Behandlung zerebraler Sehstörungen. Klin. Mbl. Augenheilkunde 56 (1916) 176

Hirsch, O.: Demonstration eines nach einer neuen Methode operierten Hypophysentumors. Verh. dtsch. Ges. Chir. 39 (1910) 51

Hitselberger, W. E., W. F. House: Surgical approaches to acoustic tumors. Arch. Otolaryng. 84 (1966) 286

Hitselberger, W. E., W. F. House: Diagnosis and Treatment of Acoustic Tumors. In: Otolaryngology 2 (1968) 1—40

House, W. F.: Surgical exposure of the internal auditory canal and its contents through the middle, cranial fossa. Laryngoscope (St. Louis) 71 (1961) 1363

House, W. F.: Transtemporal bone microsurgical removal of acoustic neurinomas. Arch. Otolaryng. 80 (1964) 599

House, H. P., W. F. House: Historical review and problem of acoustic neurinoma. Arch. Otolaryng. 80 (1964) 601

Kanavel, A. B.: The removal of tumors of the pituitary body by an infranasal route. J. amer. med. Ass. 53 (1909) 1704

Klingler: Personal communication (1960)

Kümmel, W.: Diskussionsbemerkung. Verh. Ges. dtsch. Hals-Nas.-Ohrenärzte (1912) 253

Kurze, T.: Microtechnique in neurological surgery. Proceeding of Congress of Neurological Surgery. Clin. Neurosurg. 11 (1963/64) 128

Kurze, T., J. B. Doyle, Jr.: Extradural intracranial (middle fossa) approach to the internal auditory canal. J. Neurosurg. 19 (1962) 1033

Martel, T., De: Surgical treatment of cerebral tumors. Technical consideration. Surg. Gynec. Obstet. 52 (1931) 381

Mayer, O.: Translabyrinthäre Entfernung von Akustikus-Neurinomen in 2 Fällen. (Diskussion S. 233). Z. Hals-Nas.-Ohrenheilk. 36 (1934) 233

McKenzie, K. G., E. Alexander: Acoustic neurinoma. Clin. Neurosurg. 2 (1955) 21

Mixter, S. J., A. Quackenbass: Tumor of the hypophysis with infantilism. Ann. Surg. 52 (1910) 12

Mullan, S., R. Naunton, J. Hekmat-Panah, G. Vailati: The use of the anterior approach to ventrally placed tumors in the foramen magnum and vertebral column. J. Neurosurg. 24 (1966) 536

Ojemann, R. G., W. W. Montgomery, A. D. Weiss: Suboccipital translabyrinthine approach for acoustic neurinomas. Arch. Otolaryng. 83 (1966) 566

Olivecrona, H.: Acoustic tumors. J. Neurol. Psychiat. 3 (1940) 141

Olivecrona, H.: Acoustic tumors. In: Handbuch der Neurochirurgie, Vol. IV/4, Ed. by H. Olivecrona, W. Tönnis. Springer, Berlin 1967, pp. 192—222

Panse, R.: Ein Gliom des Akustikus. Arch. Ohrenheilk. 61 (1904) 251

Pool, J. L.: Suboccipital surgery for acoustic neurinomas: advantages and disadvantages. J. Neurosurg. 24 (1966) 483

Quix, F. H.: Ein Fall von translabyrinthärisch operiertem Tumor acusticus. Verh. Ges. dtsch. Hals-Nas.-Ohrenärzte 21 (1912) 245

Quix, F. H.: Ein operierter Fall mit Geschwulst des Hörnerven mit Darstellung mikrophotographischer Lichtbilder und Besprechung der Operationstechnik. Hals-Nas.-Ohrenheilk. 21. und 22. Nov. 1914. Zbl. Hals-Nas.-Ohrenheilk. 13 (1915) 208

Rand, R. W., T. Kurze: Facial nerve preservation by posterior fossa transmeatal microdissection in total removal of acoustic tumors. J. Neurol. Neurosurg. Psychiat. 28 (1965) 311

Rand, R. W., T. Kurze: Microneurosurgical resection of acoustic tumors by a transmeatal posterior fossa approach. Bull. Los Angeles neurol. Soc. 30 (1965) 17

Rand, R. W., T. Kurze: Preservation of vestibular, cochlear and facial nerves during microsurgical removal of acoustic tumors. Case report. J. Neurosurg. 28 (1968) 158

Scanlan, R. L.: Positive contrast medium (Iophendylate) in diagnosis of acoustic neurinoma. Archs. Otolaryng. 80 (1964) 698

Schloffer, H.: Erfolgreiche Operation eines Hypophysentumors auf nasalem Wege. Wien. klin. Wschr. 20 (1907) 621

Schmiegelow, E.: Beitrag zur translabyrinthären Entfernung der Akustikustumoren. Z. Ohrenheilk. 73 (1915)

Stevenson, G. C., J. J. Stoney, R. K. Perkins, J. E. Adams: A transcervical transclival approach to the ventral surface of the brain stem for removal of a clivus chordoma. J. Neurosurg. 24 (1966) 544

Zange: Translabyrinthäre Operationen von Acusticus- und Kleinhirnbrücken-Winkel-Tumoren. Berl. klin. Wschr. 52 (1915) 1334

Zange, J.: Erkennung und Behandlung der Geschwülste des Kleinhirns. Z. Hals-Nas.-Ohrenheilk. 36 (1934) 227

Ziedses des Plantes, B. G.: X-ray examination in cerebellopontine angle tumors. Psychiat. Neurol. Neurochir. (Amst.) 71 (1968) 133

B. Cranial Nerve Lesions

(For operations on the cochlear, vestibular and facial nerves, see Chapter VIII.)

Trigeminal Neuralgia

The simple operative technique of Spiller and Frazier of blunt sectioning of the retroganglionic trigeminal fibers in Meckel's cave is well known to neurosurgeons. The uncertainty of whether all the fibers have been sectioned, with or without sparing of the motor root, is also well known. After subtemporal extradural exploration of the middle cranial fossa and slitting of the dura under the operating microscope, Meckel's cave is opened and both the sensory and the motor roots completely and convincinly visualized. Sectioning of the appropriate root presents no difficulty. In this way the vessels hidden behind and beneath the root are spared, and undesirable hemorrhage can be avoided (Figs. 100a—b).

Transtentorial Approach

Jannetta (1967) and Janetta, Rand (1966 and 1967) showed that subtemporo-occipital craniotomy and opening of the tentorium parallel to the rim of the petrous bone allows the trigeminal roots to be examined in the infratentorial compartment, where the individual roots can be more easily defined. He reported selective division of those fibers transmitting pain without loss of the sensation of touch.

The patient under general endotracheal anesthesia is placed in the lateral decubitus position and the side of the head shaved and prepared in the usual fashion. The ear is sutured down. A small skin flap is fashioned with the anterior limb one centimeter in front of the tragus and the posterior limb 2 cm. behind the pinna over the mastoid prominence. Using 4 burr holes a 4 cm. square bone flap is turned anterior-temporally attached to temporalis muscle. The lower edge of the craniotomy is rongeured away down to the floor of the middle fossa. The dura is opened along a line parallel to and 2 cm. above the inferior margin of the craniotomy opening. The superior dural flap is then left to cover and protect the temporal lobe.

The temporal lobe is elevated gently with a spatula inserted anterior to the attachment of the vein of Labbé to the sinus. Care must be taken to identify, coagulate and divide the frequent small draining veins which pass between lateral basal surface of the temporal lobe and the superior surface of the tentorium.

Although many authors advocate division of the tentorium parallel to the petrosal ridge, the authors feel this is a hazardous and troublesome approach. We favour the opening of a triangular window in the tentorium placed so that one limb is parallel to the petrosal ridge and another parallel

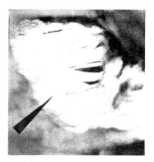

Fig. 100a. Exposure of Meckel's cave (arrow) on the right side with the operating microscope. Demonstration of the sensory roots of the trigeminal nerve.

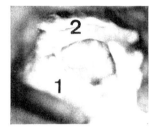

Fig. 100b. After sectioning of the sensory roots I/II with preservation of 2, root I and 1, the motor root.

to and 2—3 mm. away from the free edge of the tentorium. This tentorial window permits good exposure of the fifth nerve and minimizes the inadvertent destruction of the fourth nerve at the free edge of the tentorium or by compressing this nerve against the tentorial branch of the superior cerebellar artery when a large flap of tentorium is turned back.

Viewed from the operators position one sees at the bottom of the tentorial flap a rather large vein, the anastomotic lateral mesencephalic vein. Running parallel to the vein and above it is the portio minor of the fifth nerve which arises most dorsally of all of the trigeminal complex. The point of origin of the portio minor is just hidden under the cerebellum. Above the portio minor the small round intermediate root

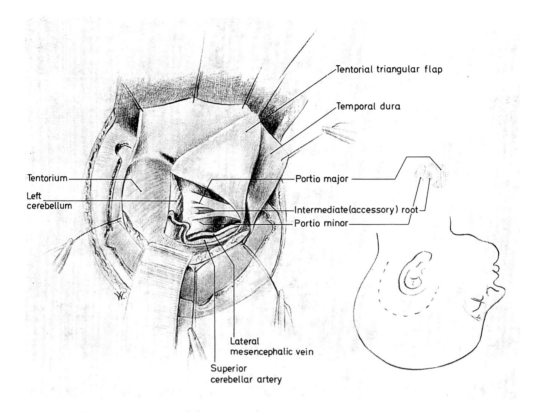

Fig. 100c. Shows the transtentorial approach for selective root section in left trigeminal neuralgia.

and above this again is the very large portio major partly wrapped around the intermediate root. It is possible to easily separate the portio major from the other roots of the complex, coagulate and divide it. In this way pain sensibility is entirely lost with preservation of touch and corneal sensation. The superior cerebellar artery has a variable course through the nerve complex; running above, below and occasionally through the roots. Great care must be taken to identify and preserve this vessel.

In our experience in four cases we have had difficulty distinguishing the 3 divisions of the major root. It is our impression that the 3rd or mandibular division is the most superior and the 1st or ophthalmic division inferior with the maxillary division occupying an intermediate position.

Spasmodic Torticollis:
Sectioning of the Spinal Accessory and the Upper Cervical Nerves

The skin incision for high cervical laminectomy in sitting position of the patient extends from the external occipital protuberance to the level of the spinous process of C5—6. After dissection and lateral spreading of the neck muscles by means of a self-retaining retractor, the spinous processes and posterior arches of C2, C3 and C4, together with the posterior arch of the atlas, are removed. The dura is incised lengthwise from C1 to C4, tethered laterally to the muscles. This exposure affords an excellent view of the spinal accessory nerves and the anterior and posterior roots of C1, 2 and 3. Exposure and sectioning of the spinal parts of the accessory nerve presents no technical difficulties. The C1 root, on the contrary is buried under the attachment of the first dentate ligament, which lies immediately over the vertebral artery at this level. The anatomical relations are easier to identify under the operating microscope. After sectioning of the dentate ligament, the root of C1 is sectioned, with sparing of the arterioles accompanying the nerve fibers (Fig. 101). Next the spinal parts of the accessory nerves and the sensory and motor root fibers of C2 and 3 are sectioned on both sides. Under the operating microscope it is possible to spare the very fine arteries and veins accompanying the nerves. In order to prevent a defect of swallowing and speech care must be taken to avoid sectioning the fine bulbar tributaries of the vagus nerve which may travel with the accessory nerves. They are easily recognizable since they lie above the vertebral artery.

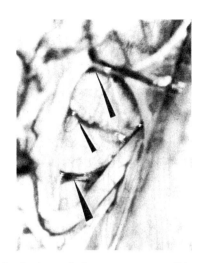

Fig. 101. Sectioning of the motor roots C1, C2, C3 with sparing of the accompanying blood vessels (arrows) for spasmodic torticollis.

References

Jannetta, P. J.: Arterial compression of the trigeminal nerve at the pons in patients with trigeminal neuralgia. J. Neurosurg. 26 (1967) 159
Jannetta, P. J., R. W. Rand: Microanatomy of the trigeminal nerve. Anat. Rec. 154 (1966) 362

Jannetta, P. J., R. W. Rand: Transtentorial retrogasserian rhizotomy in trigeminal neuralgia by microsurgical technique. Bull. Los Angeles Neurol. Soc. 31 (1966) 93
Jannetta, P. J., R. W. Rand: Vascular compression of the trigeminal nerve at the pons in patients with trigeminal neuralgia. In: Micro-Vascular Surgery. Ed. by R. M. P. Donaghy, M. G. Yaşargil. Thieme, Stuttgart 1967, pp. 140—150

CHAPTER 6

A. Vertebral Column and Spinal Cord Lesions

Spinal Arteriovenous Malformation

The typical racemose arteriovenous angioma lies on the posterior surface of the cervical and more frequently the thoracic spinal cord. For their radical removal it is essential to determine the length of the malformation preoperatively, either by positive-contrast myelography or by selective aortography and vertebral angiography. Djindjian et al. (1963, 1966), Doppman, Di Chiro (1965) Di Chiro et al. (1967) and Baker et al. (1967) have described this delicate technique of selective aortography. They were able in their cases to demonstrate the length and extend of the malformation and the number and precise level of the supplying radicular arteries. It is clearly ideal to undertake this type of angiography preoperatively in every case, so that the operation can be more accurately planned (Fig. 102).

Positive-contrast myelography is useful, particularly when performed with the patient both prone and supine, as the malformation is situated mainly on the posterior surface of the spinal cord. If this is done, the length and extent of the pathological vessels can be determined from the myelogram (Figs. 103, 104, 105).

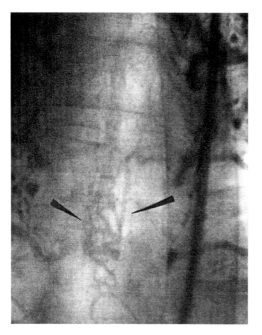

Fig. 102. A racemose angioma of the thoraco-lumbar region on the posterior surface of the spinal cord, demonstrated by upper-limb aorto-graphy (arrows).

Not infrequently the malformation extends for a considerable length, particularly those in the thoracolumbar region, so that an extensive laminectomy is often required. Personal experience has shown that the removal of the spinous processes and posterior arches of 8 or 9 thoracic vertebrae causes no instability of the vertebral column. After carrying out the laminectomy according to the usual technique, the operating microscope is attached as soon as the dura is opened, and a 10-fold magnification used. Extensive adhesions are usually present between the thickened arachnoid and the inner surface of the dura, which require very careful separation.

The appearances of these malformations vary from case to case. They usually consist of a pathological vessel with a diameter of 0.8—1.5 mm. which courses over the surface of the spinal cord in wide and narrow loops and presents as a series of small or large vessel knots (see Figs. 108a—c). The malformation usually lies within a dense network of thickened arachnoid. These abnormal arachnoid fibers surround and enclose the pathological vessels, penetrating between the loops and coils and adhering to them. As well, this reactive arachnoid is usually interposed between the malformation and the spinal pia mater which in turn covers the spinal vessels.

The malformation has numerous connections with the spinal vessels, with the pial vascular network on the posterolateral and lateral surface of the cord, and to the larger reticular vessels (0.4—1.0 mm. diameter). Solitary radicular trunks have been seen with an outer diameter of 1.0—3.0 mm. and it is not always possible in situ to decide whether they are supplying or draining vessels. The similar morphological appearance of both types of vessel is due not only to the quality of the arterial blood but also to their similar histological structure; they represent a primitive phase of development, a stage before differentiation into veins and arteries. The direction of the blood flow can only rarely be determined by temporary clamping of an individual large-caliber radicular vessel. Congestion or collapse of a convolution upon clamping is seen only exceptionally, usually with primitive angiomata: in most cases clamping of the main feeding trunks produces no effect. The malformation shows an unbelievably rich collateral circulation over its entire extent. It is clear that these hundreds of collateral pathways, some very small and some very thick, have to be sectioned individually throughout the whole length of the malformation before it can be radically removed.

Djindjian et al. (1966), Houdart et al. (1966), Baker et al. (1967) and Di Chiro et al. (1967), Ommaya et. al. (1969) have described patients in whom the main feeding vessel of the malformation was identified preoperatively and then ligated extradurally or intradurally whereupon the malformation collapsed. It is quite possible to come across rare individual cases of this type in which a solitary vessel is the source of the blood supply. However, most

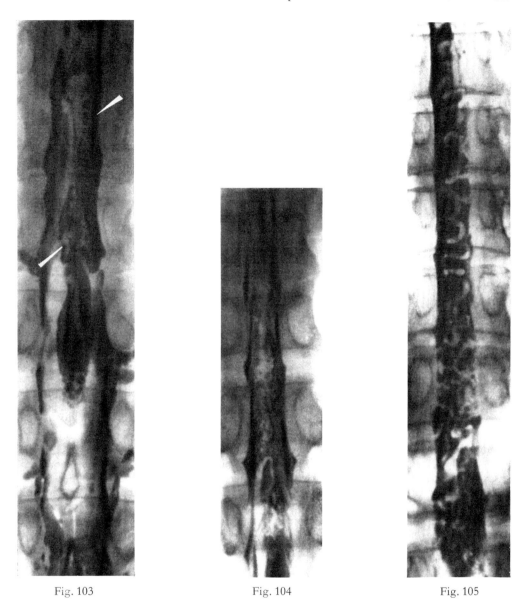

Fig. 103   Fig. 104   Fig. 105

Fig. 103. Extensive spinal angioma demonstrated by positive-contrast myelography. The notches in the contrast column are typical of a malformation (arrows); patient prone.

Fig. 104. Spinal angioma demonstrated by positive-contrast myelography. The pattern of defects in the contrast medium suggests the pressure of an arteriovenous malformation; patient supine.

Fig. 105. Extensive spinal angioma in the thoracic region, the coiled vessels of the malformation forming a characteristic pattern, in the contrast medium; patient supine.

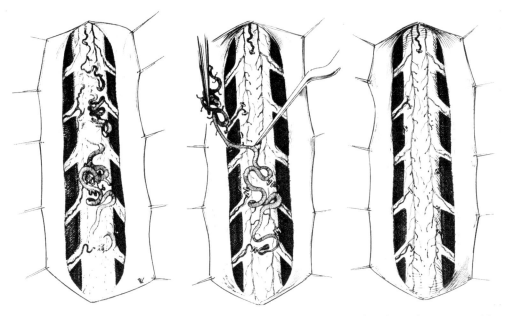

Fig. 106. Diagram of the appearances and technique of removal of a dorsal arteriovenous malformation.

cases of spinal cord arteriovenous malformation possess a very complicated structure, with numerous feeding and draining vessels, so that only radical extirpation leads to a lasting symptomatic improvement. Krause (1911) and Elsberg (1916) removed spinal vascular malformations, found incidentally at laminectomy. In 1927 Perthes diagnosed an arteriovenous malformation by means of Lipiodol myelography in a young man, and then radically resected it. Since that time various neurosurgeons have attempted radical or at least subtotal resection of such lesions, and reported good results. The author himself in the pre-microsurgery era operated successfully upon eight patients. The delicate dissection that is necessary is facilitated by the use of the operating microscope and bipolar microcoagulation in that it is more precise and less damaging to the surrounding normal tissues.

It is advisable first to deal with the cranial segment of the malformation where the pathological vessels lie in great loops; the arachnoid layer surrounding the pathological vessels is opened under the 16-fold magnification of the operating microscope. Since the vessels of the malformation are very thin-walled, they should not be handled with forceps. Instead the arachnoid membrane covering the vessels is grasped and raised with the microforceps, so that the vessels are put on the stretch (Fig. 106). Numerous fine arachnoid fibers connect the undersurface of the malformation with the upper surface of the spinal cord, as well as stretched blood vessels which anastomose with the spinal arteries. These vessels are grasped individually with a very fine forceps for bipolar coagulation and then sectioned with the microscissors. After mobilization of the vessels for a length of 1 cm., silk ligatures are applied to each vessel, which is then divided between them. In this way, the main vessel is dissected free, millimeter by millimeter, in a caudal direction; the arachnoid fibers lying posterior, posterolateral and anterolateral to the malformation being sectioned first, then the anterior fibers and small vessels. (It is interesting to note that the dissection of the malformed

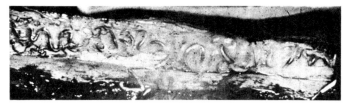

Fig. 107a. Extensive spinal angioma on the posterior surface of the spinal cord in the thoracolumbar region.

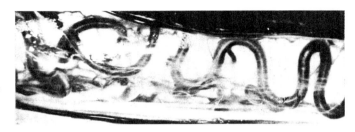

Fig. 107b. Magnified view of the malformation in the subarachnoid space.

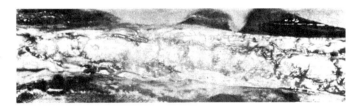

Fig. 107c. Appearance of the spinal cord after removal of the arteriovenous malformation, with sparing of the blood vessels of the spinal cord.

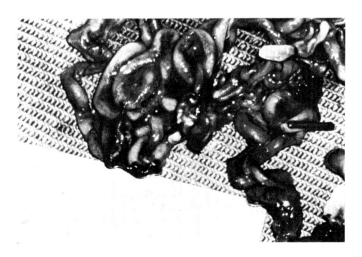

Fig. 107d. The resected specimen of the arteriovenous malformation.

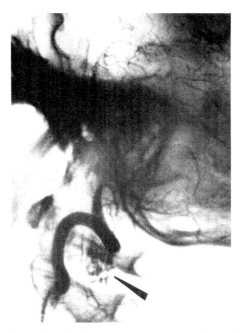

Fig. 108a. Left vertebral angiogram in a 37-year-old male presenting with subarachnoid hemorrhage: a small arteriovenous malformation (arrow) is shown at the C1—C2 level.

vessel in the thickened arachnoid is analogous to the surgery of the small intestine and its mesentery; during resection of the latter, the supplying and draining vessels in the mesentery are ligated and sectioned in turn.) The dissection and mobilization of uncoiled vessels is much easier than that of vessels in the vicinity of the coils. Here also, the same principle applies: the arachnoid fibers are sectioned between individual loops and coils with the microscissors, so that after successful radical extirpation of a 20—25 cm. long malformation, it may be pulled out to a length of 40—50 cm. Figs. 107a—d. It is not essential to remove the malformation in one piece: the lesion may be extirpated segment by segment through ligation or coagulation, particularly when the adhesions around the coiled parts are too dense and firm and lead to bleeding. Of great practical advantage is the fact that the arterial pressure in the spinal arteries and in

those of the malformation is never above 20—30 mm. Hg, so that in the event of a small vessel being damaged good hemostasis can be achieved by light compression with a cotton-wool pledget. Hemorrhage from larger arteries is controlled by coagulation of the bleeding point, its localization being aided by pledget to soak up the blood. The presence of numerous draining vessels flowing in all directions also helps to minimize the blood loss, following damage to a vessel wall. On the other hand, the blood pressure in the radicular vessels is 70—80 mm. Hg, so that they have to be doubly-ligated before sectioning. The dilated and coiled vessels accompanying the fibers of the cauda equina are left alone, since they do not actually form part of the malformation but appear enlarged as a result of engorgement. Only their direct connections with the malformation are severed. In one patient the distal end of the malformation terminated as an aneurysm about the size of a grape, which split the conus terminalis in two and displaced it anteriorly as in the case of Scoville (1948). With 16-fold magnification of the operating microscope, it was possible to define accurately a layer of pial tissue between the convolutions of the vascular malformation and the cord substance itself. In this case the malformation was dissected anteriorly and a feeding artery (diameter 5 mm.) ligated. Thereafter, the malformation could be removed in toto. The such dreaded postoperative complication of sacral anesthesia did not occur.

In sixteen other patients operated upon with the aid of the microscope since January 1967 and in eight in which it was not used between 1960—1965, no thickened intramedullary vessels were encountered (see Table XVII). One intramedullary malformation was situated in the lateral aspect of the cervical cord (C3) (Figs. 109a—d) and one in the ventrolateral aspect of the thoracic cord (T8—9). No case has yet been seen in which the malformation lay anterior to the cord.

A spinal arteriovenous malformation may be erroneously suggested by the dilated supplying and draining vessels of an intramedullary tumor (ependymoma, astrocytoma, hem-

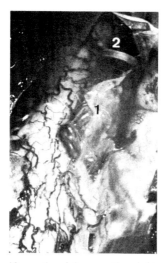

Fig. 108b. The malformation lying on the right side postero-lateral to the spinal cord 1, and supplied by branches of the 2, posterior inferior cerebellar artery.

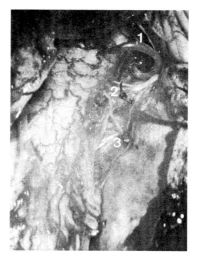

Fig. 108c. Removal of the malformation with sparing of 1, the posterior inferior cerebellar artery and 2, ligation of the feeding arteries, and 3, draining veins.

angioendothelioma). In arteriovenous malformations, the spinal cord itself is not enlarged, whereas in tumors, it is enlarged.

Spinal Tumors

Extradural Tumors

A 15-year-old youth presented with an hourglass extradural tumor at the C4—6 level, which upon laminectomy proved to be an unusually well-vascularized meningioma. The posterior and posterolateral surface of the tumor could be resected without the microtechnique, but the lateral and anterolateral surface were completely interwined with the nerve roots and had displaced them laterally in the direction to the costotransverse foramina, where it abutted directly on the vertebral artery.

With the aid of the microtechnique it was possible to dissect the tumor free from the nerve roots and remove it completely.

Intradural-Extramedullary Tumors

Lipomas, meningiomas and neurinomas that are embedded in the cord substance can be extirpated without tissue damage. The tumor deposits are isolated adjacent to the spinal

Table XVII. Results of Operated Spinal Intradural Arteriovenous Malformations

	No neuro-logical deficit	Marked improvement	Moderate improvement	No improvement	Impairment
Radical extirpation	2	11	—	—	—
Partial extirpation and obliteration through coagulation	—	4	4	3 (3)	—
	2	15	4	3 (3)	—

( ) preoperative paraplegia lasting for a long time

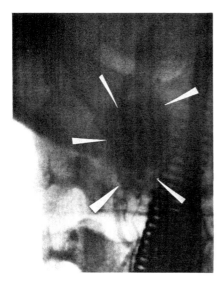

cord and nerve roots, the arachnoid fibers are sectioned with the microscissors and the anastomosis between the tumor vessels and the spinal vessels coagulated with bipolar cautery. After carefully inserting cotton-wool pledgets between the tumor and the spinal cord as well as the individual nerve roots, the tumor vessels are surface coagulated and the tumor, much reduced in size, is removed *in toto* or piecemeal. In large tumors an attempt should be made to core it out — a procedure that provides valuable space when the

Fig. 109a. Extensive racemose angioma at the level of C2—3 antero-lateral to the cord as well as within it, producing repeated attacks of subarachnoid hemorrhage and leading to significant paresis of the left arm and both lower limbs.

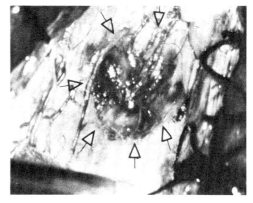

Fig. 109c. Operative exposure. Arrows indicate extent of angioma.

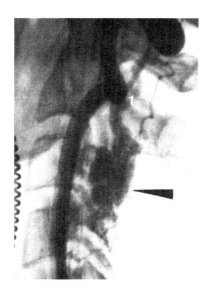

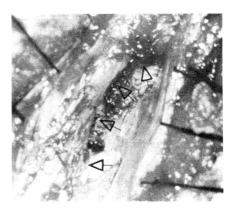

Fig. 109b. Lateral view of the angioma (vertebral angiogram). The feeding arteries arose from 1, the posterior inferior cerebellar artery.

Fig. 109d. Following removal of angioma (arrows).

tumor walls collapse, and protective cotton-wool pledgets can then be inserted between the tumor and the nerve fibers, before the last of the adhesions are freed. One of the great advantages of the operating micro-scope lies in its facility of angulation around the optical axis, which enables structures lying anteriorly and anterolaterally to be viewed stereoscopically under ideal condi-tions of illumination. This makes more precise dissection possible and minimizes or elimi-nates the necessity of retraction of the spinal cord and nerve roots.

Cauda Equina Tumors

All cauda equina tumors, particularly those that spread diffusely (ependymomas) are suitable for dissection under the operating microscope. Through patient and delicate dissection and with the aid of microinstru-ments, attempts are made to sever the ad-hesions between the tumor and the nerve fibers, while preserving the nerves and vessels. The vessels are usually densely bound to the tumor and supply it with many branches. One may then divide the adhesions and ves-sels carefully and thereby cut off the tumor blood supply without damaging the major vessel trunks. The outcome of the operation can be significantly influenced by the sur-geon exercising the greatest possible respect for microstructures, which without magni-fication cannot always be seen and are, therefore, often ignored. In each instance the extended duration of the operation is justified by the improved stereoscopic vis-ualization of all the details in the operating field.

Meningocele-Meningomyelocele

In this field the aid of the microscope and the use of microinstruments are invaluable. While the technique of freeing adhesions, dissecting the various layers of the theca, exposing nerve bundles and closing the dura are already well-established in neurosurgery, each can be more precisely and safely carried out under 10—16-fold magnification with the micro-scope. This is especially true in regard to

manipulation of the nerve fibers. We have had exceptionally good results using these techniques in 2 cases.

Intramedullary Tumors

Fenger's attempt in 1890 to remove an intra-medullary tumor was a failure. Cushing (1905) recommended the posterior midline incision for operations on the spinal cord. Von Eisels-berg and Ranzi (1913) first totally removed an intramedullary tumor in 1907. Elsberg and Beer (1911) next carried out a decom-pression, and in the absence of any improve-ment they removed the tumor. Cushing in 1928 resected a tumor extending from the medulla oblongata to the midthoracic level of the cord in two sessions. The case of Horrax and Henderson in 1936, in which they were able to remove a tumor that extended from the medulla oblongata to the conus medullaris, remains unique.

It remains to be seen whether the improved view and illumination of the operating field afforded by the use of the operating micro-scope and microcoagulation can lead to better results in the removal of intramedullary tu-mors (Slooff et al. 1964). The following tech-nique, used in the author's cases, is a modi-fication to Greenwood's method (1967).

After laminectomy of the area to be explored, the dura is split longitudinally under the operating microscope (6-fold magnification) and sutured laterally to the adjacent muscles. It is advisable to use the operating micro-scope at this stage, because the intraspinal cavity is usually filled with tumor and the dura is tightly applied to the spinal cord with dense vascular adhesions. After inspection, palpation and puncture on suspicion of a cyst, the vessels lying in the region of the planned midline incision are grasped with the micro-forceps and bipolarly coagulated; the greatest possible care is taken to preserve the para-median vessels. The longitudinal incision into the spinal cord is made in the dorsal midline with a razor blade (Figs. 110a–c). Any remaining individual bleeding points on the edge of the incision are bipolarly coagulated. The next steps depend on its size,

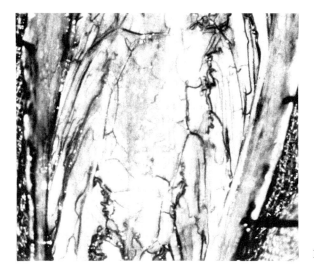

Fig. 110a. Cervical intramedullary tumor.

blood supply, consistency and histological nature. If a relatively sharply-defined tumor mass (ependymoma) is present, showing a cystic structure, the tumor is freed in a dorsal paramedian direction from the overlying cord substance by the insertion of a microdissector and cotton-wool pledgets between them and the center of the mass sucked or scooped out. This allows the lateral and anterolateral surface to be defined with microdissectors and further cotton-wool pledgets to be inserted. It is not possible to prevent operative deformity of normal nerve tissue without removing the core of the tumor. Occasionally ependymomas grow in an anterior direction, producing a factitious diplomyelia. Here the anterior spinal artery is to be recognized and spared from damage. The small arteries which can scarcely be identified with the naked eye on the boundary surface between the spinal cord and the tumor, are easily recognizable with the operating microscope, and can be microcoagulated.

If a diffuse and less well-defined tumor is present, the boundary between tumor tissue and normal nerve tissue may be impossible to discern, even under 16—25-fold magnification. If an spongioblastoma is suspected macroscopically immediate biopsy should be obtained before any attempted excision. In three proven cases of spongio-

blastoma the long term results were disappointing. An attempt should be made in such cases to core out the tumor and to leave the peripheral parts of it undisturbed. The ependymomas (2 cases) and hemangioendothelioma (1 case) are ideally situated for complete extirpation in that they are frequently associated with a welldefined cyst and their margins are clearly demarcated.

Spinal Arteriovenous Malformations

References

Baker, H., G. Love, D. Layton: Angiographic and surgical aspects of spinal cord vascular abnormalities. Radiology 88 (1967) 1078

Chiro, G. Di, J. Doppman, A. K. Ommaya: Selective arteriography of arteriovenous aneurysm of spinal cord. Radiology 88 (1967) 1065

Djindjian, R., C. Faure: Investigations neuroradiologiques (artériographie et phlébographie) dans les malformations vasculaires médullaires. Roentgen-Europ. 6—7 (1963) 171

Djindjian, R., C. Faure, M. Hurth: Explorations artériographiques des anévrismes artério-veineux de la moelle épinière. Dans: Les Monographies des Annales de Radiologie. Exp. Scient. Française, Paris 1966

Doppman, J., G. di Chiro: Subtraction angiography of spinal cord vascular malformations. Report of a case. J. Neurosurg. 23 (1965) 440

Elsberg, C. A.: The surgical significance and operative treatment of enlarged and varicose veins of the spinal cord. Amer. J. med. Sci. 151 (1916) 642

Houdart, R., R. Djindjian, M. Hurth: Vascular malformations of the spinal cord. The anatomic and therapeutic significance of arteriography. J. Neurosurg. 24 (1966) 583

Krause, F.: Chirurgie des Gehirns und Rückenmarkes. Urban und Schwarzenberg II, Berlin 1911. p. 775

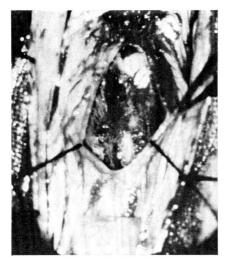

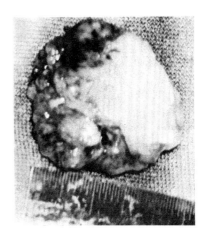

Fig. 110b. After incision of cord and removal of tumor (astrocytoma).

Fig. 110c. Tumor.

Krayenbühl, H., M. G. Yaşargil: Die Varicosis spinalis und ihre Behandlung. Schweiz. Arch. Neurol. Psychiat. 92 (1963) 74

Krayenbühl, H., M. G. Yaşargil: Die Anwendung des binokularen Mikroskopes in der Neurochirurgie. Wien. Z. Nervenheilk. 25 (1967) 268

Krayenbühl, H., M. G. Yaşargil, H. G. McClintock: Treatment of spinal cord vascular malformations by surgical excision. J. Neurosurg. 30 (1969) 427

Ommaya, A. K., G. Di Chiro, J. Doppman: Ligation of arterial supply in the treatment of spinal cord arteriovenous malformation. J. Neurosurg. 30 (1969) 679

Perthes, G.: Über das Rankenangiom der weichen Häute des Gehirns und Rückenmarks. Dtsch. Z. Chir. 203 (1927) 93

Scoville, W. B.: Intramedullary arteriovenous aneurysm of the spinal cord. Case report with operative removal from the conus medullaris. J. Neurosurg. 5 (1948) 307

Yaşargil, M. G.: Diagnosis and treatment of intradural spinal arteriovenous malformations. In Progress in Neurological surgery. (in press) 1969

Intramedullary Tumors

Church, A., D. W. Eisendrath: A contribution to spinal cord surgery. Amer. J. med. Sci. 103 (1892) 395

Cushing, H.: The special field of neurological surgery. Bull. Johns Hopk. Hosp. 16 (1905) 77

Cushing, H.: The special field of neurological surgery. Bull. Johns Hopk. Hosp. 21 (1950) 325

Eiselsberg, A. F. von, E. Ranzi: Über die chirurgische Behandlung der Hirn- und Rückenmarkstumoren. Arch. klin. Chir. 102 (1913) 309

Elsberg, C. A., E. Beer: The operability of intramedullary tumors of the spinal cord. A report of two operations with remarks upon the extension of intraspinal tumors. Amer. J. med. Sci. 142 (1911) 636

Fenger: Quoted by A. Church, D. W. Eisendrath (1892)

Greenwood, J.: Surgical removal of intramedullary tumors. J. Neurosurg. 26 (1967) 276

Horrax, G., D. G. Henderson: Encapsulated intramedullary tumor involving the whole spinal cord from medulla to conus: complete enucleation with recovery. Surg. Gynec. Obstet. 68 (1939) 814

Slooff, J. L., J. W. Kernohan, C. S. McCarty: Primary Intramedullary Tumors of the Spinal Cord and Filum Terminale. Saunders, Philadelphia 1964

Cervical Disc Herniation

In two patients the diagnosis of intramedullary tumor was made on the basis of the neurological findings. At operation however, a central disc herniation protruding directly backwards was found. In both patients the herniation was removed transdurally by the posterior route. The disc space could be freed from disc remnants with great accuracy by means of the operating microscope. The anterior as well as the posterior surface of the dura was closed. Both patients withstood the operation well and lost all neurological deficits (Figs. 111a—d).

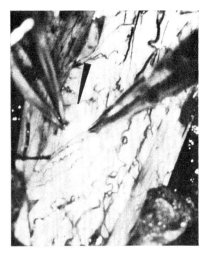

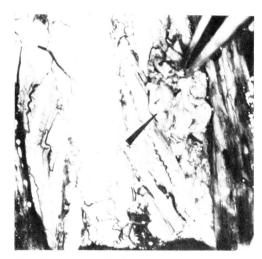

Fig. 111a. Exploration of the cervical spine for a suspected intramedullary tumor (spastic tetraparesis). Finding of a left-sided C5/6 disc herniation (arrow).

Fig. 111b. Removal of the prolapsed part of the disc, following incision of the posterior longitudinal ligament.

However, in a third case inadvertent displacement of rongeur resulted in contusion of the spinal cord with tetraplegia. In cases of undoubted disc herniation we believe that the anterior approach offers considerable advantages over the posterior approach. For anterior approach the microsurgery could bring some additional help as for example the exposure of the anterior aspect of cervical cord anterolateral cordotomy is greatly facilitated by the use of microsurgical technique (Dinning, 1969).

References

Dinning, T. A. R.: Personal communication 1969.

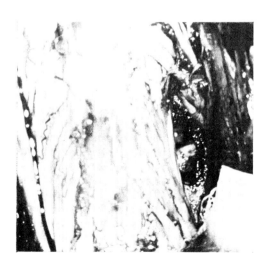

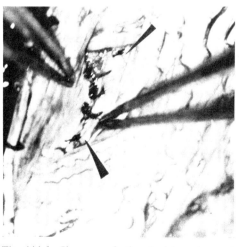

Fig. 111c. Removal of the disc tissue from the disc space.

Fig. 111d. Closure of the incision into the posterior longitudinal ligament.

B. Peripheral Nerve Lesions

Between 1962 and 1965 the diploscope was used in fourteen patients in the Neurosurgical Department of Zürich to anastomose the facial nerve to the descending branch of the hypoglossal nerve (following operation for acoustic neurinomas). The author has not performed animal experiments in order to develop microsurgical techniques on peripheral nerves.

However, plastic surgeons, who are concerned with the experimental and clinical problems of skin, finger and tendon transplantation, have developed similar microsurgical techniques.

The advantages of using a binocular operating microscope for reconstructive and constructive peripheral-nerve surgery are considerable (Smith 1964, 1966). In traumatic lesions the retracted nerve endings are easily and confidently identified under 4—40-fold magnification. The extent of the lesion on the nerve can be better determined and dissection and mobilization of the various nerve layers and adhesions to adjacent tissues accurately performed. Retraction of the perineurium in the region of the incision or axial bulging (danger of neuroma formation) is prevented by precision suturing (7.0—8.0 monofilament nylon). The interested reader is referred to the important work of Basset, Campbell (1959), Campbell, Luzio (1964) Perl, Wagner (1965), Faul et al. (1965), Ducker, Hayes (1967 and 1968) and Hirasawa, Marmor (1967) for details of peripheral nerve repair and regeneration.

References

Basset, C. A., J. B. Campbell: Peripheral nerve and spinal cord regeneration; factors leading to success of a tubulation technique employing millipore. Expl. Neurol. 1 (1959) 386

Campbell, J. B., J. Luzio: Symposium: facial nerve rehabilitation. Facial nerve repair; new surgical techniques. Trans. amer. Acad. Ophthal. Otolaryng. 68 (1964) 1068

Ducker, T. B., G. T. Hayes: A comparative study of the technique of nerve repair. Surg. Forum 18 (1967) 443

Ducker, T. B., G. T. Hayes: Experimental improvement in the use of Silastic cuff for peripheral nerve repair. J. Neurosurg. 28 (1968) 582

Faul, P., W. Heiss, A. Struppler, W. Brendel: Ersatz der chirurgischen Nervennaht durch Klebstoff. Zbl. Neurochir. 26 (1965) 3

Hirasawa ,Y., L. Marmor: The protective effect of irradiation combined with sheating methods on experimental nerve hetergraft: Silastic, autogenous veins, and heterogenous arteries. J. Neurosurg. 27 (1967) 401

Perl, J. I., R. S. Wagner: Intrathoracic phrenic nerve repair: An experimental comparison of a suture and a non-suture method. J. Int. Coll. Surg. 44 (1965) 171

Smith, J. W.: Microsurgery of pereiphal nerves. Plast. reconstr. Surg. 33 (1964) 317

Smith, J. W.: Microsurgical repair of nerves. In: Reconstructive Plastic Surgery. Ed. by J. M. Converse, Saunders, Philadelphia 1964, pp. 2246—2253

Smith, J. W.: Microsurgery: Review of the literature and discussion of microtechniques. Plast. reconstr. Surg. 37 (1966) 227

Smith, J. W., J. H. Jacobson: In: Surgery of the Hand. Ed. by J. E. Flynn, Williams and Wilkins, Baltimore 1966, pp. 729—738

CHAPTER 7

Transnasal-Transsphenoidal Approach to the Pituitary Gland

Introduction

Significant progress has been achieved in the modern neurosurgery of the hypophysis through the combination of the transsphenoidal approach to the sella turcica with televised radiofluoroscopic control and the microsurgical method of dissection.

The open transsphenoidal approach to the sella turcica has the advantage of producing relatively little trauma, providing easy and rapid access to the region and carrying a minimal risk of mortality, since it is an extracranial procedure which entails no manipulation of the intracranial structures.

Televised radiofluoroscopic control permits rapid and accurate localization of the instruments during the operative maneuver at the base of the skull and it eliminates the time usually wasted in repeated verification by conventional radiography. In addition, selective cisternal pneumography, carried out during the operation, allows the superior surface of an expanded pituitary lesion to be clearly defined. The tumor can be completely removed under continuous observation on the television screen, as well as the return of the third ventricle to its normal position as shown by refilling of the chiasmatic cistern after tumor removal (Hardy, Wigser 1965).

On the other hand, due to considerable magnification of relatively small structures, the use of the binocular operating microscope allows the precise morphology of the various structures to be clearly recognized, and incidental anatomical variations of anomalies to be itendified (Bergland, Ray, Torack 1968). It increases the precision and refinement of the surgical manipulations and, therefore, reduces the hazards of unpredictable difficulties. It even permits certain tissues which are different but intimately attached to each other, to be differentiated, so that a selective removal can be achieved. The various technical modalities of pituitary surgery that will be described in this chapter have been acquired through experience with more than 200 operations.

This chapter is limited to the surgical aspects only, and all further considerations of the clinical problems are purposely omitted.

Preoperative Radiological Study

Tomographic studies of the sella turcica are essential before operation. There are three anatomical types of sphenoid sinus, which have been classified and studied by Hamberger et al. (1961) (Fig. 112).

The Sellar Type

This type of sinus is completely pneumatized and extends backwards under the sella turcica as far as the anterior aspect of the clivus. The sellar floor is usually very thin (0.5 mm.) and bulges into the sphenoid cavity. This variety is the most common type and is ideally situated for the transsphenoidal approach and fenestration of the sellar floor. It is encountered in 86% of cases.

The presellar Type

This type of sinus is partially pneumatized, since the basis sphenoid extends forward under

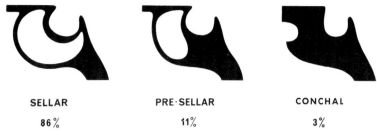

SELLAR   PRE·SELLAR   CONCHAL

86%   11%   3%

Fig. 112. Various types of sphenoid sinus.

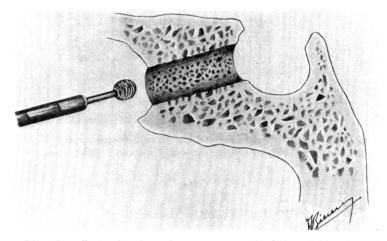

Fig. 113. Method of approaching the sella turcica through a non-pneumatized "conchal" sphenoid bone by first making a tunnel with an air-driven diamond drill.

the sella turcica so that the anterior aspect of the floor is in line with the tuberculum sellae. Since the floor does not bulge into the sphenoid cavity, it has to be located indirectly with the aid of the televised radiofluoroscopic control. It is encountered in 11% of cases.

The "Conchal" Type

This type of sinus is not pneumatized at all the sphenoid cavity being completely filled with cancellous bone. This rare variety is encountered in 3% of cases and presents a theoretical contraindication to the trans-sphenoidal approach to the sella turcica. The autor has encountered this variety in 6 patients, and has overcome the problem as follows: a tunnel was first made through the cancellous bone with a diamond drill until the sella region was reached (Fig. 113);

thereafter, the hypophysectomy could be performed in the usual manner.

It is important also to make frontal tomograms in order to study the width of the floor of the sella and to identify the position of the intra-sphenoidal septum relative to the midline.

Since direct visualization of the intrasellar contents is accomplished through the *open* procedure with the operating microscope, it is not considered necessary to perform pre-operative angiograms (carotid or retrograde jugular injection) (Rand, Hanafee 1967). However, when the operation entails the insertion of probes into the wound, it would be important to recognize incidental anatomical variations of malpositioning of the surrounding vascular structures (Forrest et al. 1959, Rand et al. 1962 and 1964, Talairach et al. 1962 and 1966, Zervas 1965, Bergland et al. 1968).

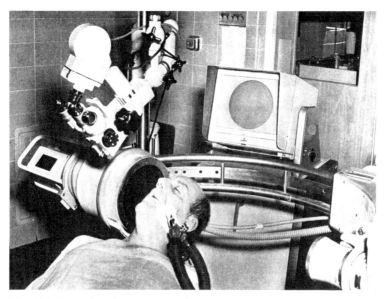

Fig. 114. Operating theater prepared for transsphenoidal surgery with the combined use of televised radiofluoroscopic control and the binocular operating microscope.

Preparation and Positioning

After Pentothal induction, light general anesthesia is maintained, with the endotracheal tube placed in the angle of the mouth. The pharyngeal cavity is packed with moist sponges in order to prevent aspiration into the bronchial tree.

The patient is placed in a semi-sitting position on the operating table and the head is firmly attached to the occipital rest. A mobile image amplifier is then positioned at the side of the head, so that the horizontal beam is centered on the sella turcica (Fig. 114). The television screen is placed just behind and above the head of the patient so that the surgeon can view it in line with the eyepiece of the microscope (Fig. 115). A video-tape recording may be obtained directly from the image intensifier for record purposes. Radiofluoroscopic control is utilized as required during the operative procedure; this is monitored with a foot pedal by the surgeon or his assistant. No more than a few seconds of radiation ex-posure are necessary at each stage of the operation, in order to ensure accurate placement of the instruments in the sella turcica. The staff in the operating theater are protected by appropriate lead shielding and aprons.

Next the patient's face, mouth and nasal cavity are prepared with an aqueous antiseptic solution (Zephiran). Infiltration of the nasal mucosa and the upper alveolar surface with 0.5% procaine containing adrenaline 1:2000 is useful for initiating the submucosal elevation as well as in reducing oozing from the mucosa.

An adhesive Vidrape covers the entire face and further sterile draping of the operative field ensures complete isolation and sterility of the procedure. A button-hole is made in the Vidrape at the level of the upper lip and sterile sponges are introduced into the mouth, so that only the upper alveolar margin is exposed.

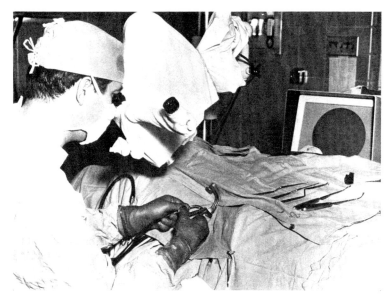

Fig. 115. Position of the surgeon for simultaneous viewing through the microscope and on the television screen.

Techniques:

The Subnasal Midline Transsphenoidal Approach

Of the various transsphenoidal procedures described e.g. transmaxillary, orbito-ethmoidal, lateral endonasal, the author has adopted the direct midline subnasal rhinoseptal route because of the definitive advantages that it offers (Guiot 1958). The main reason is that it respects a fundamental principle of surgical anatomy which obliges the surgeon to approach the sella turcica in the median sagittal plane. Adequate exposure and symmetrical visualization of the intrasellar contents enables the safest dissection to be carried out and avoids the risks of trauma to the surrounding neurovascular structures; the risks are greater with an oblique route. The most accurate description of this procedure is "The Oronasal-rhinoseptal-Transsphenoidal Approach to the Sella Turcica". Each of these terms is relevant, and corresponds to a definite step in the procedure (Figs. 116a—b):

ORAL: horizontal incision beneath the upper lip at the junction of the alveolar margin, extending to the canine fossa on either side.

NASAL: elevation of the incised upper lip and exposure of the nasal bony cavum. A sharp ridge of the upper maxilla is removed as well as the ascending rami in order to enlarge the nasal bony orifice. This ensures a better grip for the serrated nasal speculum.

RHINAL: after removal of the anterior nasal spinous process, the mucosa of the floor of the nose is elevated and reflected from both sides of the nasal septum as well. This is quick and easy to perform, since the mucosa has already been partially detached by previous procaine infiltration. A special serrated bivalve speculum is now inserted into the submucosal cavity thus formed, and after it has been opened up laterally it holds the elevated nasal mucosa apart.

SEPTAL: the inferior third of the anterior cartilaginous septum is resected with a swivelled-knife exposing the vomer bone which has the appearance of the keel of a

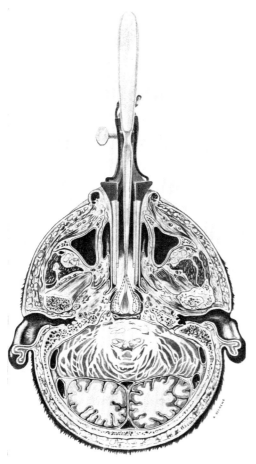

Fig. 116a

Fig. 116a—b. The subnasal midline rhinoseptal transsphenoidal approach to the sella turcica; a) horizontal section; b) sagittal section.

boat. Occasional septal deviation would thus be corrected at this step.

TRANSSPHENOIDAL: the vomer is then detached and removed. When occasionally a thick or "acromegalic" vomer is encountered, it has to be resected piecemeal with a gouge. Further resection of the anterior aspect of the sphenoid floor gives a wide exposure of the entire sinus cavity.

The mucosa is pierced and deflected. If bony septa are encountered, they are removed, until the entire posterior aspect of the sinus

has been widely exposed and the floor of the sella identified. Its boundaries are carefully located under direct vision as well as by means of fluoroscopic control. The upper recess underneath the tuberculum sellae defines the upper limit of the opening. Laterally, the use of a blunt instrument allows the groove formed by the bulging carotid artery within the carotid canal to be defined.

The sellar floor is opened first in the midline and then resected piecemeal with small angled rongeurs until a window of about one square centimeter in area has been achieved.

The binocular operating microscope is then positioned so that the operative cavity can be directly and well illuminated (see Fig. 114). The additional eyepiece of the microscope may be used by the assistant, as well as attachments for photographic and cine cameras. A television optical camera can also be attached to the eyepiece so that the magnified operative field can be transmitted simultaneously on the television screen in the operating theater and to a large screen in an amphitheatre for teaching purposes.

Total Hypophysectomy

After the defect in the floor of the sella has been enlarged to an adequate size, the dural sheath is now exposed. A cruciate incision is made in the dura strictly in the midline and special care is taken not to enter the hypophyseal capsule (Fig. 117a).

By gentle pressure on the gland, the *extracapsular* plane of cleavage can be identified. Dissection is commenced on the superior surface of the pituitary until the stalk and the diaphragmatic orifice are encountered (Fig. 117b). If the latter is large (6×6 mm.), there is often a diverticulum of the arachnoid within the sellar cavity which can be seen well and protected with a cotton-wool pledget — tearing of this diverticulum is followed by leakage of cerebrospinal fluid. A "sickle" knife with an inner cutting edge was developed especially to perform a low stalk section

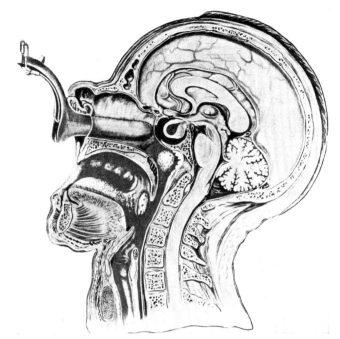

Fig. 116 b.

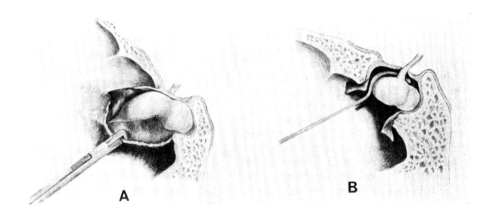

Fig. 117A—F. Technique of total extracapsular enucleation of the normal pituitary with low stalk section. For details, see description in text.

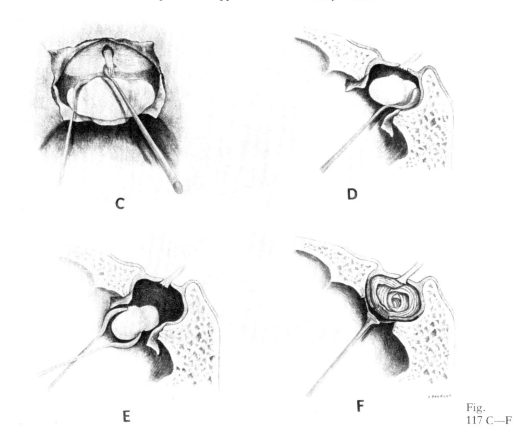

C

D

E

F

Fig.
117 C—F

at its junction with the gland (Fig. 117c). After separation, the stalk retracts upwards to hang freely.

Dissection is now continued laterally, anteriorly and posteriorly with an enucleator, in order to separate the entire surface of the pituitary capsule from its dural attachments (Fig. 117d). Each step requiring the introduction of instruments into the sella is television monitored for a few seconds at the time (see Figs. 118a—c). This is very useful, especially in patients in whom the dorsum sellae is soft and decalcified. Moreover, when the orifice of the pituitary diaphragm is wide open, radiological control prevents the surgeon from introducing his instruments above the theoretical limit of the diaphragm sellae. After the whole gland has been enucleated *extracapsularly*, it herniates into the sellar window and is removed intact in one piece

(Fig. 117e). Slight oozing from detachment of the inferior hypophyseal veins is easily controlled with Gelfoam.

The sellar cavity is then packed with a piece of muscle previously taken from the patient's thigh; this is introduced with gentle pressure. When fluid leakage takes place in the presence of a large diaphragmatic orifice, a patch of fascia lata is applied beneath the diaphragm before the muscle is inserted.

Adequate sealing is further accomplished by inserting cartilaginous graft from the previously removed septum. Being carved a little larger than the opening, it remains trapped against the inner rim of the floor of the sella. This technical refinement is necessary to prevent herniation of the muscle pack and postoperative fluid leakage (Hardy 1967).

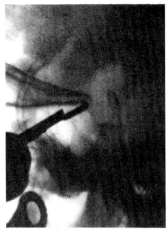 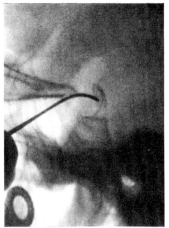 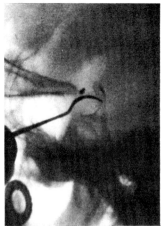

Fig. 118a   Fig. 118b   Fig. 118c

Fig. 118a—c. Steps in the televised radiofluoroscopic control during microsurgical dissection; a, opening the floor of the sella; b, commencing the extracapsular dissection of the gland on its upper surface; c, the marker indicates the position of the cotton-wool pledget inserted to protect the stalk.

Selective Anterior Pituitary Ablation

The excellent view obtained with the operating microscope has permitted a further refinement in technique making it possible, in several cases, to achieve a selective and complete ablation of the anterior pituitary (Hardy, Ciric 1968). This method was attempted in a selected series of patients suffering from diabetic retinopathy, in order to provide further information about the basic physiopathogenic mechanism of the condition. The project was suggested by the case of Poulsen (1953), a patient with selective necrosis of the anterior pituitary which was followed by complete remission of the diabetic retinopathy, and which was confirmed at autopsy 15 years later (Poulsen, 1966).

Pertinent remarks concerning the possibility of achieving a selective anterior hypophysectomy are based on histological studies of frozen sphenoid blocks from cadavers (Hardy, Schaub) correlated with the anatomical findings in operated patients. These are:

a) The anterior pituitary lobe is surrounded in life by a virtual space. In the cadaver this can be easily identified as a real space filled with venous capillaries between the dural sheath and the hypophyseal capsule (Fig. 119 A). This constant anatomical finding is the basis for the important technical detail of identifying the *extracapsular plane of cleavage* in order to initiate the dissection of the anterior lobe. The hypophyseal capsule is well recognized under the microscope because of its glistening appearance. Any disruption of this capsule may lead to false dissection, resulting in hypophyseal fragments remaining in the sella turcica.

b) The posterior lobe in contrast, both in life and in cadavers is usually firmly adherent to the posterior wall of the sella turcica, being embedded in a shallow depression on the anterior aspect of the dorsum sellae (Fig. 119 B). The line of cleavage between the anterior and the posterior lobe is provided by the intermediate lobe, which is a strip of tissue containing many vacuoles filled with colloid substance and venous capillaries (Fig. 119 C). Its loose attachment permits separation between the glandular and the neural lobe.

Dissection of the anterior pituitary is commenced along its superior surface and continued until the stalk and the orifice of the

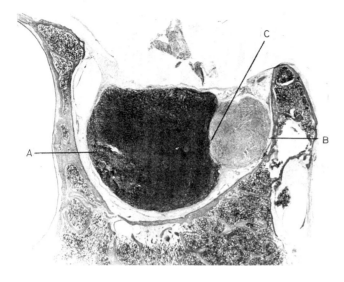

Fig. 119. Microsurgical anatomy of the pituitary fossa: A, extra-capsular plane of cleavage surrounding the anterior lobe; B, adherence of the posterior lobe to the posterior aspect of the sella turcica; C, line of cleavage between the anterior and posterior lobes.

diaphragma sellae are encountered. A small cotton-wool pledget is then applied against the stalk which is depressed backwards while the anterior lobe is pressed downwards, in order to initiate the separation of the two lobes (Fig. 120a). The cotton-wool pledget is then inserted further between the two lobes, thus protecting the posterior lobe. The dissection is continued laterally on either side and inferiorly until the whole anterior lobe is completely detached and enucleated (Fig. 120b).

When viewed through the operating microscope (16-fold magnification), the two lobes of the hypophysis possess completely different colors. While the anterior lobe is yellowish through its glistening capsule and becomes white under pressure, the posterior lobe is more gelatinous and with the stalk appears reddish-grey due to their rich capillary network. Any remaining fragments are, therefore, clearly visible and easily detached. The pars tuberalis sometimes surrounds the pituitary stalk like a collar. In some of the author's own cases it was possible to peel it off easily: in other cases, in which both lobes were firmly adherent, it was not possible to perform a selective anterior hypophysectomy. In these cases a low stalk section was then carried out with total extracapsular pituitary ablation as described above (see Fig. 117).

This method of selective anterior ablation has been attempted in a series of thirty patients and could be successfully accomplished with histological verification in nineteen (Fig. 121). In the remaining eleven a complete pituitary ablation was carried out after sectioning of the pituitary stalk. In the group of diabetic patients who underwent selective anterior pituitary ablation, this experimental clinical investigation supports the theory of a purely hormonal anterior pituitary mechanism rather than a neural mechanism involved in the pathophysiology of the diabetic retinopathy (Wolter, Knoblich 1965). The details of the authors' series are published elsewhere (Hardy 1968).

Microsurgical Selective Removal of Pituitary Adenoma with Preservation of the Normal Hypophysis

In previous papers (Hardy 1962, Hardy, Wigser 1965) the relative indications for transsphenoidal removal of pituitary fossa tumors have been discussed in detail. In particular, the indispensable role of televised radiofluoroscopic control for the adequate removal of midline suprasellar expansions has been stressed, combined with peroperative pneumoencephalography. These are neces-

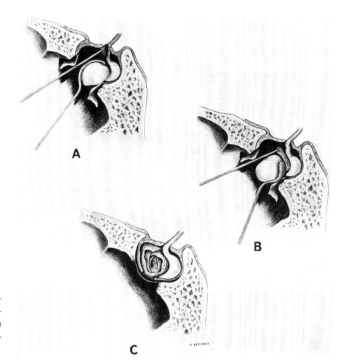

Fig. 120 A—C. Technique of microsurgical selective anterior pituitary ablation with preservation of the neurohypophysis. For details, see description in text.

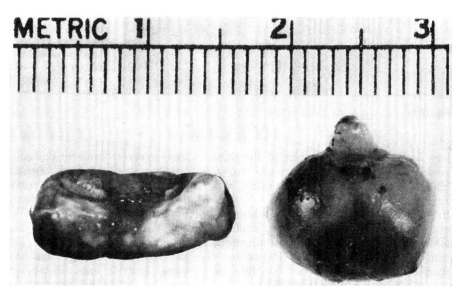

Fig. 121. Surgical specimens of: a, selective anterior lobe removal; b, total extracapsular pituitary ablation with low stalk section.

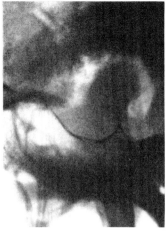

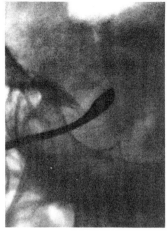

Fig. 122a — b. Televised radio-fluoroscopic monitoring performed during removal of a pituitary tumor with a suprasellar expansion.

Fig. 122a   Fig. 122b

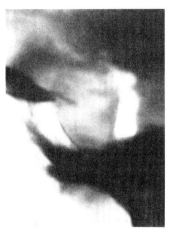

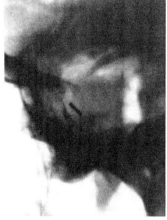

Fig. 123a. Preoperative pneumogram showing a large suprasellar tumor expansion.

Fig. 123b. Postoperative pneumogram confirming the complete removal by refilling of the chiasmatic cistern with air and the clip marker attached to the collapsed diaphragma sellae.

Fig. 123a   Fig. 123b

sary for visualizing the return of the third ventricle to its normal position and the refilling of the suprachiasmatic cistern with air (Figs. 122, 123).

In some of the large pituitary adenomas, even the tumor cavity has been explored under the microscope. This has permitted further curetting of residual fragments of neoplastic tissue to be carried out, thus ensuring a more complete removal.

It has also been possible, with the microscopical method of dissection, to distinguish clearly in several cases the remnant of normal hypophyseal tissue from the pathological adenomatous tissue. During removal of the adenoma by fragments with blunt dissecting instruments and aspiration, grey-reddish soft tissue, white gelatinous or dark purple necrotic material can easily be differentiated from the yellow-orange firm tissue of the normal anterior lobe. Usually the normal tissue lies in the posterior part of the enlarged sella, having the appearance of a thin tongue of tissue, or the entire lobe may have retained its nodular appearance. A correlation between the size and shape of the remnant of normal pituitary tissue and the preoperative endocrine deficit was possible in some cases. For example: the patient illustrated in Fig. 123 presented with a visual defect but no hormonal insufficiency. At operation a normal pear-shaped anterior lobe was found lying posterolaterally in the sella (Fig. 124), embedded in a mass of pathological adenomatous tissue which was completely excised. Postoperatively, normal vision returned within three days and the patient required no hormonal substitutes. Endocrine studies twelve days later were entirely normal.

Of eleven cases submitted to microsurgical dissection and tumor removal, normal pituitary glandular tissue was identified and preserved in ten cases. None of these patients required hormonal substitutes. The eleventh patient subsequently showed a pituitary insufficiency requiring replacement therapy; during the operation in this case, the normal pituitary tissue had been recognized but accidently aspirated during the dissection.

Microsurgical Selective Removal of Intrapituitary Microadenoma

In three cases of acromegaly without detectable radiological adenoma and with elevated growth hormone levels, the microsurgical exploration of the sella turcica revealed the presence of a small intrapituitary microadenoma which could be selectively removed, resulting in clinical improvement of the acromegaly, reduction of the growth hormone levels and the development of no other pituitary disturbance.

One of these patients presented with severe and advanced skeletal deformities af acromegaly. The sella turcica was apparently only slightly enlarged. A fractional pneumoencephalogram and cisternogram revealed a large diaphragmatic orifice and the air actually entered the sella turcica, ruling out the presence of an expanding pituitary adenoma (Fig. 125). A transsphenoidal microsurgical exploration revealed a microadenoma, 5 mm. in diameter, sharply delineated at the antero-inferior pole of the anterior lobe. It was

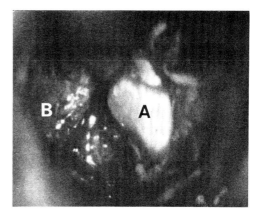

Fig. 124. Operative magnified view of: A, the normal anterior pituitary which was found intact and preserved, during selective microsurgical removal of B, the chromophobe adenomatous tissue.

selectively removed. The preoperative growth hormone level of 32 ngr. dropped to 5 ngr. after the operation. The patient was clinically improved and required no hormonal substitution.

Another interesting case that illustrates the value of microsurgical exploration of the sella turcica, is that of a 39-year-old woman with thyrotoxic exophthalmos. Following thyroidectomy, the exophthalmos grew worse and endocrinological assays demonstrated a persistently high level of the long-action thyroid factor. The endocrinologist recommended operation, and within the normal sella turcica a very small cystic adenoma was found which could be well identified and selectively removed from the surrounding normal pituitary tissue. The patient presented no pituitary deficit postoperatively and within a few months the exophthalmos had diminished.

Another patient, suffering from Cushing's syndrome, underwent microsurgical exploration of the sella turcica, and a microadenoma was removed with preservation of the normal pituitary tissue. The clinical features of Cushing's syndrome regressed completely. Two years later the patient married, and has subsequently successfully conceived.

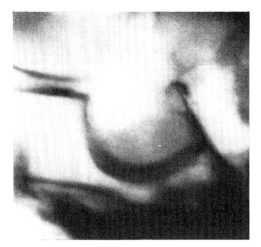

Fig. 125a. A case of acromegaly. Preoperative cisternography, ruling out the presence of an expanding pituitary adenoma.

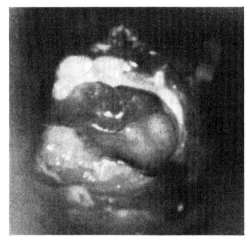

Fig. 125b. Operative magnified view of an eosinophilic microadenoma herniating from the normal-sized pituitary during microsurgical selective removal.

These cases illustrate the possibility of obtaining a clinical cure of hyperpituitarism without inducing pituitary insufficiency. On the basis of this limited experience of microsurgical exploration of the sella turcica, it would seem that hyperpituitarism is associated with a well circumscribed nodular microadenoma (O'Neal 1968) in the pituitary parenchyma rather than with diffuse hyperplasia of the pituitary glandular tissue. Early microsurgical removal of the microadenomas responsible for hyperpituitarism represents the ideal treatment of this pathological entity (Fig. 126). Also the fact that amenorrhoea-galactorrhoea is often associated with a normal sella turcica, does not rule out the presence of an intrapituitary microadenoma. It would, therefore, be logical to include microsurgical exploration of the sella as an additional diagnostic procedure in cases of well-documented clinical pituitary disorders. The early detection and selective removal of an intrapituitary microadenoma would prevent further pituitary insufficiency and even favour the restoration of function.

Provided the microsurgical removal of the pituitary adenoma has been complete, the author does not routinely sumbit the patients to radiotherapy postoperatively.

However, in view of the risk of possible recurrence of the tumor, advantage is taken of the transsphenoidal approach and of collapse of the diaphragma sellae. A metallic clip is left attached as a marker for repeated follow up plain radiography of the pituitary fossa (see Fig. 123).

In the event of a recurrence, the earliest sign would be elevation of the clip, even before the defect of vision. Radiotherapy would then be given at once. In this series, none of the cases of benign pituitary adenoma which have undergone a verified complete radical microsurgical extirpation have so far presented evidence of tumor recurrence.

Summary

The microsurgical technique has contributed to significant progress in the modern neurosurgery of the pituitary gland, when combined with the extracranial transsphenoidal approach and televised radiofluoroscopic control.

The magnified view obtained with the binocular operating microscope allows anatomical variants of the intrasellar contents to be identified and reduces the risk of trauma of the surrounding anatomical structures.

The microscopic dissection of the pituitary with special instruments confirms the completeness of the extracapsular pituitary to the surgeon. It also permits a more precise identification of the two lobes of the hypophysis, so that a more selective ablation of the anterior pituitary becomes possible in the treatment of diabetic retinopathy.

In the treatment of pituitary adenoma, the radical removal of the tumor can be accomplished with identification and preservation of the normal glandular pituitary remnant, occasionally leading to complete restoration of the pituitary function.

By microsurgical exploration of the sella turcica, it is even possible to identify and remove selectively an intrapituitary microadenoma with preservation of the normal hypophysis, as applied in the treatment of hyperpituitarism.

Because of the relatively harmless nature of the transsphenoidal procedure, the rapidity and accuracy of the technique, the adequacy of the surgical exposure and visualization of the intrasellar contents with the binocular operating microscope, it is forecast that microsurgical exploration of the sella turcica will eventually become an additional diagnostic procedure in cases of welldocumented clinical pituitary disorder. The early detection and selective removal of an intrapituitary microadenoma with preservation of the normal anterior pituitary confirms a fundamental principle in the therapeutic management of analogous benign lesions elsewhere in the human body.

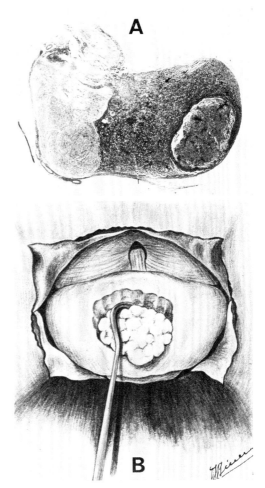

Fig. 126. A) Pathological specimen, a chance finding in a cadaver, showing a well circumscribed nodular intrapituitary microadenoma. B) selective microsurgical removal of an intrapituitary microadenoma.

References

Bergland, R. M., B. S. Ray, R. M. Torack: Anatomical variations in the pituitary gland and adjacent structures in 225 human autopsy cases. J. Neurosurg. 28 (1968) 93

Forrest, A. P., D. W. Blair, D. A. Brown, H. J. Stewart, A. T. Sandison, R. W. Harrington, J. M. Valentine, P. T. Carter: Radioactive implantation of pituitary. Brit. J. Surg. 47 (1959) 61

Guiot, G. et al.: Adénomes Hypophysaires. Masson, Paris 1958

Hamberger, C. A., G. Hammer, G. Norlén, B. Siögren: Transsphenoidal hypophysectomy. Arch. Otolaryng. 74 (1961) 2

Hardy, J.: L'exérèse des adénomes hypophysaires par voie trans-sphénoidale. Un. méd. Canada 91 (1962) 933

Hardy, J., S. M. Wigser: Transsphenoidal surgery of pituitary fossa tumours with televised radiofluoroscopic control. J. Neurosurg. 23 (1965) 612

Hardy, J.: La chirurgie de l'hypophyse par voie transsphénoidale ouverte. Étude comparative de deux modalités techniques. Ann. Chir. 21 (1967) 1011

Hardy, J., I. Ciric: Selective anterior hypophysectomy for treatment of diabetic retinopathy: A transsphenoidal microsurgical technique. J. amer. med. Ass. 203 (1968) 73

Hardy, J., A. Panisset, A. Marchildon, A. Lanthier: Transsphenoidal microsurgical selective anterior pituitary ablation: a pathophysiological investigation of diabetic retinopathy. Presented at the Airlie Symposium on Diabetic Retinopathy, Warrenton, Va. 1—2 Oct. 1968 (in press).

Hardy, J., C. Schaub: Microsurgical anatomy of the pituiarty fossa (in press).

O'Neal, L. W.: Correlation between clinical pattern and pathological findings in Cushing's syndrome. Med. Clin. N. Amer. 52 (1968) 313

Poulsen, J. E.: Houssay's phenomenon in man; recovery from retinopathy in a case of diabetes with Simmond's disease. Diabetes 2 (1953) 7

Poulsen, J. E.: Diabetes and anterior pituitary insufficiency: Final course and post-mortem study of a diabetic patient with Sheehan's syndrome. Diabetes 15 (1966) 73

Rand, R. W., W. N. Hanafee: Cavernous sinus venography and stereotaxic cryo-hypophysectomy. J. Neurosurg. 26 (1967) 521

Rand, R. W., A. M. Dashe, D. H. Solomon, J. L. Westover, P. H. Crandall, J. Brown, R. Tranquada: Stereotaxic Yttrium-90 hypophysectomy for metastatic mammary carcinoma. Ann. Surg. 156 (1962) 986

Rand, R. W., A. M. Dashe, D. E. Paglia: Stereotaxic cryo-hypophysectomy. J. amer. med. Ass. 189 (1964) 255

Talairach, J. et al: La chirurgie stéréotaxique hypophysaire. Confin. neurol. (Basel) 22 (1962) 204

Talairach, J., R. Sedan, G. Szikla, A. Bonis, C. Schaub, M. Harder: La chirurgie stéréotaxique de l'hypophyse non-tumorale par les radioisotopes. Neuro-chir. Paris 12 (1966) 141

Wolter, J. R., R. R. Knoblich: Pathway of centrifugal fibres in the human optic nerve, chiasm and tract. Brit. J. ophthal. 49 (1965) 246

Zervas, N. T.: Technique of radiofrequency hypophysectomy. Confin. neurol. (Basel) 26 (1965) 157

CHAPTER 8

Oto-Neurosurgical Operations

Transtemporal Extralabyrinthine Operations on the Internal Auditory Canal, the Eighth and the Seventh Cranial Nerves

The transtemporal Extralabyrinthine Approach to the Internal Auditory Canal

Exposure of the superior surface of the petrous pyramid by elevation of the temporal dura after removing the squamous part of the temporal bone has been carried out by otologists since the turn of the century. It has been used for the evacuation of purulent material from the apex of the petrous pyramid (Eagleton 1930, Hilgermann 1933, Streit 1938, Unterberger 1938), also in the operative treatment of otosclerosis (dural elevation over the tegmen tympani, Wittmaack 1933) and for the extrapyramidal fenestration of the superior semicircular canal (Wullstein 1952). By the same route the Glasgow surgeon Parry (1904) exposed the internal auditory canal in a patient with severe Menière's disease and sectioned the auditory nerve. During the course of this operation Parry inadvertently damaged the facial nerve. This unfortunate incident is probably why the transtemporal approach to the internal auditory canal was then abandoned. Until quite recently the approach to the eighth nerve has been exclusively through the transoccipital intracranial route described by the American neurosurgeon Dandy.

It is to the credit of William F. House (1961) to have demonstrated that with the aid of microsurgical techniques the internal auditory canal can be reached from the middle cranial fossa, without damaging the facial nerve. Since 1962 this operative approach has been utilized by neurosurgeons as well

(Kurze, Doyle 1962). Its potential scope is still partly unexplored.

The principle of the transtemporal or middle cranial fossa approach to the internal auditory canal is illustrated diagrammatically in Fig. 127.

The internal auditory meatus is exposed through the bone after a temporal craniotomy and elevation of the dura from the floor of the middle cranial fossa. The technical details are illustrated in Fig. 128. The patient is placed supine with the head rotated. The surgeon is seated at the head of the operating table. The squamous temporal bone is exposed by a preauricular skin incision extending from the base of the zygomatic arch to the upper margin of the temporalis muscle (Fig. 128a). The squamous portion of the temporal bone is exposed through a cross incision of the temporalis muscle (Fig. 128b). A 4×3 cm. craniotomy flap is then prepared with the aid of a cutting drill, so that the base of the zygomatic arch lies in the middle of its lower rim (Fig. 128c). The lower edge of the craniotomy is carried as deep as possible with a bone rongeur to the level of the floor of the middle cranial fossa (Fig. 128d). After this, the dura can be elevated step by step with the aid of the operating microscope from the superior surface of the petrous pyramid as far as its posterior rim, until the space between the arcuate eminence and the hiatus of the facial canal is exposed. Dural detachment should be undertaken from behind forwards in order to avoid damage to the greater superficial petrosal nerve which is closely attached to the dura.

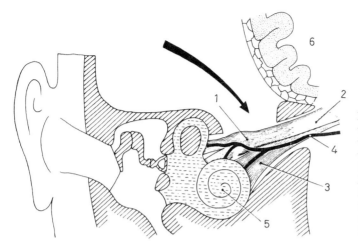

Fig. 127. Schematic illustration of the transtemporal extralabyrinthine approach to the internal auditory meatus. 1 = vestibular (Scarpa's ganglion) 2 = vestibular nerve, 3 = cochlear nerve, 4 = arterial system of the internal auditory canal, 5 = cochlea, 6 = temporal lobe.

Particular care should be also taken in the region of the geniculate ganglion. This structure was found to lie free under the dura in 3 out of 70 cases (see also House 1963 and Rhoton et al. 1968). The blood vessels running between the upper surface of the petrous pyramid and the dura are cauterized using bipolar coagulation. Retraction of the temporal lobe is facilitated by drainage of the cerebrospinal fluid through a small incision in the temporal dura, as well as by the use of a selfretaining mechanical retractor with a Cushing spatula (Fig. 128e).

House (1963 and 1964) uses the facial nerve as the landmark to locate the internal auditory canal through the hard compact bone of the labyrinthine capsule. For this purpose the facial nerve must be identified after removal of the bone overlaying the proximal part of the greater superficial petrosal nerve and the geniculate ganglion, and then exposed proximally to the level of the fundus of the internal auditory meatus. The bone work is performed with a diamond drill under continuous irrigation with Ringer's solution. Accidental opening into the cavities of the inner ear (basal turn of the cochlea, vestibule or superior semicircular canal) is to be avoided, since it may lead to loss of function of the inner ear (House 1963)

The author uses a modification of the technique described by House. It is preferable to identify the internal auditory canal following exposure of the superior semicircular canal and thus avoid extensive dissection of the facial nerve (Figs. 129, 130). The superior semicircular canal is exposed with a diamond drill (under continuous irrigation) its position being easily recognized through the thin transparent layer of bone as a faint greyish-blue line (Figs. 129a, 130a). The arcuate eminence is used as landmark for the localization of the blue line of the superior semicircular canal. The latter lies, however, somewhat further forwards and medially, against the tip of the petrous pyramid, rather than directly under it. The continuous irrigation-suction during the bone work is essential and invaluable for removing particles of bone dust as they are produced by the diamond burr and in order to give to the bone the necessary transparency. During drilling the hard compact bone of the labyrinthine capsule surrounding the superior semicircular canal is easily distinguished from the remaining lamellar, mostly pneumatized bone (Fig. 130a). In some rare instances — 2 per cent of the cases — the blue line of the superior semicircular canal is visible through the intact bone immediately after reflection of the dura. The blue line of the superior semicircular canal is the *only landmark* necessary for locating the internal auditory canal. The internal auditory meatus is situated immediately in front of the superior semicircular canal under a layer of

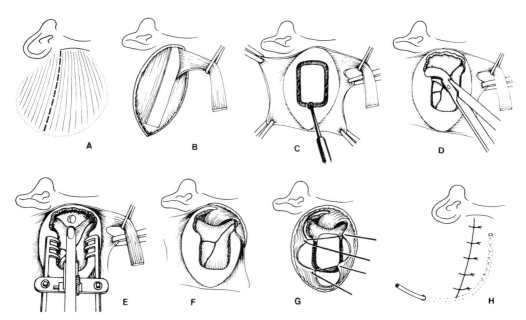

Fig. 128. Surgical stages of the transtemporal extralabyrinthine approach to the internal auditory meatus. A, skin incision. B, exposure of the squamous part of the temporal bone through a cross incision in the temporalis muscle. C, the craniotomy is performed with the cutting drill. D, extension of the craniotomy to the floor of the middle cranial fossa with bone rongeur. E, retraction of the temporal dura with a mechanical selfretaining retractor and exposure of the internal auditory canal. F, the craniotomy flap is replaced. G, closure of the skin incision after the introduction of a suction drain (Redon).

bone varying in thickness and in degree of pneumatization. In searching for it, it is best to drill a bony sector centered over the superior ampulla and limited posteriorly by the exposed blue line of the superior semicircular canal and anteriorly by an imaginary line forming an angle of 60° with it (Fig. 129). The bone is carefully removed in this area with the diamond drill staying as close as possible to the blue line until the dural sheath of the meatus becomes visible. Again, the meatal dural sac appears through the last thin layer of bone as a greyish-blue area. Starting from this point the entire roof of the meatal dural sac is then exposed from the fundus to the region of the porus (Fig. 130b). A bony rim is left in the region of the porus in order to support the tip of the retractor blade. It is usually possible at this stage to identify through the thin dural sheath the contents of the internal auditory canal

(Figs. 129c, 130b). The vestibular and facial nerves lie in the superior half of the meatus very close to one another. The vestibular nerve is posterior taking a straight course forward in the direction of the superior ampulla. The facial nerve runs just anterior and closely applied to the vestibular nerve bending forward at the meatal fundus in order to reach the entrance of the Fallopian canal. The vestibular and facial nerves can be differentiated with certainty when they are exposed for a short distance through the bone distal to the region of the meatal fundus.

It is now possible to proceed with the *intradural part* of the operation, i. e. to the opening of the meatal dural sac (Fig. 129c). The incision into the dura is made along the posterior (dorsal) rim of the meatus, since the risk of damaging underlying nerves and vessels is least at this site. The bulging

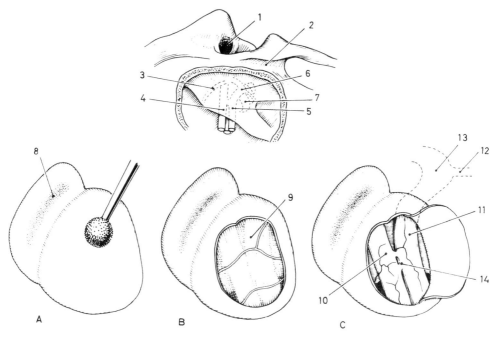

Fig. 129. Identification of the internal auditory canal by the transtemporal extralabyrinthine approach using the superior semicircular canal as unique landmark. On the top of the figure the relationship of the external auditory canal (1), the root of the zygomatic arch (2), the superior semicircular canal (3), the vestibular nerve (4), the facial nerve (5), the geniculate ganglion (6), and the basal turn of the cochlea (7) are demonstrated. A, location of the blue line (8) of the superior semicircular canal and removal of the bone laying in a sector of 60° anterior and medial to it with the diamond drill. B, exposure of the dural sac (9) of the internal auditory meatus. C, view of the content of the internal canal. The auditory vestibular nerve (10), the facial nerve (11) and the vestibulo-facial anastomosis (14) are exposed. The position of the geniculate ganglion (13) and of the greater superficial petrosal nerve (12) is given by the dotted line.

arachnoid is then pierced to release the cerebrospinal fluid from the cerebellopontine cistern. Damage to the arachnoid attachement fixing the vestibular and facial nerves to the roof of the meatus should be avoided, to prevent these nerves sinking on to the floor of the canal. When the dural sac is open the structures within the auditory canal are inspected (Figs. 131, 132). The vestibular and facial nerves as well as the anastomotic fibers between them, the so-called vestibulo-facial anastomoses (Penzo 1893, Shute 1951, House 1964) are clearly seen. In the region of the fundus the vestibular and facial nerves diverge making it easier to find a plane of cleavage between them. The larger superior ramus of the vestibular nerve completely covers the two smaller inferior divisions, the posterior ampullar and the saccular nerves (Figs. 131, 132). The vestibular ganglion (Scarpa's) in contrast to most anatomical drawings and in spite of the use of the operating microscope is difficult to distinguish from the vestibular trunk (Fig. 131). The cochlear nerve is covered by the facial nerve and with its accompanying arteries follows an anterior course entering the modiolus of the cochlear at the level of the transverse crest. In order to expose the cochlear nerve it is, therefore, necessary to apply gentle retraction on the facial nerve as it passes over the entrance of the modiolus (Fig. 132). Knowledge of the arrangement of the arterial system of the internal auditory canal

(Fisch 1968) is essential in order to avoid loss of hearing during manipulations in this area. The arterial topography is illustrated in Fig. 133.

The operations performed on the exposed internal auditory canal will be discussed in detail later. At the end of each procedure the dura is sutured to the temporalis muscle, the bone flap of the craniotomy is replaced (Fig. 128f) a suction-drain (Redon) is introduced and the wound is closed in a single layer (Fig. 128g).

Conclusion

The use of the operating microscope and diamond drill dissection under continuous irrigation permits exposure of the internal auditory canal extradurally, through the middle cranial fossa, without damage to the facial nerve or the inner ear structures.

The choice of the superior semicircular canal as the sole essential landmark to identify the internal auditory canal through the petrous pyramid has proven quick and safe. Anatom-

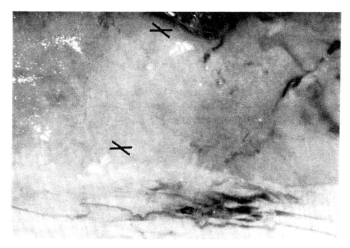

Fig. 130a—b.   Identification and exposure of the internal auditory meatus using the blue line of the superior semicircular canal as unique landmark (left side). A, demonstration of the blue line of the superior semicircular canal (X-X) following removal of the surrounding compact labyrinthine bone. B, the bone situated in a sector of 60°, centered over the superior ampulla has been removed staying very close to the blue line of the superior semicircular canal exposing the dural lining of the internal auditory meatus. Through the thin dural sac the vestibular (V) and facial (F) nerves are visible. Note the relationship between the exposed blue line and the vestibular nerve. The vestibular and facial nerves diverge in the region of the meatal fundus. The greater superficial petrosal nerve (npsm) is seen in the upper right corner of the figure.

Fig. 130a

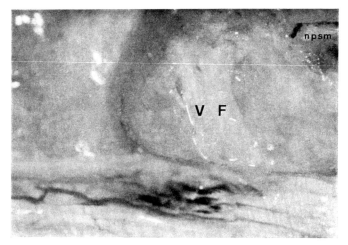

Fig. 130b

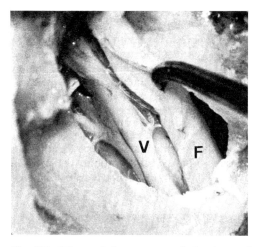

Fig. 131. View of the content of the internal auditory canal (left side). The facial nerve (F) has been gently reflected forwards. The superior branch of the vestibular nerve (V) lays over the transverse crest. The inferior branch divides under the crest into the saccular and posterior ampullary (singular) nerves.

ical studies have shown and surgical experience has confirmed that there is a constant relation between the superior semicircular canal and the vestibular nerve in its intrameatal course. With the present technique unnecessary exposure of the facial nerve is avoided and the risk of inadvertent damage to these structures is minimized. If the blue line of the semicircular canal is used as the unique landmark to identify the internal auditory canal the greater superficial petrosal nerve becomes a useful but not essential point of reference. In this way, elevation of the dura in the vicinity of the foramen spinosum (middle meningeal artery) and the sphenopetrous synchondrosis — which always causes bothersome bleeding — may be restricted to a minimum.

To date seventy* patients have been submitted to operation by the transtemporal extralabyrinthine route in Zürich. The details that are now given of the individual transtemporal procedures used are the result of this experience.

References

Eagleton, W. P.: Osteomyelitis der Felsenbeinpyramide. Arch. Otolaryng. 13 (1930) 386

Fisch, U.: Surgical anatomy of the so-called internal auditory artery. Proc. Xth Nobel Symposium, Stockholm 1968

Hilgermann, R.: Quoted in: Die oto-rhino-laryngologischen Operationen von H. J. Denecke, Springer, Berlin 1953

House, W. F.: Middle Cranial Fossa Approach to the Petrous Pyramid. Arch. Otolaryng. 78 (1963) 460

House, W. F.: Transtemporal bone microsurgical removal of acoustic neuromas. Arch. Otolaryng. 80 (1964) 597

House, W. F.: Surgical exposure of the internal auditory canal and its contents through the middle cranial fossa. Laryngoscope (St. Louis) 71 (1961) 1363

Kurze, T., J. B. Doyle: Extradural intracranial (middle fossa) approach to the internal auditory canal. J. Neurosurg. 19 (1962) 1033

Orzalesi F., E. Pellegrini: Sui rapporti fra i nervi intermedio e vestibulare e sulla struttura del ganglio e del nervo vestibolare nell'uomo. Arch. ital. Anat. Embriol. 31 (1933) 105

Parry, R. H.: A case of tinnitus and vertigo treated by division of the auditory nerve. J. Laryng. 19 (1904) 402

Penzo, R.: Über das Ganglion geniculi und die mit demselben zusammenhängenden Nerven. Anat. Anz. 8 (1893) 738

Rhoton, A. L., J. L. Pulec, G. M. Hall, A. S. Boyd: Absence of bone over the geniculate ganglion. J. Neurosurg. 28 (1968) 48

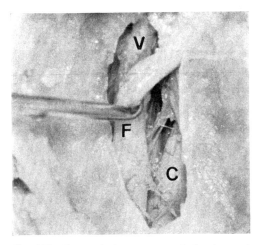

Fig. 132. View of the content of the internal auditory meatus (left side). Visualization of the cochlear nerve (C) after posterior retraction of the facial nerve (F). V, vestibular nerve.

* The first fourteen operations were performed in collaboration with Professor M. G. Yaşargil.

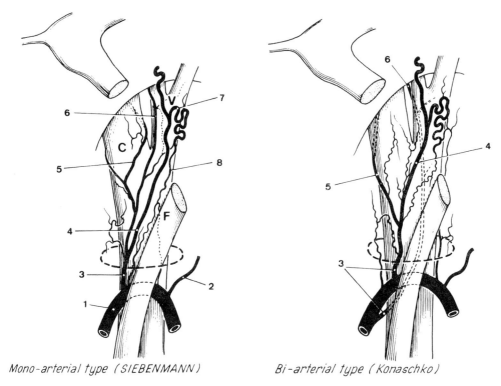

Mono-arterial type (SIEBENMANN)   *Bi-arterial type (Konaschko)*

Fig. 133. Schematic illustration of the arterial system of the internal auditory canal in man. 1, anterior inferior cerebellar artery. 2, subarcuate artery. 3, labyrinthine artery or arteries. 4, anterior vestibular artery. 5, cochlear artery. 6, vestibulocochlear artery. 7, artery of the vestibular ganglion. Two or more small arteries enter the meatus. One or two of these are the labyrinthine arteries (mono-arterial and bi-arterial type). During excision of the vestibular nerve the artery to the vestibular ganglion is sectioned. The cochlear arteries can be identified and spared.

Shute, C. C. D.: The anatomy of the eigth cranial nerve in man. Proc. Roy. Soc. Med. 44 (1951) 1013

Streit, H.: Quoted in: Hermann Beyer: Die Operationen am Ohr, 2nd Ed. Kabitzsch, Leipzig, 1938

Unterberger, S.: Quoted in: Hermann Beyer: Die Operationen am Ohr, 2nd Ed. Kabitzsch, Leipzig 1938

Wittmaack, K.: Über die operative Behandlung der Oto-sklerose mit Duralüftung am Tegmen Tympani. Klin. Wschr. 12 (1933) 658

Wullstein, H.: Die Eingriffe zur Gehörverbesserung. In: Anzeige und Ausführung der Eingriffe an Ohr, Nase und Hals, Ed. by W. Uffenorde, 2nd Ed. Thieme, Stuttgart 1952

A. Exploration of the Internal Auditory Canal in Cases of Suspected Intrameatal Acoustic Neurinoma

The transtemporal extralabyrinthine approach to the internal auditory canal is indicated when clinical and radiological evaluation suggest the presence of an intrameatal acoustic neurinoma (House 1964, Johnson, House 1964, Scanlan 1964, Ziedses des Plantes 1968, Fisch, Yaşargil 1968a and 1968b, Valvassori 1966), (Fig. 134).

During the transtemporal exploration it is particularly important to remove the roof of the internal auditory canal as far as possible from the porus acousticus inwards, in order to be able to inspect not only the contents of the meatus but also the lateral aspect of the cerebellopontine angle. An intrameatal neurinoma is particularly suitable for radical resection when it remains confined to the lateral part of the internal auditory canal (causing no great disorder of the adjacent nerves and vessels) particularly if

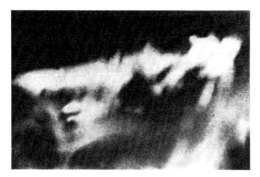

Fig. 134 a

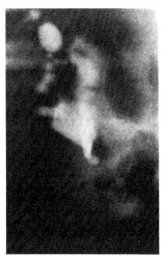

Fig. 134 b

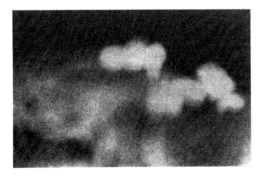

Fig. 134 c

the auditory function is still preserved. If a marked vestibular-nerve deficit is present preoperatively, it is advisable to section this nerve completely during excision of the tumor because residual vestibular function may be more troublesome to the patient than a total unilateral deficit. If the presumptive clinical diagnosis of acoustic neurinoma is not confirmed at operation, at the same sitting, a further procedure may be undertaken to relieve the vestibulo-cochlear symptoms, (see the next sections).

Conclusion

The contents of the internal auditory meatus can be easily inspected by means of transtemporal extralabyrinthine surgery. Through the described approach the risk of severe hemorrhage is practically non-existent, since the intrameatal arteries, particularly the labyrinthine arteries have a maximal diameter of 200 microns (Fisch 1968). All twelve patients submitted to transtemporal extralabyrinthine exploration experienced an uneventful postoperative course and were discharged from hospital one week after surgery. The preoperative diagnosis of an intrameatal neurinoma remains a problem. If positive contrast medium penetrates as far as the fundus of the internal auditory canal during cerebellopontine cisternography (Fig.

Fig. 134 A—C. Positive contrast visualization of the left internal auditory canal. Tomograms in Stenvers projection. A, normal filling of the internal auditory canal. Note the dye outlining portions of the facial nerve (above) and cochlear nerve (below) at the meatal fundus. B, incomplete filling of the internal auditory canal. Note the filling defect at the meatal fundus. This appearance could be produced by an early acoustic neurinoma developing from the inferior branch of the vestibular nerve. In this patient, however, at operation only a swelling in the region of the vestibular ganglion was demonstrated to cause the filling defect. C, the contrast medium has failed to enter the internal auditory canal. An acoustic neurinoma of 8 mm. length filling the entire internal auditory canal was removed at surgery.

134a), the presence of a tumor mass can be excluded. Incomplete filling, on the other hand, is not always due to an intracanalicular tumor. A very small acoustic neurinoma was suspected preoperatively in twelve personal cases. The preoperative diagnosis was confirmed surgically in only one case (Fig. 134c). In the remaining eleven cases, despite clearcut clinical and radiological signs, a swelling of the vestibular ganglion (Scarpa's) or a thickening of the arachnoid tissues ('arachnoiditis') was found (Fig. 134b) to be the cause of the filling defect observed at cisternography.

References

Fisch, U.: The surgical anatomy of the so-called internal auditory artery. Proc. Xth Nobel Symposium Stockholm 1968

Fisch, U., M. G. Yaşargil: Transtemporale, extrapyramidale Eingriffe am inneren Gehörgang. Practica oto-rhino-laryng. (Basel) 30 (1968) 377

Fisch, U., M. G. Yaşargil: Der translabyrinthäre Zugang für das Akustikus-Neurinom. Mèd. et Hyg. (Genève) 26 (1968) 1190

House, W. F.: Transtemporal bone microsurgical removal of acoustic neuromas. Arch. Otolaryng. 80 (1964) 597

House W. F., W. E. Hitselberger, B. J. Hurley: Acoustic Neuroma Diagnosis: The Adaptation of Polytomography and Iophendylate to the Early Diagnosis of Acoustic Tumors. Publ. Otol. Med. Group Los Angeles 1967

Johnson E. W., W. F. House: Auditory findings in 53 cases of acoustic neuroma. Arch. Otolaryng. 80 (1964) 667

Scanlan, R. L.: Positive contrast medium (Iophendylate) in diagnosis of acoustic neuroma. Arch. Otolaryng. 80 (1964) 698

Valvassori, G. E.: The radiological diagnosis of acoustic neuromas. Arch. Otolaryng. 83 (1966) 582

Ziedses des Plantes, B. G.: X-ray examination in cerebellopontine angle tumors. Psychiat. Neurol. Neurochir. 71 (1968) 133

B. Operations on the Vestibular Nerve

1. Selective Sectioning of the Vestibular Nerve (Vestibular Neurotomy)

Selective sectioning of both the main trunk and particularly the upper branch of the vestibular nerve has been successfully performed in the internal auditory canal by House (1961, 1963) and by Kurze, Doyle (1962) in cases of Menière's disease, as well as in cases of severe peripheral posttraumatic dizziness, Paget's disease, etc.

Conclusion

The vestibular nerve can be precisely and easily identified in the fundus of the internal auditory meatus. At this level the cochlear and vestibular fibers, which are closely applied to each other in their extramedullar course, separate, the cochlear nerve diverging anteriorly to enter the modiolus and the vestibular nerve running posteriorly to the vestibular area (Figs. 132, 135). The vestibular nerve was identified without difficulty in all 55 operations undertaken by the author with the object of sectioning these fibers. The upper branch of the vestibular nerve can be seen as soon as the meatal dura is opened. The lower branch, which divides into the saccular nerve and the posterior ampullary nerve, can be clearly identified only after sectioning of the upper branch. Relief of vertigo, and preservation or improvement of hearing in Menière's disease can only be obtained when all vestibular fibers are completely sectioned preventing their possible regeneration. This goal is best achieved if an entire segment of the vestibular nerve incl. its ganglion is removed. For this reason vestibular neurectomy was undertaken in preference to selective section of the vestibular nerve (vestibular neurotomy) after our experience with the first seven cases (Fisch, Yaşargil 1968).

2. Excision of a Segment of the Vestibular Nerve, Including the Vestibular Ganglion (Vestibular Neurectomy)

In this procedure a segment of the vestibular nerve containing the vestibular ganglion (Scarpa's) is excised within the internal auditory canal. For this purpose, the anastomoses between the vestibular and facial nerves, as well as the upper and lower branches of the vestibular nerve itself, are first sectioned as distally as possible to the meatal fundus with a fine neurotomy knife (Fig. 135).

The trunk of the vestibular nerve is reflected upwards and medially in order to enable identification and, therefore, ensure complete section of all the vestibular fibers lying underneath the transverse crest. A fine pair of

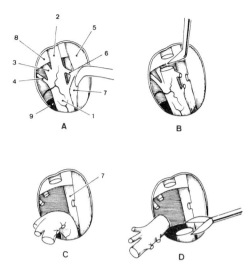

Fig. 135 A—D. Schematic illustration of the vestibular neurectomy (left side). A, identification of 1, the vestibular nerve. 2, superior branch of the vestibular nerve. 3, saccular nerve. 4, posterior ampullary (singular) nerve. 5, facial nerve, 6. vestibulo-facial anastomosis. 7, cochlear nerve. 8, transverse or falciform crest. 9, the porus acousticus internus. B, sectioning of the vestibulofacial anastomosis and the superior branch of the vestibular nerve. C, sectioning of the inferior branches of the vestibular nerve, (saccular and posterior ampullary nerves). Upward of the nerve trunk. D, excision of the dissected segment of the vestibular nerve including the vestibular ganglion.

scissors is now used to divide the dissected trunk of the vestibular nerve proximally, as close as possible to the porus. The excised segment of nerve must include the vestibular (Scarpa's) ganglion cells. The limits of the excision are then inspected again after gentle anterior reflection of the facial nerve exposing the cochlear nerve situated beneath it. The topographic arrangement of the arteries in the internal auditory canal (Fig. 133) enables one to perform a vestibular neurectomy without endangering the arteries accompanying the cochlear nerve. When the operation has been completed the exposed auditory canal is covered with a free muscle graft and with a pedicle flap from the temporalis muscle (see Section D), in order to prevent cerebrospinal fluid leakage.

Conclusion

Vestibular neurectomy was performed in forty-eight patients without complication. The indications for surgery were severe peripheral vertigo resistant to conservative treatment, particularly in patients with Menière's disease. As already mentioned, excision of a segment of the vestibular nerve is to be preferred to simple sectioning, because the improved visibility during neurectomy enables one to verify the complete division of all vestibular fibers. Vestibular neurectomy also eliminates the risk of regeneration of nerve fibers, which is possible if the section was carried out only distal to the vestibular ganglion (Wersäll 1968). Furthermore, with this procedure it is reasonable to assume that the efferent fibers of the olivo-cochlear bundle of Rasmussen (which accompany the vestibular nerve [Rasmussen 1946 and 1953]), have been included in the excised segment of nervous tissue.

The transtemporal extralabyrinthine approach is to be preferred to the transoccipital intracranial route (Dandy 1933 and 1941, McKenzie 1936, Fluur and Tovy 1965) for selective surgery on the vestibular nerve, because identification of the vestibular fibers at the fundus of the internal auditory canal is more precise than at the porus acousticus. Investigations of Rasmussen (1940) have shown that even in those few instances where two divisions of the eighth nerve may be differentiated at the porus acousticus, one nerve trunk usually consists only of vestibular fibers and the other of cochlear and vestibular fibers. Therefore, complete sectioning of the vestibular fibers by the intracranial approach implies the sacrifice of a part of the cochlear nerve (see also Dandy 1941). Moreover, the risk of damaging labyrinthine blood vessels or even the anterior inferior cerebellar artery or its branches is quite unlikely if the transtemporal extralabyrinthine approach is used (see p. and Fig. 136).

Vestibular neurectomy not only abolishes vertiginous attacks of Menière disease but also has a favourable effect on the cochlear symptoms of this disease. Thus, postoperative improvement in hearing of over 20dB for the speech frequences was recorded in thirty per cent and preservation of hearing without further fluctuations in fifty-three per cent of the patients operated upon. Relief or improvement of the tinnitus occurred in eighty-six per cent of the cases. These favorable results may be influenced by several factors. 1) The exposure of the internal auditory canal and the removal of a segment of the vestibular nerve implies a decompressing effect on the content of the internal auditory canal (drainage of cerebrospinal fluid from the cerebellopontine cistern, enlargement of the spatial relationship within the canal itself). 2) Sectioning of the olivo-cochlear bundle (Rasmussen's) along with the vestibular fibers may also influence hearing. The olivo-cochlear efferents terminate at the hair cells of the organ of Corti. Their electrical stimulation in animal experiments leads to inhibition of the action potentials of the cochlear nerve (Galambos 1956, Desmedt 1962, Fex 1962). 3) The pedicle flap of temporalis muscle laid over the internal auditory canal at the end of the operation (see Section D: Meato-myo-syn-angiosis) may improve the blood supply of the cochlea through revascularization.

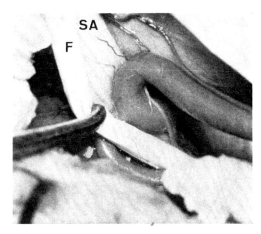

Fig. 136. View of the left porus acousticus in adult man showing the loop of the anterior inferior cerebellar artery around the eighth or statoacoustic (SA) and facial (F) nerves. Two labyrinthine arteries penetrate the porus. Note the difference in diameter between the anterior inferior cerebellar artery (diameter of 2 mm.) and the labyrinthine arteries (diameter of 0.2 mm.).

References

Dandy, E.: Treatment of Menière's disease by section of only the vestibular portion of the acoustic nerve. Bull. Johns Hopk. Hosp. 5 (1933) 52

Dandy, E.: The surgical treatment of Menière's disease. Surg. Gynec. Obstet. 72 (1941) 431

Desmedt, J. E.: Auditory-evoked potentials from cochlea to cortex as influenced by activation of the efferent olivo-cochlear bundle. J. acoust. Soc. Amer. 34 (1962) 1478

Fex, J.: Auditory activity in centrifugal and centripetal cochlear fibers in cat. Acta physiol. scand. 55 (1962) Suppl. 189

Fisch, U.: Die Vestibularis-Neurectomie mit Meato-Myosynangiose. Rev. Laryng. (In press) 1969

Fisch, U., M. G. Yaşargil: Transtemporale, extrapyramidale Eingriffe am inneren Gehörgang. Practica oto-rhino-laryng. (Basel) 30 (1968) 377

Fluur, E., D. Tovy: Microscopic intracranial section of the vestibular nerve in Menière disease. A preliminary report. Acta oto-laryng. (Stockh.) 59 (1965) 604

Galambos, R.: Suppression of auditory nerve activity by stimulation of efferent fibers to the cochlea. J. Neurophysiol. 19 (1956) 424

House, W. F.: Surgical exposure of the internal auditory canal and its contents through the middle cranial fossa. Laryngoscope. (St. Louis) 71 (1961) 1363

House, W. F.: Middle cranial fossa approach to the petrous pyramid. Arch. Otolaryng. 78 (1963) 460

Kurze, T., J. B. Doyle: Extradural intracranial (middle fossa) approach to the internal auditory canal. J. Neurosurg. 19 (1962) 1033

McKenzie, K. G.: Intracranial division of the vestibular portion of the auditory nerve for Menière' disease. Canad. med. Ass. J. 34 (1936) 369

Rasmussen, A. T.: Studies of the VIIIth cranial nerve of man. Laryngoscope. 50 (1940) 67

Rasmussen, A. T.: The olivary peduncle and other fibers projection of the superior olivary complex. J. comp. Neurol. 84 (1946) 141

Rasmussen, A. T.: Further observations of efferent cochlear bundle. J. comp. Neurol. 99 (1953) 61

Rasmussen, A. T.: Efferent fibers of the cochlear nerve and cochleanucleus. In Neural Mechanisms of the Auditory and Vestibular Systems, Ed. by G. L. Rasmussen, W. F. Windle, Ill. Thomas 1960

Wersäll, J.: Personal Communication, 1968

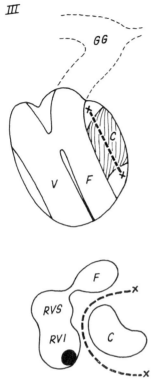

Fig. 137. Selective sectioning of the cochlear nerve (schema). The cochlear division of the eighth nerve (C) becomes visible after the drilling of the anterior rim of the internal auditory canal. F, facial nerve. G-G, geniculate ganglion. V, vestibular nerve. RVS, superior branch of the vestibular nerve. RVI, inferior branch of the vestibular nerve.

C. Operations on the Cochlear Nerve

Selective Sectioning of the Cochlear Nerve

The cochlear nerve may be exposed by the transtemporal extralabyrinthine route through careful drilling of the anterior wall of the internal auditory meatus (Fig. 137), and it can then be selectively sectioned.

Conclusion

Transtemporal selective sectioning of the cochlear nerve has been attempted in patients with severe tinnitus (House 1963,

Fisch and Yaşargil 1968). The experience of House (2 patients) and the author (3 patients) in this regard corresponds to the observations made by Dandy (1941) following intracranial sectioning of the auditory nerve in similar cases. The tinnitus is favourably influenced by sectioning of the cochlear nerve in only half of the cases. The results of vestibular neurectomy in cases of tinnitus due to Menière's disease are more encouraging with eighty-seven per cent of the patients relieved or improved. It may be worthwhile to consider vestibular nerve section (including the efferent olivo-cochlear bundle) as a therapeutic method for individuals suffering from the isolated symptom of tinnitus.

References

Dandy, W. E.: The surgical treatment of Menière's disease Surg. Gynec. Obstet. 72 (1941) 421

Fisch, U., M. G. Yaşargil: Transtemporale, extrapyramidale Eingriffe am inneren Gehörgang. Practica oto-rhino-laryng. (Basel) 30 (1968) 577

House, W. F.: Middle cranial fossa approach to the petrous pyramid. Arch. Otolaryng. 78 (1963) 460

D. Transposition of a Pedicle Flap of Temporalis Muscle over the Exposed Internal Auditory Canal (Meato-Myo-Synangiosis)

Pedicle muscular flaps have been used in order to promote the revascularization of portions of the brain that have undergone circulatory damage (Henschen 1950). The meato-myo-synangiosis is based on the same principle. (Fig. 138).

A pedicle of temporalis muscle is mobilized and rotated over the exposed internal auditory meatus, in contact with the arterial system of the meatus. In this way it may be possible to create a 'shunt' between the extracranial and intracranial blood vessels, i.e. a meato-myo-synangiosis, favoring circulation in the internal auditory canal. Stages of the procedure are shown schematically in Fig. 139.

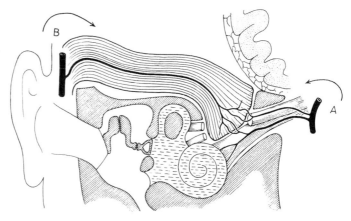

Fig. 138. The principle of meato-myo-synangiosis. A pedicle flap of temporalis muscle is rotated over the internal auditory canal in order to produce a vascular shunt between extracranial (B) and intracranial (A) vessels in the region of the exposed internal auditory canal. Meatomyo-synangiosis may be combined (Figure) with vestibular neurectomy.

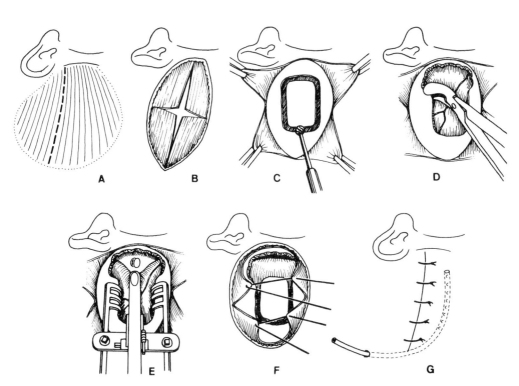

Fig. 139 A—G. Transtemporal extralabyrinthine approach to the internal auditory meatus with meato-myo-synangiosis. A, skin incision. B, preparation of a pedicle flap of temporalis muscle. C, temporal craniotomy using the cutting drill. D, extension of the craniotomy to the floor of the middle cranial fossa with bone rongeur. E, retraction of the temporal lobe and exposure of the internal auditory canal. F, the pedicle flap of temporalis muscle is rotated to cover the exposed internal auditory canal. G, replacement of the craniotomy bone flap. H, closure of the skin incision after insertion of a suction drain (Redon).

Conclusion

Meato-myo-synangiosis was carried out in combination with vestibular neurectomy in fifty patients presenting with various inner ear disturbances of the peripheral type. After the encouraging experience of improvement or stabilization of hearing obtained by the author in cases of Menière's disease, the meato-myo-synangiosis was also utilized in cases of progressive sensory-neural hearing loss of probable vascular origin. Patients who experienced transient benefit to their hearing from vasodilator therapy (Papaverine) are particularly suited to this type of surgery. The preliminary results achieved with meato-myo-synangiosis have been very promising (Fisch 1969). — This is in contrast to similar but disappointing experiences of Kurze and Doyle (1962), who did not use a pedicle flap of muscle.

References

Fisch, U.: Die transtemporale, extralabyrinthäre Chirurgie des inneren Gehörganges. Arch. Ohr.-Nas.-Kehlk.-Heilk. (In press) 1969

Henschen, C.: Operative Revaskularisation des zirkulatorisch gschädigten Gehirnes durch Auflage gestielter Muskellappen (Encephalo-myo-synangiose). Langenbecks Arch. klin. Chir. 264 (1950) 392

Kurze, T., J. B. Doyle: Extradural intracranial (middle fossa) approach to the internal auditory canal. J. Neurosurg. 19 (1962) 1033

E. Operations on the Facial Nerve

The intratemporal course of the facial nerve may be divided into four segments:

1. the *meatal segment*, from the porus acousticus to the fundus of the internal auditory canal.

2. the *labyrinthine segment*, from the fundus of the internal auditory canal to the medial wall of the tympanic cavity. This segment runs first to the geniculate ganglion where it bends backwards forming almost a right angle before reaching the medial wall of the middle ear cleft.

3. the *tympanic or horizontal segment*, running parallel to the axis of the pyramid shortly beyond the geniculate ganglion, then along the medial wall of the tympanic cavity to reach the lateral semicircular canal above the oval window; and

4. the *mastoid or vertical segment*, running from the posterior part of the later semicircular canal to the stylomastoid foramen.

The labyrinthine, tympanic and mastoid segments of the facial nerve lie in a special bony canal, the facial or Fallopian canal. The labyrinthine segment of the nerve contains the geniculate ganglion and gives off the greater superficial petrosal nerve as well as a communicating branch to the lesser superficial petrosal nerve. The transtemporal extradural approach is particularly suited for surgery on the labyrinthine and meatal portions of the facial nerve.

Exposure of the Meatal and Labyrinthine Segments of the Facial Nerve

If the internal auditory canal is exposed (see p. 195) it is possible for one to inspect the facial nerve from the porus acousticus to the meatal fundus. Through the transtemporal approach the bony roof of the facial (or Fallopian) canal can be removed with the microscope and diamond drill as far as the tympanic cavity, thus exposing the entire labyrinthine segment of the nerve (Figs. 140, 141).

In order to avoid damage from heat, the bony roof of the facial canal is removed under continuous irrigation with Ringer's solution. The last thin transparent layer of bone covering the facial nerve is finally removed with a fine excavator. Bleeding may occur following exposure of the geniculate ganglion and of the greater superficial petrosal nerve because of the extensive vascularization of these structures. Disturbing bleeding from larger vessels in this area is controlled by bipolar coagulation. Bone hemorrhage is best dealt with using bone wax. Exposure of the facial nerve is extended from the beginning of the Fallopian canal to the cochleariform process which gives origin to the tendon of the tensor tympani muscle (Figs. 140, 141). To achieve this dissection, the tegmen tympani must be opened between the medial wall of the tympanic cavity and the ossicular chain, care being taken to avoid damaging the incudo-malleolar joint with the drill. At the end of the procedure the opening into the tegmen tympani is covered with a fragment of bone removed from the craniotomy flap. This will prevent post-operative prolapse of the dura resulting in limitation of the mobility of the auditory ossicles (Fig. 140).

If the entire intratemporal course of the facial nerve needs to be exposed, the operation is pursued beyond the cochleariform process using a mastoidectomy approach through a second separate retroauricular skin incision. In this way the mastoid and tympanic portions of the facial nerve are easily approached. Together with Miehlke (1960), the author utilizes Wullstein's (1958) posterior tympanotomy approach exposing the tympanic segment of the facial nerve: this method provides the working space necessary to expose the facial nerve under the short and long processes of the incus. Using the finest diamond drill and excavator it is now possible to link up with the part of the nerve already exposed from above.

Conclusion

Transtemporal operative exposure of the labyrinthine segment of the facial nerve was successfully used by Clerc and Batisse (one case — 1954), House (three cases — 1963, 1966), Pulec (one case — 1966) and Miehlke and Bushe (one case — 1967) in cases of facial palsy following fractures of the petrous pyramid and herpes zoster. Total exposure of the facial nerve has so far been performed by the author in six patients. In three patients peripheral facial palsy occurred immediately following pyramidal fracture with involvement of the greater superficial petrosal nerve. A comminuted fracture of the bony (Fallopian) canal was found in the region of the geniculate ganglion impinging upon the nerve fibers. In a case of Melkersson-Rosenthal syndrome a marked swelling of the trunk of the facial nerve was demonstrated in its meatal segment just proximal to the beginning of the facial canal. A similar finding was present in a patient with otic herpes

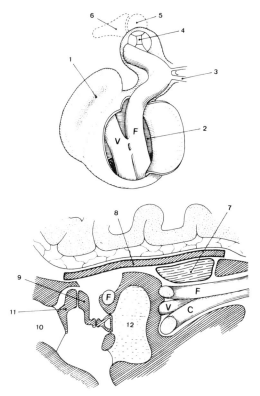

Fig. 140. Exposure of the meatal and labyrinthine segments of the facial nerve. The facial nerve (F) is exposed from the porus acousticus to the level of the tendon of the tensor tympani muscle (top of the figure). 1, blue line of the semicircular canal, 2, internal auditory meatus, 3, greater superficial petrosal nerve. 4, Tendon of the tensor tympani muscle. 5, head of the malleus. 6, body of the incus. After the exposure the roof of the internal auditory canal is closed with a free muscle graft and the opening in the tegmen tympani is covered with a bone fragment from the craniotomy flap (bottom of the figure). In this way the prolaps of the dura over the incudomalleolar joint is prevented. 7, free graft of temporalis muscle. 8, bony fragment of the craniotomy flap. 9, incus. 10, external auditory meatus. 11, malleus. 12, vestibule.

zoster with a facial palsy of six days' duration. In a patient with post-traumatic facial spasm, however, no abnormality was found in any part of the exposed intratemporal segment of the nerve.

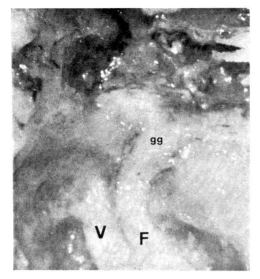

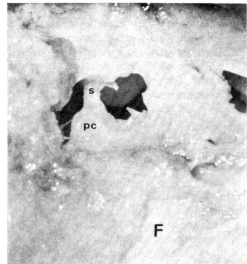

Fig. 141 a   Fig. 141 b

Fig. 141 a—b. Exposure of the labyrinthine segment of the facial nerve (left side). A, exposure of the facial canal between the meatal fundus and the tympanic cavity. The knee of the facial nerve is clearly visible at the level of the geniculate ganglion (gg) and the greater superficial petrosal nerve. F, facial nerve. V, vestibular nerve. B, the tegmen tympani is laid open. The facial nerve has been freed as far as the cochleariform process (pc). S, tendon of the tensor tympani muscle.

References

Clerc, P., R. Batisse: Abord des organes intrapétreux par voie endocranienne (greffe du nerf facial). Ann. Oto-laryng. (Paris) 71 (1954) 20

House, W. F.: Surgery of the petrous portion of the VIIth nerve. Ann. Otol. (St. Louis) 72 (1963) 802

House, W. F., J. A. Crabtree: Surgical exposure of petrous portion of seventh nerve. Arch. Otolaryng. 81 (1966) 506

Miehlke, A.: Die Chirurgie des Nervus facialis. Urban und Schwarzenberg, Munich 1960

Miehlke, A., K. A. Bushe: Die operative Freilegung der mittleren Schädelgrube und des Porus acusticus internus zur Behandlung interlabyrinthärer Läsionen des N. facialis. Chir. Plast. Reconstr. 3 (1967) 37

Pulec, J. L.: Total decompression of the facial nerve. Laryngoscope. (St. Louis) 76 (1966) 1015

Schiff, M., M. Magi, A. M. Warner: Transtemporale facial nerve decompression. Arch. Otolaryng. 77 (1963) 595

Wullstein, H.: Die Methode der Dekompression des N. facialis vom Austritt aus dem Labyrinth bis zu dem aus dem Foramen stylomastoideum ohne Beeinträchtigung des Mittelohres. Ohr.-Nas.-Kehlk.-Heilk. 172 (1958) 582

CHAPTER 9

Anesthesia in Microsurgical Operations on the Central Nervous System

The development of microsurgical techniques of operating on the central nervous system has involved the neuroanesthetist in a new field of activity (Table XVIII). Apart from the actual anesthetics, the pre- and postoperative periods call for special additional investigations and measures.

Table XVIII. Microsurgical Procedures

	No. of cases				No. of cases	
Cerebrovascular Diseases				*Rhizotomies*		
Stenosis and occlusions				Trigeminal Neuralgia	5	
Int. carotid artery	11			Spasmodic Torticollis	11	30
Middle cerebral art.	11			Menière disease	14	
Extra-intracranial Anastomosis	9	32		*Spinal Cord*		
Anastomosis between anterior				Intradural spinal AV-Mal-		
cerebral arteries	1			formation	16	
Saccular Aneurysms	109			Epidural tumor (Meningioma,		
Arteriovenous malformations	14	126		Neurinoma, Neuroblastoma)	3	
Carotid-cavernous Fistula	3			Extramedullary tumor (Meningio-		
				ma, Neurinoma, Lipoma)	8	43
Tumors:				Cauda equina tumor		
Basal Meningiomas	5			(Ependymoma, Neurinoma)	3	
Basal Chordomas	6			Intramedullary tumor (Astro-		
Pituitary Adenomas	1			zytoma, Ependymoma, Hem-		
Craniopharyngiomas	4			angioblastoma)	13	
Orbital Neurinoma	1			Meningomyelocele occipital	1	
Acoustic Neurinomas	29	54		Meningomyelocele lumbar	2	
Cerebellopontine angle				Cervical herniated disc	3	7
Meningiomas	2			Hydromyelia	1	
Cerebellar tumors (Astrocytoma,				*Peripheral Nerve Anastomosis*		
Medulloblastoma, Hämangio-				N. facialis	15	
blastoma)	6					

A. General

Heart and Circulation

The type of patients undergoing cerebrovascular surgery commonly possesses similar lesions elsewhere in the circulatory system. Hypertension, a postmyocardial infarction state, phlebitides and thromboses are not uncommon. Hypertension should be treated according to its grade of severity: hypertensive crises (over 200 mm. Hg) must be dealt with by appropriate drug treatment, while values under 200 mm. Hg frequently return to normal with bed rest, analgesics and hypnotics.

Hypotension is no less serious than hypertension in neurosurgical patients, and it may exert a deleterious effect on a deficient cerebral circulation. Low-molecular Dextran

(Rheomacrodex, 500—1000 ml. per 24 hr.) may be of value in the management of low blood pressure (Bergentz et al. 1963, Eiken 1961).

The Prevention of Edema

As a prophylactic measure to overcome the deleterious effects of cerebral edema the corticosteroid Decadron (dexamethasone phosphate) is started the day before operation and maintained for 5 days postoperatively.

However, in the last 50 cases Decadron has not been used, but the postoperative course has been equally satisfactory.

During the operation the occurrence of cerebral edema can be counteracted by the use of positive pressure respiration and hyperventilation (Hayes, Slocum 1962, Zingg 1962).

Preoperative Prevention of Recurrent Hemorrhage from Aneurysms and Vascular Malformations

Recurrent hemorrhage from a vascular lesion may be minimized by pharmalogical reduction of elevated blood pressure. Although the anti-plasmin Epsamon (epsilon amino caproic acid) has been used in doses of 20—25 g. daily by mouth or as a slow drip infusion we have not been convinced of its efficacy as has been suggested by the experimental work of Mullan, Dawley (1968). In patients in whom there is a Vitamin K deficiency as shown by a prolonged prothrombin time, Konakion (Vitamin K) 10—20 mg. a day is given.

The headaches following cerebral hemorrhage produces restlessness, which itself may increase the risk of hemorrhage and this should be dealt with by the use of effective analgesics (morphine derivates).

B. Anesthetic Techniques

As is shown in table XVIII, microsurgical operations involve the most diverse parts of the central nervous system. For the anesthetist, there is a considerable difference between an intracranial operation and one performed on the spinal cord. With craniotomies, pain is usually minimal and the duration of painful episodes brief, but variations and stress on hormone metabolism and respiratory and circulatory mechanisms — depending on the site of the malformation or tumor — are severe. Lamin-

ectomy may occasionally be accompanied by prolonged and severe attacks of pain, and the position of the patient during the operation is an additional burden. Three anesthetic techniques are required to give the best results:
a) Neuroleptanalgesia (Brown et al. 1963),
b) Mixed inhalation anesthesia with Penthrane (Zingg 1968),
c) Valium and nitrous oxide anesthesia (with or without Penthrane), (Marrubini et al. 1965, McClish 1966).

C. Special Tasks for the Anesthetist

Apart from the actual anesthetic techniques, special procedures in microsurgical operations demand the attention of the anesthetist and these will be briefly discussed. They are:
a) Induced hypotension (Hunter 1953, Saunders 1954),
b) Induced hypertension (Moyer et al. 1954) and

c) Induced hypothermia (Meyer, Hunter 1957, Posnikoff et al. 1960, Rosomoff 1965).

Induced Hypotension

Artificial induced hypotension is used in operations on aneurysms, arteriovenous malformations and highly vascular tumors as the lowered intravascular tension reduces the risk of hemorrhage and facilitates the manipulation of the aneurysm and vessels. Arfonad (trimetaphan), as so-called short-acting ganglion-blocking agent (maximum duration of action between 5 and 10 minutes) is the drug of choice.

Essential preliminary investigations are listed in Table XIX. The contraindications for the use of induced hypotension are summarized in Table XX.

Table XIX

1. ECG
2. Complete blood picture
3. Blood groups and rhesus factor
4. State of nutrition
5. Renal function tests (clearance, urea and urinanalysis)
6. Liver function tests (bilirubin, transaminases)
7. Half-hourly blood pressure check for at least 24 hours

Table XX

1. Central as well as peripheral arteriosclerosis
2. Myocardial infarction
3. Uncorrected anemia or hypovolemia
4. Renal disease with reduced clearance
5. Primary idiopathic hypertension
6. Pregnancy
7. Small children and senile individuals

Arfonad is given as a two per cent solution (in five per cent glucose) by slow drip infusion. The initial dose in patients with circulatory damage and hypertension is 30—60 drops/minute (10—20 mg. Arfonad/minute); in patients with a normal circulatory system the blood pressure is lowered to about 20 mm. Hg above the described level by 60—12 drops/minute. Thereafter, the number of drops is reduced with careful monitoring of the blood pressure until the desired level is reached. In general, twenty-five per cent of the initial dose is adequate to maintain the hypotension. A rise in blood pressure should be prevented because significantly higher doses of Arfonad are required to reduce it for the second time (due to phenomenon of tachyphylaxis).

The amount of Arfonad required varies from patient to patient and cannot be predetermined. On the whole hypertensive and poor risk patients react more rapidly to Arfonad. The depth of the hypotension required is determined by the nature and the technical difficulty of the operation. In hypertensives the level of the blood pressure should not be lowered below fifty per cent of the systolic value. Normotensives tolerate lowering of the systolic blood pressure to levels of 50—60 mm. Hg well, but for prolonged periods of hypotension it should be maintained at 70 mm. Hg to safeguard renal perfusion.

After clipping of the aneurysm or extirpation of the malformation the Arfonad infusion is discontinued. As a rule the blood pressure returns to a normal level within the same period of time that it took to fall (5—10 minutes).

If the blood pressure cannot be reduced to the desired level, despite large doses of Arfonad, the addition of 0.5—1 per cent Halothane to the gas mixture for a few minutes will ensure it.

If the blood pressure drops below the desired level and shows no signs of reverting to normal after withdrawal of Arfonad, the patient is given a 100—200 ml. transfusion of blood or plasma. At the same time, hypoxia is countered by administering oxygen and the renal circulation is protected by infusing 25 g. Mannitol. Prolonged unwanted hypotension is seen in poor risk and elderly subjects. Its treatment depends on the circumstances, but elevation of the lower extremities and the pelvis may counteract the low pressure increasing the cardiac return by autotransfusion. One must remember that the risk of hemorrhage is present whenever the wound is closed before the blood pressure has been restored to normal.

Induced Hypertension

In special individual cases (occlusions of the carotid or middle cerebral arteries) an attempt should be made to prevent cerebral ischemia by maintaining normal the systemic blood pressure.

Aramine (metaraminol) enables a well-controlled artificial hypertension to be achieved. It may be given intramuscularly or intravenously. Not only does Aramine raise the blood pressure but it also maintains the cerebral, renal and myocardial circulation. Sloughing of the tissues seldom appears after Aramine but to prevent tissue necrosis following its prolonged use, the infusion should be administered through a large vein — preferably by caval catheter.

During the operation the induced hypertension is controlled by administering the Aramine in a slow drip infusion (100 mg. of stock solution in 500 ml. glucose). While constantly monitoring the blood pressure the infusion is initially run at 30—50 drops/minute, then slowed to 10—20 drops/minute when the blood pressure begins to rise.

When the desired level has been reached, the drip is turned off for 2—3 minutes to test the reaction time of the vasopressors (usually 2—3 minutes). The duration of action of Aramine is between 20—60 minutes. If fluctuations in the blood pressure occur when the infusion is discontinued and there is a tendency for it to fall, the Aramine is restarted: otherwise the initial dose is adequate to ensure an increased cerebral circulation for the duration of the procedure. A risk of cumulative side effects exists with the prolonged administration of Aramine.

Absolute contraindications for the use of Aramine are hypovolemia, hypertension and cardiac and thyroid disorders. A relative contraindication is diabetes mellitus.

This technique has not been used in this clinic.

Induced Hypothermia

Generalized hypothermia (whole body cooling) to moderate or intermediate levels (reduction of the body temperature to the 28—30° range) is used for microsurgical operations. Esophageal and rectal temperature leads coupled to an electrical thermometer are attached to the anesthetized, intubated and artificially respirated patient. The desired temperature level is obtained by special cooling mattresses which surround the patient and through which cold water circulates. The skin and surface of the tissues of the body are utilized in this method for thermal conduction. The time taken to cool a normothermic patient to 28—30° varies, depending not least on the patient's state of nutrition.

When cooling process is complete, a compensatory mechanism comes into play, through which the body temperature is stabilized. Of importance to the surgeon is the fact that the temperature recorded from the nasopharyngeal lead corresponds to the temperature at the base of the brain, while the temperature of the cerebral cortex is about 3° higher. Hypothermia can be combined with any of the anesthetic techniques described here.

The most feared complication with surface cooling is ventricular fibrillation. This event must be anticipated whenever the temperature drops below 30°.

This technique has been used in only one instance in this clinic during the transclival approach to a basilar aneurysm.

Until the patient becomes normothermic postoperatively, the endotracheal tube is left in situ and oxygen is administered during the rewarming process in order to prevent hypoxemia. Re-warming should proceed slowly, like cooling, so that no acidosis develops.

D. Special Subjects

Aneurysms

The anesthetic of choice in patients with aneurysms is NLA in association with intermittent positive pressure respiration.

As soon as the patient is anesthetized, two transfusions are commenced, one through a caval catheter. Two transfusions are necessary, in order to be able to obtain blood samples, administer drugs and monitor the central venous pressure simultaneously while infusing Arfonad during the period of induced hypotension. The bladder is catheterized, a tube is placed in the stomach and a lumbar puncture is performed for drainage of cerebrospinal fluid. ECG monitoring apparatus should be used in case of cardiac disease. If the aneurysm is situated on the basilar artery or prolonged circulatory interruption of functionally important arteries is anticipated the patient is cooled to $28-30°C$. Of course, accurate replacement of blood and fluids and the addition of Mannitol, sodium bicarbonate, and fibrinogen if this is lacking, are also necessary.

After the dura has been opened, a striking release in intracranial volume can be achieved by drainage of the cerebrospinal fluid.

Induced hypotension (Arfonad) is indicated during dissection of the aneurysms and the adjacent blood vessels. The Arfonad infusion time should be kept to a minimum. The dura should be closed only after the blood pressure has returned to normal.

Postoperatively the anesthetist is responsible for maintaining a clear airway by repeated laryngoscopic and bronchoscopic suction, and for correcting any anemia and fluid and electrolyte disturbances.

Arteriovenous Malformations

The type of premedication used depends on the drug history of the patient and on his mental state.

The NLA anesthetic technique and its administration during the operation in aneurysm patients corresponds to the procedure being utilized. The increased anesthetic requirement in drug-treated patients may be met by altering the ration of nitrous oxide to oxygen in the mixture from 3:2 to 2:1. A period of hypotension may be of value during the dissection of the lesion.

The postoperative measures are dictated by the postoperative state of the patient.

Acoustic Neurinomas

A patient with an acoustic neurinoma may be an anesthetic problem. The giddiness, vomiting and swallowing disturbances produced by the tumor may prevent the patient from being adequately nourished by mouth. Thus, a poor state of nutrition may be present, with marked fluid and electrolyte imbalance, and protein and vitamin deficiency. The patient's initial condition may require combined peroral and parenteral alimentation (gastric tube and caval catheter).

In other respects, the patient is prepared for operation in the same way as an aneurysm patient.

Usually the patient is placed in an erect sitting position for the operation, and the additional strain entailed by this position merits special attention. Elderly subjects and hypertensives react to this severe alteration in posture with a drop in blood pressure. Thus, it appears logical to employ the anesthetic agent that is least likely to embarrass the circulation. Since circulation stability is the anesthetist's primary concern, Penthrane or an intravenous barbiturate combined with the NLA is the procedure of choice.

The second problem presented by the sitting position of the patient during the operation is air embolism (Hunter 1962). The risk of air embolism (due to the negative pressure in the thorax) is particularly high when large venous sinuses are opened. It is reduced to a minimum by positive pressure respiration i.e. omission of the negative suction phase during maintenance of the hyperventilation. Continuous ECG monitoring is advisable in order to ensure the early diagnosis of this serious complication. Air embolism is most effectively treated by advancing the caval catheter into the right auricle and aspirating the gas and in addition keeping the patient on his left side.

Children are anesthetized with Penthrane, adults with NLA.

Craniopharyngioma

Substitution therapy with cortisone is commenced during the induction. Once commenced, it must under no circumstances be interrupted: blood and other infusion mixtures must be administered through a second vein.

Blood pressure variations and irregularities of pulse may occur when the brainstem is compressed or deflected in the course of dissection, but these changes usually disappear upon removal of the cause and do not involve the anesthetist. In rare instances — particularly with small children — attacks of bradycardia must be countered with the administration of intravenous Atropine (0.125–0.25 mg.).

The postoperative course of a case of craniopharyngioma may be complicated by diabetes insipidus. Careful fluid balance studies and twice-daily checks of the body weight are essential. Electrolyte disturbances should be corrected immediately, particularly in children. Patients who are awake present no problem, in that they are able to compensate for the increased excretion by taking more fluids by mouth. In somnolent or comatose patients, in whom the fluid balance has to be maintained by infusions, it may be necessary to compute the total glucose intake in insulin units.

Occlusive Cerebrovascular Disease

The preoperative measures in patients with occlusions of the cerebral arteries depend on the site and extent of the lesions. In general, the same schedule can be applied as is used in aneurysm patients. In reconstructive surgery of the cerebral vessels (thrombectomy, embolectomy and creation of an anastomotic channel) the most satisfactory anesthesia appears to be a combination of Valium and nitrous oxide. One of the principal objectives is to maintain a stable circulation and prevent changes in blood pressure, especially hypotension.

Since the operation is usually fairly free from pain, anesthetic agents may be used sparingly, so that the patient is awake at its conclusion.

Spasmodic Torticollis

The anesthetist is presented with a particular challenge in these patients because of the complicated response of these individuals to narcotics, neuroleptics and analgesics. Haloperidol is poorly tolerated so that Penthrane-inhalation anesthesia is used instead.

The endotracheal tube is left in place at the end of the operation, until the patient regains consciousness and his cough reflex.

Postoperative anesthetic management corresponds to the measures already discussed for acoustic neurinomas.

Spinal Arteriovenous Malformations and Intramedullary Tumors

No special demands are made on the anesthetist in microsurgical operations on the spinal canal and cord.

Patients with lesions of the cervical spinal cord are managed in the same way as patients with acoustic neurinomas. Lesions situated more distally present anesthetic problems only in so far as the general condition of the patient (spasticity, paresis) may present difficulties.

Measures aimed at preventing hemorrhage, as discussed in the general section above, are important in patients with arteriovenous malformations.

The anesthetic of choice is a Penthrane-inhalation mixture, because episodes of severe pain are to be expected during the laminectomy.

References

Bergentz, S. E., L. E. Gelin, O. Eiken: Rheomacrodex in vascular surgery. J. cardiovasc. Surg. (Torino) 4 (1963) 388

Brown, A. S., I. M. Horton, W. R. McRae: Anaesthesia for neurosurgery: the use of the haloperidol and phenoperidine with light general anaesthesia. Anaesthesia 10 (1963) 143

Eiken, O.: Thrombotic occlusion of experimental grafts as a function of the regional blood flow. Acta chir. scand. 121 (1961) 410

Hayes, G. J., H. C. Slocum: The achievement of optimal brain relaxation by hyperventilation techniques of anesthesia. J. Neurosurg. 19 (1962) 65

Hunter, A. R.: Air embolism in the sitting position. Anaesthesia 17 (1962) 455

Hunter, A. R.: Discussion on hypotension during anaesthesia. Proc. roy. Soc. Med. 46 (1953) 612

Lougheed, W. M., D. S. Kahn: Circumvention of anoxia during arrest of cerebral circulation for intracranial surgery. J. Neurosurg. 12 (1955) 226

Marrubini, M., L. Tretola: Diazepam as a preoperative tranquillizer in anaesthesia (a preliminary note). Brit. J. Anaesth. 37 (1965) 934

McClish, A.: Diazepam as an intravenous induction agent for general anaesthesia. Canad. Anaesth. Soc. J. 13 (1966) 562

Meyer, J. S., L. Hunter: Effect of hypothermia on local blood flow and metabolism during cerebral ischemia and hypoxia. J. Neurosurg. 14 (1957) 210

Moyer, J. H., C. A. Handley, G. Morris, H. Snyder: A comparison of a cerebral-hemodynamic response to aramine and norepinephrine in the normotensive and the hypotensive subject. Circulation 10 (1954) 265

Mullan, S., J. Dawley: Antifibrinolytic therapy for intracranial aneurysms. J. Neurosurg. 28 (1968) 21

Posnikoff, J., J. Stratford, W. Feindel: The effect of hypothermia and other factors on cerebrospinal fluid pressure. Canad. Anaesth. Soc. J. 7 (1960) 429

Rosomoff, H. L.: Adjuncts to neurosurgical anaesthesia. Brit. J. Anaesth. 37 (1965) 246

Saunders, J. W.: Effect of controlled hypotension of cerebral function and circulation. Lancet 1 (1954) 1156

Zingg, M.: Erfahrungen mit der Penthraneanästhesie bei neurochirurgischen Eingriffen. Z. prakt. Anästh. 3 (1968) 168

Zingg, M.: Blood gas analysis studies wit hyperventilation in neuroleptanalgesia. Proc. First European Congress of Anaesthetists, Vienna (Sept. 1962)

List of Drugs

Aramine	Metaraminol	Merck/Sharp
Arfonad	Trimetaphan Camphosulfon	Roche
Biobond	EDH-Adhesive	Yoshitomi
Combélène	Dimethylaminopropyl-phenothiazine	Bayer Leverkusen
Decadron	Dexamethasone phosphate	Merck/Sharp
Epsamon	Epsilon aminocaproic acid	Emser Werke
Hypnorm	Fluanisone and phentanyl	N. V. Philips-Duphar
Konakion (Synkavit)	Vitamin K	Roche
Merfen	Phenylmercurum boric	Zyma
Nobecutan	Acrylacetat	Bofors Nobelkut
Penthrane	Metoxyfluranum	Abbott
Pentothal	Thiobarbiturate	Abbott
Polamivet	Analgesic	Hoechst
Rheomacrodex	L. M. W. Dextran	Pharmacia
Valium	Diazepamum Benzodiazepin derivative	Roche

Manufacturers and Suppliers of Microsurgical Equipment

Microscope

Carl Zeiss
Postfach 35/36
D-7082 Oberkochen/Germany

Automatic Microscope Stand

Dr. Ing. Hans R. Voellmy
Contraves AG
Schaffhauser Straße 580
CH-8052 Zürich/Switzerland

Microsurgical Instruments

Aesculap-Werke
Postfach 40
D-72 Tuttlingen/Germany

> *American Distributor*
>
> Holco Instrument Corporation
> 257 Park Avenue South
> New York, N. Y. 10010

F. L. Fischer: MET
Guntramstraße 14
Postfach 529
D-78 Freiburg i. Br./Germany

> *American Distributor*
>
> Holco Instrument Corporation
> 257 Park Avenue South
> New York, N. Y. 10010

V. Mueller & Co.
6600 West Touhy Avenue
Chicago, Ill. 60648/USA

Codman & Shurtleff, Inc.
Randolph, Mass. 02368/USA

Storz Instrument Co.
4570 Audubon Avenue
St. Louis, Missouri 63110/USA

Instruments for Transsphenoidal Hypophysectomy (J. Hardy)

Down Bros. and Mayer & Phelps Ltd.
Church Path
Mitcham, Surrey/England

Otoneurosurgical Instruments (U. Fisch)

F. L. Fischer: MET
Guntramstraße 14
Postfach 529
D-78 Freiburg i. Br./Germany

> *American Distributor*
>
> Holco Instrument Corporation
> 257 Park Avenue South
> New York, N. Y. 10010

Micro-Coagulator

Malis-Coagulator:
Codman & Shurtleff, Inc.
Randolph, Mass. 02368/USA

Fischer-Coagulator:
F. L. Fischer: MET
Guntramstraße 14
Postfach 529
D-78 Freiburg i. Br./Germany

Bipolar Forceps for Malis-Coagulator

Mathys & Sohn
Arzt- und Spitalbedarf
Gerbergasse
CH-8001 Zürich/Switzerland

Scoville-Clips

Down Bros. and Mayer & Phelps Ltd.
Church Path
Mitcham, Surrey/England

Scoville-Clip Applier (long armed)

Aesculap-Werke
Postfach 40
D-72 Tuttlingen/Germany

Hemostasis Clip (Samuel Clip)

Ed. Weck & Co. Inc.
49—33 31st Place
Long Island City 1, N. Y./USA

Bayonet-shaped Applying Forceps for Hemoclips

Aesculap-Werke
Postfach 40
D-72 Tuttlingen/Germany

Heifetz-Clip

Mfg. Flex-Bild Inc.
2214 Euclid Street
Santa Monica, Calif./USA

Silastic Nerve Cuff

Dow Corning
International Limited
Medical Products
Midland, Michigan 48640/USA

Paddies, Swab

American Silk Sutures Inc.
20 Roosevelt Street
Roslyn Heights, N. Y./USA

Microvascular Injection Compounds

Canton Bio-Medical Products
1803 Washington Street
Canton, Mass./USA

Tubes

Dow Corning
International Limited
Medical Products
Midland, Michigan 48640/USA

Electro-Drill

Kerr Surgical Electro Torque Motor with surgical Electro Torque Foot Control
Kerr Manufacturing Company, Detroit, USA

European Distributor
A. Koelliker & Co. A. G.
Löwenstraße 1
8021 Zürich/Switzerland

T-Tubes

The Holter Company
3rd and Mill Streets
Box 100
Bridgeport, Penna. 19405/USA

Suture Material

S & T, Springler-Tritt
Chirurgische Nadeln
Postfach 93
Schaffhauser Straße 40
D-7893 Jestetten/Germany

European Distributor
F. L. Fischer: MET
Guntramstraße 14
Postfach 529
D-78 Freiburg i. Br./Germany

Davis & Geck Department
Cyanamid International
Wayne, New Jersey/USA

Ethicon Inc.
405 High Street
Hampton, N. H./USA

Watchmaker Forceps

Jules Saumon
Rennweg 35
CH-8001 Zürich/Switzerland

Television

Autophon
Industriefernsehen
Zürcher Straße 137
CH-8952 Schlieren/ZH/Switzerland

Film-Material

Slides: Kodak (Type B)
Highspeed Ektachrome EHB 135-20
Movies: Ektachrome,
Type 7242 B, 16 mm. EFB 449.

Urban Cine Camera

Urban Engineering Company,
Burbank, Calif., USA

Microsurgical Outfit

Peripheral Vessel Carotid and Femoral Arteries Rat, Cat, and Rabbit	Brain Arteries Dog and Monkey	Human Occlusive Vascular Disease

Forceps 1 ⎫
Scalpel 1 ⎪
Dissectors 2—4 ⎬ Macro
Clamps 2 ⎪
Scissors 1 ⎭
Forceps (jeweler) 30 0—5
Scissors 1 Meso
Microclamps
Razor blades
Silastic tube 1 cm.
Probes 1
Dams
Paddies
Sutures 2/0, 7/0, 8/0, 9/0
Needle holder Meso
Saline, Papaverine
Cups
	Forceps 1 ⎫
	Scalpel 1 ⎪
	Scissors 1 ⎪
	Dissectors 2 ⎬ Macro
	Retractor 1 ⎪
	Coagulator 1 ⎪
	Sucker 1 ⎭
	Drill 1
	Wax
	Paddies
	Hook 1 ⎫ Micro
	Scissors 1 ⎬ Bajonet
	Forceps 2 ⎭
	Microclamp 1
	Razor blades
	T-tube
	Malis coagulator and forceps
	Sutures 8/0—10/0
	Needle holder Micro, Bajonet
	Saline, Papaverine
	Gel-foam, Oxycel
		Malis coagulator
		Forceps 1—2 Meso
		Scissors 1—2 ⎫
		  straight ⎪
		  curved ⎬ Micro
		Dissectors 1—2 ⎭
		Arachnoid knives
		Razor blades
		Silastic tube 0.8—5.0 mm.
		T-tube
		Needle holder Micro
		Sutures 8/0—10/0
		Paddies
		Dam
		
		Aneurysm (like above)
		and
		Weck-Hemo clip
		Clip applier 3
		Scoville 2
		Microclips (Aesculap) 2

Author Index

Index